Eating and Moving For Your Cycle

Understanding Your Cycle to Live and Feel Your Best

BY HEATHER EVANS, MS
&
KAILEE KARST, DPT

KWE PUBLISHING

A big thank you to all of our friends and family who made writing this book possible! A special thank you to Debi Karst for all of her hard work behind the scenes and our team for their patience in this journey. It's been a heck of a ride, and we're so excited to share the transformative information and research we've compiled.

Evans, Heather, Karst, Kailee. *Eating and Moving for Your Cycle: Uanderstanding Your Cycle to Live and Feel Your Best*

You can contact Kailee and Heather at eating-moving.com.
You can reach out to the KWE Publishing team at kwepub.com.
Cover image and illustrations by Carly Teigler. You can reach Carly at schematicdesigncompany.com.

Table of
CONTENTS

INTRODUCTION

Are you ready to make changes that will positively impact your health and how you feel *throughout* your cycle? Do you have painful periods, polycystic ovary syndrome, or endometriosis? Do you feel confused and overwhelmed with all of the contradicting health information available and are not sure where to start?

You are not alone, and we're so glad you're here!

> This book is written to empower you to understand how daily decisions can create greater physical and mental well-being and radically impact how you feel. Citing over 800 peer-reviewed sources, this book is based on current science to promote evidence-based recommendations, emphasizing a holistic approach to health and well-being for individuals with a menstrual cycle. Our goal is to present information in a way that is easy to understand and integrate into your life.

While we focus on eating and moving to optimize your cycle and overall health, we want to remind you this information is meant to be educational and not diagnostic. We hope to help you become aware of which issues need to be addressed with your healthcare team and what questions may be relevant to ask.

This book focuses on the typical hormonal changes occurring on a monthly basis for individuals with a menstrual cycle, and we believe this information is useful for anyone and everyone!

If you have a menstrual cycle and want to use the information in this book, great! If you don't have a menstrual cycle, there is still some research you might find interesting, and it may give you some ideas for healthy lifestyle hacks for you and your loved ones (because who doesn't love a good bio-hack?). This book may also help you understand the physical and emotional fluctuations of your friends, family, and loved ones with menstrual cycles.

HOW TO USE THIS BOOK

We wrote this book to answer the questions we've found to be common among individuals with a cycle and to give an explanation of why you might experience period problems, sometimes without even realizing it. The book is divided into sections to help answer your questions about your cycle.

- **Part 1 – The Science:** This section focuses on the nervous system, sex hormones, and stress hormones.

- **Part 2 – Your Cycle Explained:** This section dives into the specifics of the menstrual cycle and is the foundational information about the monthly changes occurring in your body.

- **Part 3 – Period Problems:** This section covers topics including cramps, premenstrual syndrome (also known as PMS), estrogen dominance, polycystic ovary syndrome (also known as PCOS), endometriosis, and much more.

- **Part 4 – Restoring Your Cycle:** This section gives insight into healing our hormones with proper nourishment and healthy movement.

THE HEALTH PYRAMID

You will notice we *love* nerding out about science and the body, but it's important to view health as a pyramid. Each person's body and health needs are specific and unique, but there are general principles that play a role in establishing a foundation of health.

The bottom of the pyramid includes the basics: movement, nutrition, hydration, sleep, stress management, and community. All of these are vital aspects of health and well-being, and you may find it challenging to heal if each is not addressed.

So, before you reach for external answers (supplements, strict diet plans, cleanses, and detoxes) for your health problems, ask yourself these quick, simple questions:

- Am I getting some sort of movement each day, or at least three thirty-minute movement sessions per week?
- Am I getting five servings of fruits and veggies each day?
- Am I drinking half of my body weight in ounces of water each day?
- Am I getting a baseline of seven to nine hours of sleep per night?
- Am I able to handle the daily stress in my life?
- Do I have a good emotional and mental support system?

Once you have answered these questions honestly, you will hopefully have a better understanding of what your specific well-being needs are. You may want to start with some basic practices before reaching for flashy "wellness" gimmicks.

GIVE YOURSELF A YEAR

It's important to remember that with all things, change takes time. When we realize the way we treat our bodies influences how we feel, it creates a mental framework, helping us make better choices for our bodies on a daily basis. These changes accumulate over time, affecting our overall health and well-being. If you started today, imagine how much progress you could make in one year. In the long term, think about what a difference it could make in *ten* years! When you start making small, positive decisions for your health by exercising, eating well, and maintaining healthy relationships, you will feel your very best.

So put away your scales, friends. Start thinking about how you feel on the inside instead of how you look on the outside. *Weight does not define health or happiness.* We celebrate all bodies as beautiful bodies, worthy of healthy nourishment, movement, and love. You'll be surprised how this shift in mindset can help shape a healthy, happy life.

A NOTE FROM THE AUTHORS

New science is always emerging, and the research referenced in this book is by no means a *complete* overview of all the research conducted over the years. This is a compilation of some of the science we found to be relevant to hormone health and general well-being. We included the sources of our information and encourage you to look up any articles you think are relevant to you. It's important to investigate when it comes to the questions you have about your health.

This book is full of general information and is in no way meant to diagnose or treat pre-existing conditions. If you relate to any of the problems we mention, please speak with a healthcare provider, and remember to consult with a provider before making changes to your current diet or exercise routine.

THE SCIENCE BEHIND YOUR CYCLE

FIVE MISCONCEPTIONS ABOUT YOUR CYCLE

Misconception 1: Birth control pills, also known as hormonal contraception, are the only option for treatment of polycystic ovary syndrome (PCOS), endometriosis, and irregular periods.

- We'll talk all about birth control and how it affects the body, as well as other symptom management strategies, later in this book.

Misconception 2: You have a normal menstrual cycle if you're on the pill.

- If you're on hormonal contraception, you actually don't have a true cycle!

Misconception 3: Bleeding through a super tampon or overnight pad in one to two hours is normal.

- This is actually not normal. You should let a medical provider know if you frequently bleed through your pads or tampons, or wear pads "just in case" when you're using a tampon.

Misconception 4: It's normal for healthy athletes to miss periods regularly.

- While some athletes do have healthy menstrual cycles, this isn't always the case. Missing your period for any reason besides pregnancy is a sign that something is not right.

Misconception 5: PMS is a normal part of life.

- We'll debunk this myth about PMS in the PMS chapter!

The goal of this book is to describe the best practices of eating and moving for a "normal" cycle, meaning one without the inhibition of cycling caused by hormonal contraceptives. Once you start paying attention to your body and using your cycle as a tool to optimize your well-being rather than inhibit it, you will be amazed at your hidden potential for living your best life. A big part of the process of transformation is listening to your body and making informed decisions about what is best for *you* when it comes to nourishing your body with food and movement and maintaining healthy relationships.

It's important to understand the science behind the inner workings of your body so you can make the best, most educated decisions about how you take care of yourself. The ways in which you eat and move have an impact on your nervous system and hormone production, which both play a large role in just about every process in your body!

Note: If you're not into science, you can skip straight to page 99, which focuses specifically on the menstrual cycle. We encourage you to read the following sections as we discuss the nervous system, hormones, and how these systems are intricately connected. If you're like us and enjoy biology and anatomy, the Khan Academy has excellent videos on basic biology, anatomy, and neuroscience. TeachMeAnatomy.com has great review materials for human anatomy—and they're both free! We encourage readers to learn as much about their bodies as they can. We all live in one, so the more you know, the better you can understand yourself.

HORMONES: OUR BODIES' CHEMICAL MESSENGERS

Hormones are responsible for the changes occurring in our bodies during the menstrual cycle. While we usually think about messages being transmitted throughout the body by the nervous system, did you know hormones play a role in relaying messages, too?

> Hormone production and activation is a dynamic system responsible for facilitating communication between different areas and systems within the body and creating physiological changes based on this communication. This system is known as the endocrine system.

You can think of hormones as little keys traveling throughout the body. They bind to specific proteins known as receptors, which are like locks. The matching receptors allow hormones to be effective and "unlock" actions in the body. Hormones can create an action in the location where they are made, or they can be secreted into the bloodstream to produce actions in other areas of the body.[1] Hormones influence systems such as the reproductive, skeletal, muscular, cardiac, digestive, and immune systems.[2]

We will go into the specific hormones of the menstrual cycle in the chapter Your Cycle Explained. For now, let's take a look at our nervous system and how it plays an integral role in the health of our menstrual cycle.

YOUR CYCLE AND NERVOUS SYSTEM: WHY THE NERVOUS SYSTEM IS VITAL TO WELL-BEING

Nerves relay messages to different parts of the body, but unlike hormones, which create chemical messages, nerves transmit messages based on electrical impulses.[3] The nervous system plays a key role in transmitting and processing information in the body and includes the brain, spinal cord, and all the nerves running throughout the body.

The nervous system is constantly adapting to what's happening in and around our bodies. The ability of the brain to adjust to the world around us is known as neuroplasticity. Our brains and bodies are constantly changing, so why not shift this change in a positive direction?

> Creating changes in our nervous system can be as simple as adjusting our daily habits. Research has shown variables such as diet and physical activity can produce changes in our brain and nervous system,[4] meaning the choices we make regarding food and exercise can influence our nervous system response! This shows we do have some control over how we feel, and health is not something that happens "to us" but is a lifestyle we play an active role in every day.

In order to better understand the concept of neuroplasticity, it is important to understand the nervous system. Let's start with the basics.

DIVISIONS OF THE NERVOUS SYSTEM

The nervous system is divided into the central nervous system and peripheral nervous system. The central nervous system is located in the center of the body and includes the brain and spinal cord. The peripheral nervous system is composed of the nerves throughout the rest of the body, which can control both voluntary and automatic processes.

The somatic nervous system is the part of the peripheral nervous system that controls voluntary actions, like running down a soccer field or doing a warrior pose in yoga. These are actions requiring active thought.

The autonomic nervous system is the part of the peripheral nervous system that controls all of our basic and involuntary functions, including breathing, heart rate, and digestion. Thankfully, we don't have to actively think about these processes all day long!

PRO TIP

While the autonomic nervous system functions without us thinking about it, one way to influence our autonomic nervous system response is by changing our breathing patterns.

THE LIMBIC SYSTEM: EMOTIONAL REGULATION AND THE NERVOUS SYSTEM

Did you know there are specific areas of the brain responsible for regulating emotional response, behavior, memory, and smell? And guess what? These areas of the brain are constantly adapting and changing the signals they send based on the environment inside and outside of our body. This system is known as the limbic system.

Estrogen is one of the primary hormones involved in the menstrual cycle, and certain parts of the brain involved in our emotional response have a high presence of estrogen receptors. This relationship between our brain and estrogen receptors may explain some of the differences in stress-coping mechanisms, learning, anxiety, and mood in menstruating people.

THE HPA AXIS: OUR MIND-BODY CONNECTION

While the limbic system is composed of the specific parts of the brain associated with emotion, smell, and memory, the Hypothalamic-

Pituitary-Adrenal axis, also referred to as the HPA axis, is the link between our nervous system, hormone system and stress response. The HPA axis connects the hypothalamus in the brain with the pituitary and adrenal glands, which are part of the endocrine system. This allows these systems to coordinate and create physiological changes in the body based on what's happening in our internal and external environment.

The hypothalamus is responsible for merging information from the brain, spinal cord, and brainstem and relaying this information to the pituitary gland.[5] The pituitary gland, known as our master gland, communicates with other glands to specify which hormones they should release.[6] Glands create hormones that can be released into the bloodstream to be transferred throughout the body.[7] The adrenal glands influence our response to stress, which we will talk about in the next section of this chapter.

FASCINATING FACT

A 1995 review found the HPA axis is heavily influenced by limbic system structures.[8] If you feel afraid or think you're in danger, this will affect the physiological processes in the body, including those that influence the menstrual cycle.

THE HPA AXIS IN ACTION

Let's take a look at the limbic system and HPA axis in action. Imagine you are at the start of a trail that divides into two paths. One path leads you to a gigantic grizzly bear, which triggers your body's fight/flight/freeze/fawn* response.[9] The second path leads you past a peaceful meadow, which triggers your body's rest-and-digest response.

While most of us have heard of fight/flight/freeze, the fawn response is when individuals in high stress situations immediately try to please the people around them in order to avoid conflict.

The body sends signals to parts of the limbic system in the brain, such as the amygdala. The amygdala is a key player in our emotional response and is well known for its role in our perception of fear and response to perceived threats. The amygdala and other areas of the brain then send signals to the hypothalamus, which initiates communication with the pituitary gland to release different hormones, setting our body's response into action. Do you need to run quickly away from immediate danger, or can you walk slowly, relaxing and enjoying the sunshine?

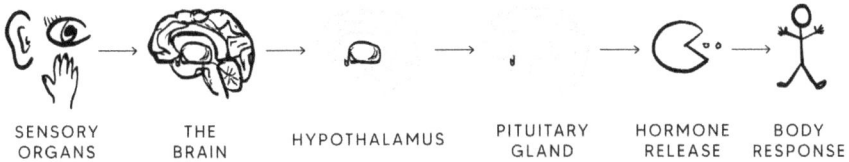

| SENSORY ORGANS | THE BRAIN | HYPOTHALAMUS | PITUITARY GLAND | HORMONE RELEASE | BODY RESPONSE |

FASCINATING FACT

There is evidence that oral contraceptives and other medications may cause dysregulation of the HPA axis and lead to increased cortisol levels.[10] Cortisol is one of our main stress hormones, which we'll discuss in the next few sections. We want you to feel comfortable asking questions when it comes to what you are putting into your body because medications can have more consequences than just the desired effect.

STRESS AND YOUR CYCLE

Stress is a word commonly used in our modern culture, but what does it actually mean? Stress is how our body responds to changes in our internal or external environments. This response can be based on previous experience or our perception of safety. The concept of stress is particularly interesting in the present day because most aspects of our life are "safe," but psychosocial and emotional situations can create feelings of unease and fear.

OUR CHEMICAL RESPONSE TO STRESS

Our biochemical response to stress can affect our cycles, which is one of the reasons we focus so much on addressing stress!

Stress can influence levels of gonadotropin-releasing hormone (GnRH), luteinizing hormone (LH), and follicle-stimulating hormone (FSH), potentially affecting menstrual problems like missing periods and lack of ovulation.[11]

TYPES OF STRESS

We all experience stress as part of our normal lives. Daily activities such as caregiving, commuting and work, life changes including moving, marriage, or divorce, and things out of our control like natural disasters (and pandemics!) can all initiate our stress response. There may also be other things happening in the background, for instance, noise pollution, crowding, and air quality that may contribute to high stress levels without you even realizing it!

Short-term stress affects the body differently than chronic, long-term stress. The longer a person experiences high levels of stress, the greater the harmful consequences in the body.

Prolonged stress can increase risk of issues with your cardiovascular and immune systems and can negatively impact the gastrointestinal system, causing inefficient digestion of food, poor metabolism of nutrients, and bowel problems including constipation or diarrhea.

The good news is that there are a variety of tools we can use to change how we perceive and manage the stress we encounter.

CHANGING HOW OUR BODIES REACT TO STRESS AND FEAR

Did you know we can actively change how our bodies respond to stress and fear? Our bodies respond to stress as we perceive the environment around us. Changing how we view and internalize what's happening in our surroundings can influence how our bodies physiologically respond to stress. This is why mindfulness practices can be so beneficial.

We often hear about mindfulness—but what is it? Mindfulness is simply paying attention to the present moment. One of the easiest ways to practice mindfulness is to be aware of your breathing or any physical sensations you're experiencing in a given moment. Examples of mindfulness include:

- Taking a long breath in through the nose and exhaling through the mouth or nose, feeling the air as it moves in and out of the body
- Feeling sensations on your skin, such as the wind or air on your skin or the clothes on your body, like an itchy sweater or a soft cotton shirt
- Observing the smell of your environment, such as the essential oils in a diffuser, the woods you're walking in, or the flowers nearby

One of the reasons we talk about mindfulness and yoga in detail is because these practices influence the nervous system. Something as simple as paying attention to your breathing can help regulate emotions through its effects on the amygdala and the prefrontal cortex, which are part of the limbic system.[12] This may be why treatments including mindfulness have been associated with improvements in symptoms related to depression![13]

Along with creating positive changes in the areas of the brain responsible for emotional reactions, breathing exercises can also stimulate your vagus nerve, which aids in creating a relaxation response in the body. This means there are multiple benefits in the body when incorporating mindfulness and relaxation techniques into your routine. Keep reading to learn more about the vagus nerve!

THE VAGUS NERVE: THE BIGGEST PLAYER IN OUR REST-AND-DIGEST RESPONSE

The vagus nerve plays a key role in our parasympathetic nervous system, which is responsible for our rest-and-digest response.[14]

The primary role of the vagus nerve is to sense the internal environment in the body. It has more sensory fibers than responsive fibers, which means it plays a huge role in our awareness about the internal environment in our body and gut.[15]

The vagus nerve starts at the brainstem and has nerve endings in various organs in the body, allowing these organs to communicate back and forth with the brain.[16] It has branches in the abdomen, influencing digestion and GI functions[17] and may be one of the ways the gut and brain communicate, influencing the positive psychological effects of a healthy gut.[18] Because of its positive influence on GI function, vagus nerve stimulation has even been proposed as a treatment strategy for irritable bowel syndrome, also known as IBS![19]

FASCINATING FACT

For those of you interested in current research, vagal tone is a measurement of the activity of the vagus nerve. Increased vagal tone is associated with our parasympathetic or rest-and-digest response. This means that by stimulating the vagus nerve, we can transition ourselves out of our fight/flight/freeze/fawn response and into our rest-and-digest response.

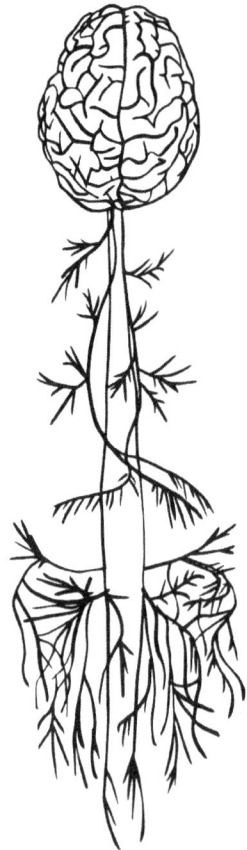

We are passionate about sharing the information in this book because simply changing the way we breathe can optimize our nervous system, leading to greater health. While medical treatments have been created to stimulate the vagus nerve by sending impulses through a medical device, we want you to understand that there are ways to naturally stimulate the vagus nerve. Check out our section Restoring Your Cycle to learn more.

THE GUT: A NEW DIVISION OF THE NERVOUS SYSTEM

Gut health is a major factor contributing to overall health and well-being, and it plays a critical role in every system of the body.

FASCINATING FACT

Did you know the gut has over 100 million neurons, which is more than the spinal cord and peripheral nervous system? These neurons can act independently of the rest of the nervous system, and because of this, it is now considered to be its own division of the autonomic nervous system! This new division is called the enteric nervous system. Some researchers have even nicknamed the gut as our "second brain" due to its influence on physical and mental health.[20]

Your gut holds a collection of bacteria, viruses, and fungi collectively known as the gut microbiome. The gut microbiome plays an important role in the internal environment of your body, making it a vital player in how you feel.

Along with aiding in digestion, the gut microbiome influences the release of chemical messengers and markers of inflammation, and it may even impact cognition and mood through its influence on neurotransmitters. Neurotransmitters are chemical messengers that allow nerves to pass signals to each other.

Serotonin is a particularly important neurotransmitter due to its role in mood, behavior, and memory.[21] It's estimated that ninety-five percent of serotonin is found in the gut,[22] making gut health vital for emotional regulation and behavior.

This is particularly relevant to menstruating people because of serotonin's role in mood and premenstrual symptoms. We'll talk about serotonin and your cycle in our chapter on premenstrual dysphoric disorder (PMDD), but if you're taking antidepressants in the selective serotonin reuptake inhibitor family, known as SSRIs, it may be beneficial to add addressing gut health into your treatment plan. As always, talk with a medical provider about any changes you make, especially if you are on medications.

Another neurotransmitter relevant to mental and physical health is dopamine, and it's estimated that fifty percent of dopamine is produced in the gut.[23] Dopamine is associated with processes like cognition, motivation, reward responses, motor control, and reproductive behaviors,[24] and may even play a role in the regulation of inflammation in the body.[25]

Our gut influences the production of these key neurotransmitters and other chemicals associated with mood, cognition, and inflammation. A healthy enteric nervous system is vital to how we feel in both body and mind!

YOUR CYCLE AND DISEASES OF THE GUT

Gut health and mental health are intricately linked, making diseases of the gut important to understand and address. Irritable bowel syndrome (known as IBS) and inflammatory bowel disease (known as IBD) are two common diagnoses among menstruating people, and according to a 2018 review IBS is more common in menstruating people.[26]

Irritable Bowel Syndrome (IBS) is a condition defined by abdominal pain or discomfort and changes in bowel habits with no known medical cause,[27] making it a very frustrating diagnosis! Common symptoms of IBS include abdominal discomfort, bowel problems, bloating, and distention, and symptoms may worsen after eating. IBS can be characterized by loose stools and diarrhea, known as IBS-D; constipation, known as IBS-C; or both. IBS-C is more common in individuals who cycle,[28] and we want you to know constipation is not normal or healthy, especially if you have a menstrual cycle or hormone problems.

IBS has been linked with anxiety, depression, and fatigue, which can negatively influence quality of life.[29] Individuals with IBS may also be at a higher risk of developing psychiatric disorders, including depressive and sleep disorders, bipolar disorder, and anxiety within the first five years of diagnosis.[30]

Because of the interplay between gut and psychological health, treating IBS may involve more than just treating the GI tract. A 2019 study found cognitive behavioral therapy, which is therapy focused on emotional regulation and behavioral changes, and Qigong-based exercises, which involve slow, mindful movement, may be a beneficial treatment strategy for management of IBS-D symptoms.[31]

Who would have thought addressing mental health could be the first step towards creating a healthy gut? We are big fans of licensed clinical social workers, counselors, therapists, psychiatrists, and psychologists. We're passionate about what we're writing because physical and mental health go hand in hand, and both should be taken into consideration.

Inflammatory Bowel Disease (IBD) is a group of disorders related to inflammation in the GI tract. The most common forms of IBD are Crohn's disease and ulcerative colitis. A 2013 study looking at patients receiving military-based health care found IBD to be more common in menstruating versus non-menstruating people,[32] and a 2021 review found higher rates of Crohn's disease in menstruating people, while ulcerative colitis rates seem to be similar between the groups.[33]

Why does this matter? IBD may influence how you feel throughout your cycle. A 2020 study found higher rates of premenstrual and menstrual symptoms in individuals with IBD.[34]

The good news? Sleep and physical activity may help with IBD symptoms! According to the CDC, low physical activity and sleeping less than seven hours per night may *increase* risk of developing IBD, so if you start to manage these health factors, you may positively influence your gut health and maybe even your menstrual health! Stress and smoking may also increase risk of developing IBD, making these important aspects of health to manage as well.[35]

One of the goals of this book is to help menstruating people understand how menstrual health and overall well-being are intricately linked. Our nervous system, hormones, gut, and overall health are delicately intertwined, and what is healthy for those of us with a menstrual cycle may be different from what is healthiest for our non-cycling counterparts. We want to celebrate our uniqueness and give space to educate ourselves on how to best serve our bodies—they're the only ones we get!

EXERCISE AND YOUR GUT

You're probably starting to realize the importance of good nutrition. But guess what? There's new research coming out about the positive effects of exercise on gut health.

According to a 2017 review, exercise may increase the total number and types of good bacteria in the gut while creating a better environment for beneficial bacteria to thrive. These changes in the gut microbiome can improve overall health and may even help slow the progression of certain diseases.[36]

Cardiorespiratory fitness has also been linked to increased gut microbiome diversity, which means improving your fitness may improve your gut health. Because of this, exercise has been proposed as an effective adjunct therapy in combating health problems associated with microbial imbalances in the gut.[37]

FASCINATING FACT

While many of us relate body mass index (BMI) with health status, we would be remiss not to mention our belief that BMI is not a good representation of overall health. In regards to the gut microbiome, a 2018 study analyzing first-year college students found BMI did not affect the number and diversity of bacteria in the gut. What did positively affect the gut microbiome was differences in physical activity and fiber consumption, both of which we address in this book.[38]

Even though it's easy to have a "go-hard-or-go-home" exercise mentality, even low-intensity exercise may be beneficial for gut health! A 2001 review found low-intensity exercise may have positive benefits on the GI tract, and exercise may reduce the risk of colon cancer by up to fifty percent.[39]

Exercising too hard may have temporary *negative* effects on the gut.[40] While the gut can normally meet the demands of exercise by balancing fluids, electrolytes, and nutrients, a review in 2000 found prolonged high-intensity activity may produce GI distress and tissue damage if a person is dehydrated.[41] If you're engaging in high-intensity exercise, hydration and proper nutrition are key!

To optimize the health of your enteric nervous system (and improve overall health), keep active and eat well. Remember, ninety percent of serotonin and fifty percent of dopamine are produced in the gut, so a healthy gut helps support a healthy mind. The Standard American Diet, SAD, is not ideal for gut health, which is especially important if you have a menstrual cycle since menstruating people may be more susceptible to certain diseases of the gut. Exercise may promote improved gut health, but remember, everything is best in moderation. While exercise is great, endurance exercise in the heat, especially if you're not hydrating properly, may lead to unintended GI symptoms.

INFLAMMATION AND YOUR CYCLE

Inflammation gets a bad rap; however, it actually can be beneficial! Inflammation is a sign that the body is capable of responding to tissue damage or the introduction of pathogens into the body.

Think about an ankle sprain. Acute, immediate inflammation is helpful in the initial healing process. However, chronic inflammation, which persists for months or years after the initial injury or infection, can affect the health of your cycle along with influencing the development of type II diabetes, cardiovascular disease, chronic obstructive pulmonary disease, allergies, and arthritis.[42]

FASCINATING FACT

It makes sense that lifestyle factors like the foods you eat can influence inflammation, but did you know the vagus nerve, which is involved in our rest-and-digest response, may also influence inflammation? A 2009 review found the vagus nerve may play a role in preventing excess inflammation in the body.[43]

By learning to eat well and manage stress, you may be able to positively influence your vagus nerve and gut microbiome, helping to mediate problems related to chronic inflammation.

PROSTAGLANDINS

Prostaglandins are inflammatory markers[44] created in the body that directly play a role in menstrual health.[45]

Prostaglandins promote uterine contractions, helping to shed your uterine lining during your period. In excess, prostaglandins can contribute to period woes, including cramps, nausea, and headaches.[46] Prostaglandins have even been proposed to play a role in heavy menstrual bleeding.[47]

> The reason non-steroidal anti-inflammatory drugs like Advil (ibuprofen) and Aleve (naproxen) are commonly used for menstrual symptoms is because they inhibit the production of prostaglandins. We'll talk more about NSAIDS after our chapter on PMDD.

If you're suffering from period problems, inflammation and prostaglandins may be playing a role in your symptoms! Reaching for pain meds, whether over-the-counter or prescribed, doesn't have to be your go-to. We hope to teach you how to naturally manage symptoms like period pain, heavy bleeding, and inflammation through strategies including nutrition, exercise, and stress management—because let's face it, small positive choices over time make a big difference. We will talk more about these solutions in the section Restoring Your Cycle.

BODY FAT, HORMONES, AND INFLAMMATION

Did you know there are several types of fat stores in the body that affect our biological processes differently?

White adipose tissue can be found around the organs in the abdominal cavity and under the skin throughout the body.[48] While the primary role of white adipose tissue is energy storage, it also has endocrine functions, meaning there is an interplay between white adipose tissue and our chemical messengers and hormones.[49] White adipose tissue has the ability to secrete different chemical messengers influencing our bodily functions.[50]

Abdominal fat stores, which have a high concentration of white adipose tissue, have been found to produce some markers of inflammation at a rate two to three times higher than fat stores found under the skin.[51] Because of the inflammatory substances produced by white adipose tissue, excess white adipose tissue has been associated with health problems related to obesity.[52]

Brown adipose tissue has different biological functions than white adipose tissue and plays a role in temperature regulation. Brown adipose tissue may even have a beneficial effect on body composition,[53] and it has been hypothesized that brown fat may influence appetite control and resting metabolism.[54] We will review ways to naturally influence our brown fat stores in the next section.

FASCINATING FACT

If you've noticed a difference between the body shapes of menstruating and non-menstruating individuals, this may be a natural occurrence based on differing hormonal profiles. Menstruating people tend to have more fat around the hips, thighs, and butt instead of in the abdomen,[55] giving individuals with a cycle more of a "pear" shape.

Estrogen may be responsible for the common "pear" shape and the tendency for menstruating people to have higher subcutaneous versus abdominal fat deposits. High levels of other sex hormones, such as androgens, may be a contributing factor in storing fat abdominally.

Remember, fat is not the enemy, and some body fat is necessary for biological functions. Menstruating people need body fat because of all the incredible things our bodies accomplish as we cycle through our hormones. We believe you can find optimum health at any size. All are welcome at our table, no matter what shape, size, or how much or how little jiggle you have!

DIET AND BROWN FAT DISTRIBUTION

The food choices we make can influence how our body uses energy. For example, certain foods can increase brown fat activation, which increases thermogenesis in the body.

A 2020 review found certain phytochemicals, including isoflavones, catechins, stilbenes, quercetin, luteolin, resveratrol, berberine, and capsaicin, may increase brown fat activation.[56]

Some natural and whole food sources of these phytochemicals include:

- Isoflavones: soybeans and soy products

- Catechins: fava beans, algae, apples, and chocolate

- Stilbenes: berries and peanuts

- Quercetin: elderberries, red onions, white onions, cranberries, hot peppers, and kale

- Luteolin: radicchio, green peppers, serrano peppers, green chili peppers, chicory greens, and celery

- Resveratrol: grape skins, wine, peanuts, cocoa beans, blueberries, bilberries, and cranberries

- Alkaloids (berberine and capsaicin): coffee, cocoa beans, tea leaves, turmeric, and nightshade vegetables such as tomatoes, eggplant, peppers, and potatoes

- Coumestrol: pinto beans, alfalfa sprouts, unfortified soy milk, and chickpeas

Well done! You've made it through some really thick science material. Here's where the real fun begins.

YOUR CYCLE EXPLAINED

Now that we've covered some of the basic science principles let's talk about the menstrual cycle.

First of all, what is the menstrual cycle?

The biological function of the menstrual cycle is to prepare an egg for fertilization and further development into a baby. Typically, the menstrual cycle lasts twenty-eight to thirty-two days, but it can be longer or shorter, varying from cycle to cycle as well as between individuals.

The menstrual cycle has four parts, each with specific biological purposes and different hormone profiles. The four stages are:

- Menstruation
- The Follicular Phase
- Ovulation
- The Luteal Phase

While your menstrual cycle revolves around reproduction, there is so much more going on than just potential baby-making!

We're passionate about this topic because there is a lack of comprehensive public education about the menstrual cycle and reproductive health.

We believe that in order to optimize your well-being throughout your cycle, it is vital to become familiar with these stages and what they indicate for your physical, emotional, and mental health. Let's dive in!

THE STAGES OF YOUR CYCLE: THE SPARKNOTES VERSION

Disclaimer: the following outline is based on a twenty-eight-day cycle. Cycles can vary month to month and person to person, and most cycles are about twenty-eight to thirty-two days long. Each individual has a unique cycle length, and the duration of each stage may vary each month. Different medical conditions may also influence the length of your cycle, making it important to keep track of your monthly rhythms and listen to *your* body.

MENSTRUATION (BLEEDING DAYS: DAY 1 – END OF BLEEDING)

Menstruation, also known as menses or your period, is the bleeding stage in which the uterine lining is shed.

During your period, estrogen and progesterone are at their lowest levels. The drop in progesterone just before your period signals decreased blood flow and oxygenation to the uterus, causing the inner wall to disintegrate. Prostaglandins stimulate muscular contractions to help remove this tissue vaginally, which is what we experience as our "bleed." Toward the end of menstruation, estrogen promotes clotting and the regrowth of the uterine lining.[1]

THE FOLLICULAR PHASE (DAY 1 – OVULATION)

The follicular phase is the first half of your cycle, which technically includes menstruation.

The function of this phase is to prepare for our fertile window and ovulation.

FASCINATING FACT

While most people are aware that ovulation is our most fertile time, you might be surprised to learn that your fertile window starts in the follicular phase, about four to five days before ovulation.[2]

The follicular phase involves the growth and maturation of follicles, which surround the eggs in the ovaries until they are ready to be released into the fallopian tube during ovulation.[3]

The follicular phase is characterized by a rise in estrogen[4] and an increase in the release of follicle-stimulating hormone, known as FSH, from the pituitary gland. The increase in estrogen signals the uterine lining to grow in preparation for potential pregnancy, and the rise of FSH stimulates the growth and maturation of follicles, which is necessary for ovulation.[5]

In the mid-follicular phase, luteinizing hormone, called LH for short, slowly rises, and FSH declines as ovulation approaches.[6] The surge in LH just before ovulation signals the follicle to release the egg into the fallopian tube.[7]

OVULATION (MID-CYCLE)

Ovulation occurs when the mature follicle releases an egg into the fallopian tube to potentially be fertilized if it comes in contact with healthy sperm. The egg then travels to the uterus. If it has been fertilized, it will implant into the uterine lining...hello, pregnancy! If it has not been fertilized, it will disintegrate.

THE LUTEAL PHASE (POST-OVULATION – DAY 28)

The luteal phase involves the maintenance of the uterine lining for potential implantation of a fertilized egg, which generally occurs five to ten days after ovulation.[8] This creates a healthy environment to sustain a viable pregnancy.

Progesterone is the primary hormone present in the luteal phase and is secreted by the empty follicle, called the corpus luteum. The corpus luteum also produces a small amount of estrogen. While estrogen promotes the growth of the uterine lining, progesterone plays an important role in keeping the uterine lining thick and healthy, which is necessary for pregnancy.[9] Progesterone continues to rise through the mid-to-late luteal phase, and both estrogen and progesterone decline just before the start of your period.[10]

THE HORMONES OF YOUR CYCLE

The menstrual cycle is a delicate and complicated process, involving communication between our nervous system and reproductive organs. Hormones play a critical role in this communication.

It is empowering to know and understand what is happening in our bodies and how the natural hormonal fluctuations in our menstrual cycle can impact our physical, emotional, and mental well-being. It's wild and amazing to think about how much our bodies are doing without us even thinking about it!

How we eat, move, and manage stress greatly impacts the hormones of our menstrual cycles, so it's important that our habits are health and hormone supportive. We will describe hormone-supportive habits in our section Restoring Your Cycle, but for now, let's review the major sex hormones involved in your cycle and how they impact you![11]

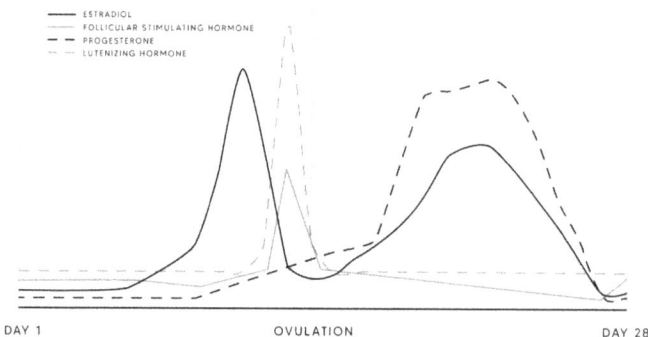

ESTROGEN

Although primarily associated with reproduction and menstruation, estrogen has multiple functions in the body and is even found in small quantities in individuals without a menstrual cycle!

Estrogen influences bone health, appetite regulation, fat metabolism, and cardiovascular function.[12] In relation to your cycle, estrogen stimulates the growth of the uterine lining to prepare for pregnancy and influences the development of breast tissue.[13]

Although estrogen is primarily found in the ovaries, it can also be produced in the adrenal glands, breast tissue, adipose tissue, and the placenta during pregnancy.

There are three types of estrogen: estrone (E1), estradiol (E2), and estriol (E3), each with specific biological functions.

- **Estrone,** although present during the reproductive years, is the primary type of estrogen present after menopause. Estrone is primarily produced in fat tissue.

- **Estradiol** is the most influential form of estrogen in our reproductive years. It is a highly potent form of estrogen, and while it is mainly secreted by our ovaries, it can also be produced in the pituitary gland and brain.

- **Estriol** is the form most prevalent during pregnancy but is also found in very small amounts during the reproductive years and transition into menopause. Estriol is primarily produced by the placenta.[14]

LUTEINIZING HORMONE (LH)

Luteinizing hormone is released by the pituitary gland, and the surge of LH in the middle of your cycle stimulates ovulation.[15]

FOLLICLE-STIMULATING HORMONE (FSH)

Follicle-stimulating hormone is also released by the pituitary gland and promotes the growth of follicles around the eggs in the ovaries in the first half of your cycle. The growth of the follicles influences the increase in estrogen production during this time.[16]

PROGESTERONE

Progesterone, the primary hormone released in the second half of our cycle, is produced by the corpus luteum, which is the empty follicle after the egg has been released during ovulation.

We'll talk all about how the ratio of estrogen to progesterone influences the health of your body and cycles in our chapter on estrogen dominance!

BONUS: GONADOTROPIN-RELEASING HORMONE (GNRH)

Gonadotropin-releasing hormone is produced by the hypothalamus and stimulates FSH and LH production and release from the pituitary gland.

Stress can greatly affect the release of GnRH, which, in turn, affects the production of FSH and LH.[17] This means stress, whether physical or psychological, can affect our hormones, which is one of the reasons we are passionate about providing education on stress management!

NUTRITION OVERVIEW

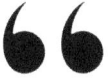

> What most people don't realize is that food is not just calories; it's information. It actually contains messages that connect to every cell in the body.

DR. MARK HYMAN

At this point, you may be wondering, *how can I eat to optimize my reproductive and hormone health?* This is one of the main questions we want to address in this section. We're delighted you've read this far—here's where the *fun* begins!

GUT HEALTH BASICS

Gut health and menstrual health are intricately linked, so improving your gut health may help alleviate some of your period problems.

Have you ever heard the statement, "You are what you eat"? Well, in a sense, this statement is true. The foods we eat are the building blocks for our body's cellular processes, meaning gut health and overall health are strongly influenced by the foods we consume.

Let's review some best practices for nourishing our bodies!

First and foremost, our bodies *thrive* on whole foods! Whole foods are any type of food that has been minimally processed or not processed at all. Think about the difference between shopping in the center aisles at a grocery store versus the produce section located on the outer edges of the store. Most of the food in the center of the grocery store is boxed, bagged, or canned. This is processed food.

When filling your pantry or freezer, reading labels is key! If you're getting frozen or canned produce, try to aim for products containing just the produce, and be mindful that some frozen options have not-so-healthy additives mixed in. Ingredients on labels are listed in order of quantity, meaning the ingredients at the beginning of the list make up a higher proportion of the food. If fats are higher on the list, it might be better to find a healthier alternative.

PRO TIP

A simple tip for optimizing your gut health is to get at least five servings of fruits and veggies per day.

Frozen veggies are better than no veggies, and cooking doesn't have to be complicated!

If you're having a really busy week, you can use frozen veggies to make sure you get some greens in. We often use frozen cauliflower, broccoli, or Brussels sprouts. And if you aren't sure what to do with your vegetables, try roasting them! Simply preheat the oven to 350 degrees Fahrenheit, toss the veggies with salt, pepper, and olive oil, put them on a baking sheet, and bake for about thirty minutes, checking occasionally during the cooking process.

If you're tired of salads, try adding veggies into smoothies, eggs, tacos, stir-fries, pasta, and sandwiches. You can also make soups with frozen veggies by blending them in a blender with different spice mixtures and heating on the stove. One of our favorite recipes is coconut milk, frozen kale, frozen cauliflower, and a mixture of coriander, ginger powder, turmeric powder, garlic powder, salt, and pepper. You can always check the web for detailed recipes!

PROBIOTICS

Now, let's talk about foods that nourish the gut microbiome.

As a review, the gut microbiome is the collection of bacteria, viruses, and fungi residing in the gut. The gut microbiome plays an important role in the internal environment of your body, making it a vital player in health and well-being. For a refresh on the gut microbiome, flip back to our section The Gut: A New Division of the Nervous System.

So, what helps with maintaining a healthy gut microbiome? Probiotics and prebiotics!

Probiotics are living microorganisms that can improve gut health and immune function, decrease risk of bowel disease, and potentially influence mental health due to the gut-brain connection.[1]

FASCINATING FACT

There are certain probiotic strains that may be beneficial for individuals struggling with psychiatric illnesses known in research as psychobiotics.[2] If you're interested in learning more about psychobiotics, check out the current research in PubMed at https://pubmed.ncbi.nlm.nih.gov/.

The two most common dietary sources of probiotics are fermented foods and probiotic supplements. As always, we recommend whole food sources unless otherwise directed by a healthcare provider.

Probiotic food sources include yogurt, kimchi, kombucha, sauerkraut, kefir, and fermented vegetables.[3]

So, how do probiotics relate to your menstrual cycle and reproductive health? Probiotics promote improved gut health, which is vital for maintaining proper metabolism of estrogen. There are even specific bacteria, collectively known as the estrobolome, that are responsible for maintaining proper metabolism of estrogen in the

GI tract.[4] We'll talk all about the estrobolome in our chapter on estrogen dominance on page 136. This is why problems with the gut may lead to larger problems, such as hormonal imbalances, and, in particular, symptoms of estrogen dominance, making probiotics even more important.[5]

FASCINATING FACT

Did you know your vagina also has a microbiome of its own? Certain probiotics, including those in the lactobacilli family, may support the health of your vaginal microbiome. Lactobacilli may even reduce the risk of sexually transmitted infections[6] and can be found in the whole food sources listed on the previous page.

Although there are many probiotic supplements on the market, a 2003 review notes that most products are not regulated by the FDA and have not been part of large-scale trials to validate efficacy.[7] This is something to consider when buying expensive supplements and is another reason to focus on consuming whole food sources of nutrients. It may be worth asking your PCP or a nutritionist what supplements, if any, they recommend for you.

PREBIOTICS

Prebiotics are the foods that fuel the good bacteria in your gut and can also improve gut health! Prebiotics are dietary fiber that cannot be digested in the small intestine, and instead get fermented in the large intestine, creating positive changes in the gut microbiome.[8]

There are three main types of prebiotics:

- fructo-oligosaccharides (FOS)
- galacto-oligosaccharides (GOS)
- trans-galacto-oligosaccharides (TOS)[9]

Prebiotics not only positively influence the gut microbiome, but they also support enhanced production of short-chain fatty acids, promote improved gut barrier function, help reduce pathogen growth, and improve micronutrient bioavailability, which is how easily the body can process and use micronutrients.[10] These positive changes can affect your immune system, bone health, and the health of your organs, including your reproductive organs!

Prebiotic food sources include bananas, cow's milk, beans, oats, apples, barley, garlic, onions, leeks, artichokes, and asparagus.[11]

NUTRIENT ABSORPTION AND THE MICROBIOME

If your gut is in a state of dysbiosis, meaning that there is an imbalance of good and bad bacteria, you will not be able to optimally digest and absorb nutrients from the foods you are eating. Gut health is truly a major determining factor in one's total health outcome. This is why it is important to talk about gut health when we're healing our hormones.

To put it succinctly: what you eat impacts the state of your gut microbiome, and your gut microbiome greatly impacts the health of your cycle!

Now, let's talk about macronutrients and how they influence health.

MACRONUTRIENTS

Macronutrients, often referred to as macros, include carbohydrates, proteins, and fats. Eating a balanced diet full of whole foods containing all three macronutrients is critical to maintaining overall health and well-being.

All, we repeat, *all* macronutrients should be included in the diets of menstruating people. Each has its essential purpose in supporting reproductive health. The necessary amount of each varies from person to person depending on factors such as physical activity and metabolic rate.

CARBOHYDRATES

Over the years, carbohydrates have acquired a not-so-healthy rap. From the Atkins diet to the Keto diet to the old-fashioned low-carb diet, there seems to be a focus on reducing the intake of carbohydrates to the smallest amount humanly possible. Our goal in this section is to provide education and help you understand that "low carb" does not necessarily mean healthy, especially if you have a menstrual cycle.

Carbohydrates are the body's preferred source of energy, and your brain and nervous system rely on carbohydrates to function optimally.[12] In the absence of carbohydrates, the body begins to break down not only fat from adipose tissue but also protein from muscle tissue for energy, which is not ideal if you're working on building strength![13]

If you've been told by an influencer, friend, or family member that you need to cut carbs completely, or that you'll be healthier if you go "keto," think again.

Decreasing carbohydrates too much may negatively impact your cycle. In a 2012 study, metabolic and hormone changes were examined in participants who followed three types of diets: low-fat, low glycemic index (low in processed sugars and refined carbohydrates), and very low carbohydrate, in which even carbohydrates from whole foods and natural sources were decreased. The very low-carbohydrate diet resulted in changes including increased markers of inflammation, increased levels of cortisol (our primary stress hormone), and issues regulating thyroid hormones, all of which are detrimental to a healthy cycle.[14]

A small 2003 study analyzing the effects of a ketogenic diet, a diet low in carbohydrates and high in fats, found that forty-five percent of those who were on the ketogenic diet suffered from menstrual disruption during the six-month study. Six participants out of the thirteen subjects on the Ketogenic diet experienced missing periods, known as amenorrhea, likely as a result of their low carbohydrate intake.[15]

You don't have to cut carbs out completely in order to have optimal health, and including whole food sources of carbohydrates, such as fruits, veggies, and whole grains can help you to maintain a hormone-supportive, balanced diet.

TYPES OF CARBOHYDRATES

It's important to note that menstruating people need carbohydrates, but not all carbohydrates are created equally.

Eating carbohydrates in their natural, whole food forms, such as fruits, veggies, and whole grains, is more beneficial for the body than eating refined, processed carbohydrates such as chips, cookies, candy, frozen desserts, and sugary drinks.

All carbohydrates are made from sugars, known as saccharides, but not all carbohydrates are processed the same way in the body!

Monosaccharides are the simplest form of carbohydrates, often found in processed foods and in smaller amounts in some natural foods, such as fruit.

- Examples of monosaccharides include glucose, fructose, and galactose.

Disaccharides are two monosaccharides linked together.

- Examples of disaccharides include sucrose, lactose, and maltose.

Polysaccharides contain three or more monosaccharides linked together.

- Examples are amylose, amylopectin, resistant starch, dextrins, and glycogen.

> **FASCINATING FACT**
>
> Did you know dietary fiber is considered a carbohydrate? Dietary fibers are polysaccharides that are not digested or absorbed in the small intestine.[16]

Besides helping you maintain healthy bowel movements, certain types of dietary fiber act as prebiotics, or food, for the good bacteria in the gut.[17]

It's recommended that menstruating people get twenty-five to twenty-eight grams of fiber per day.[18] If you're not getting enough dietary carbohydrates and fiber to support healthy bowel habits, this can lead to bacterial build-up, imbalances in the gut microbiome, and recirculation of waste products back into the body.[19]

But don't worry, if you're getting five or more servings of fruits and veggies per day, you should be meeting the dietary fiber recommendations to optimize your gut health! Sources of dietary fiber include whole grains, legumes, nuts, fruits, and vegetables.[20]

GLYCEMIC INDEX: SIMPLE AND COMPLEX CARBOHYDRATES

You've heard of simple and complex carbs, right? Well, let's break it down and explain exactly what those terms mean.

Simple carbohydrates contain monosaccharides or a combination of both mono- and disaccharides and are commonly found in foods with refined flours and added sugars. These foods have a high glycemic index, meaning they have more of an immediate impact on blood sugar.

Complex carbohydrates contain polysaccharides and are carbohydrates that are generally sourced from minimally processed foods, including whole grains and vegetables. These foods have a low glycemic index, indicating that they have less of an effect on blood sugar.[21]

Whether a carbohydrate is simple or complex is one of the most important factors to consider when consuming carbohydrates. While we need carbohydrates as a source of fuel for our bodies, in excess, carbohydrates, specifically simple carbohydrates, can negatively influence blood sugar levels. High carbohydrate intake in a short period of time can lead to quick increases in the amount of circulating glucose in the blood, known as hyperglycemia. Hyperglycemia, when present for a long time and left untreated, can cause damage to our nerves, cardiovascular system, kidneys, and eyes.[22]

Blood sugar levels can also influence reproductive health![23] A 2009 study found individuals who consumed a diet full of simple carbohydrates, such as refined flours and sugars, had a higher risk of infertility and problems with ovulation. Individuals in this study who ate a diet rich in complex carbohydrates, such as those found in fresh, whole foods and grains, had a lower risk of problems with fertility and ovulation.[24]

FASCINATING FACT

Our body is not well-equipped to process the high concentration of sugar found in high-fructose corn syrup and other refined sugars.

Fructose, commonly found in fruits, table sugar and high-fructose corn syrup, cannot be fully absorbed by the small intestine when consumed in large quantities. Instead, it continues through the large intestine to the liver where it is processed.[25]

A 2008 study found that in individuals with non-alcoholic fatty liver disease, consumption of fructose was two to three times higher than in controls,[26] and liver problems due to sugar intake are common among children.[27]

Unfortunately, high-fructose corn syrup runs rampant in our processed food system in the U.S., accounting for forty percent of added sweeteners.[28] While carbs are not the enemy, it's important to monitor processed sugar intake in order to promote optimal health.

Our advice: while carbs are a necessary part of our diet, try your best to avoid processed sugars. You can use the World Health Organization's sugar guidelines to see if you're consuming too much sugar...once you start reading labels, you might be surprised at how much sugar is in the foods we eat every day!

Remember, carbohydrates are an important source of fuel for many systems in the body. Eating carbs from whole food sources is the best rule of thumb. We'll talk more about how added sugars and low-carb diets affect the body in the chapter Fad Diets, Sugar, and Your Cycle.

PROTEINS

Proteins are necessary for growth and repair in the body. Many chemicals necessary for biological processes consist of proteins, including most enzymes, antibodies, and certain types of hormones. Neurotransmitters are made from the building blocks of protein known as amino acids.

Similar to carbohydrates, not all dietary proteins are created equally.

ESSENTIAL AMINO ACIDS

Amino acids are the building blocks of protein. While non-essential amino acids can be produced in the body, essential amino acids cannot. Because of this, essential amino acids need to be consumed in our diet.

The essential amino acids are:

- Histidine
- Isoleucine
- Leucine
- Phenylalanine
- Valine
- Lysine
- Threonine
- Methionine
- Tryptophan

COMPLETE VS. INCOMPLETE PROTEINS

A protein is labeled complete or incomplete based on its essential amino acid content.

Complete proteins contain all nine essential amino acids. Animal proteins, dairy, and eggs are all examples of complete proteins.

Incomplete proteins include some but not all of the essential amino acids. Grains, legumes, and vegetables are examples of incomplete proteins.

So, how do you know whether you're getting an adequate amount of essential amino acids in your diet?

If you're a meat-eater or a vegetarian who eats dairy and eggs, you are likely getting all nine essential amino acids through your diet. Vegans are the most at risk of missing out on some of the essential amino acids.

With this information in mind, it's important for our vegan friends to combine different types of incomplete proteins to fill the amino acid gaps. For example, combining legumes such as black beans, lentils, or peas with whole grains such as rice, quinoa, or couscous results in two incomplete proteins coming together to make a complete protein. Pretty fascinating, right?

Examples of complete protein combinations include tofu and rice, hummus and bread, nuts or seeds and beans, and tempeh and noodles.

PRO TIP

It's worth noting that most plant-based meat alternatives are highly processed in order to provide all nine essential amino acids. Because of the additives and the way these foods are processed, they aren't always the most health-supportive choices. So, when you're choosing plant-based alternatives, make sure to check the ingredient lists.

The recommended dietary allowance (RDA) for protein for menstruating people with normal activity levels is 46 grams per day. If you find yourself ravenous in the middle of the day, be sure to include adequate protein in your breakfast. A high protein breakfast may help with appetite control and blood sugar regulation, reduce the desire to use food as a reward and be a catalyst for other positive dietary changes.[29] Eggs or protein powder in a smoothie can be easy options to increase your morning protein intake!

FATS

Dietary fats contain higher amounts of energy than carbohydrates and proteins. While carbohydrates and proteins carry four calories per gram, fats contain nine calories per gram.[30]

Because fat has more than double the calories of carbs and proteins, low-fat diets used to be all the rage. However, research is catching up with the fact that fat plays a vital role in our physiology and health, and the "calories-in, calories-out" equation may not be all it's been cracked up to be.[31]

Healthy sources of dietary fat are beneficial for the body, especially if you have a menstrual cycle![32]

Dietary fats are necessary for the synthesis of hormones like estrogen, progesterone, testosterone, and vitamin D.[33] They also play a role in the utilization and storage of fat-soluble vitamins like A, D, E, and K[34] and can positively influence bone health.[35]

FASCINATING FACT

Fat stores in the body are known as adipose tissue, and different dietary fats have varying effects on the formation of adipose tissue.[36] It's interesting to know that high sugar consumption may also play a role in adipose tissue formation, so if you're worried about weight management, it may be beneficial to look at both processed fats *and* sugars as potential culprits.[37]

TYPES OF DIETARY FAT

Dietary fats are made up of several different types of fatty acids. These include saturated, unsaturated (monounsaturated and polyunsaturated), and trans-fatty acids.

Saturated fatty acids are solid at room temperature. An example of a food high in saturated fat is butter.

Unsaturated fatty acids (mono- and polyunsaturated) are liquid at room temperature. Olive oil is a type of monounsaturated fat, and sunflower oil is a type of polyunsaturated fat.

Trans-fatty acids are unsaturated fatty acids that have hydrogen added to them to give them qualities more similar to saturated fatty acids.[38] Spoiler alert: they aren't good for you, and we have a whole section on them later in this chapter.

ESSENTIAL FATTY ACIDS

Essential fatty acids are polyunsaturated fatty acids that cannot be produced in the body, meaning these nutrients are only available through your diet.

There are two types of essential fatty acids:

Omega-3: An anti-inflammatory polyunsaturated fatty acid molecule. Dietary sources of omega-3s include fatty fish like salmon, tuna, and herring, fish oil, flaxseeds, and chia seeds.

Omega-6: A pro-inflammatory polyunsaturated fatty acid molecule. Dietary sources of omega-6s include corn oil, sunflower oil, soybean oil, wheat germ oil, canola oil, and safflower oil.[39]

> The ratio of omega-3 to omega-6 is critical for managing inflammation. While omega-6 is usually deemed pro-inflammatory and omega-3 is usually thought of as anti-inflammatory, both are critical parts of your diet and should be consumed in a balanced, healthy ratio.[40]

What does a balanced ratio look like? A healthy ratio of omega-3 to omega-6 is in a range between 1:1 and 1:4.[41] In the United States, this ratio is typically between 1:20 and 1:30 due to the foods we eat and how they're processed. This high ratio is one to watch if you suffer from chronic inflammation because it lends itself to a pro-inflammatory state.[42]

When it comes to your cycle, a balanced ratio of essential fatty acids is vital for managing period symptoms like cramps and period pain, which are heavily influenced by inflammation.[43] An easy tip to improve this ratio is decreasing packaged and restaurant foods high in processed fats and omega-6.

TRANS FAT

If you've ever been told to steer clear of trans fats, we encourage you to take this advice! Trans fats negatively impact human health, and sadly, they're hidden in plain sight on the labels of many common foods! So, what are trans fats?

Trans fats are composed of hydrogenated unsaturated fatty acids. Hydrogenation is a process that helps extend the shelf life of foods[44] and is why trans fats are common in prepackaged items. Hydrogenation takes away many of the health benefits associated with unsaturated fats.

Small amounts of trans fat can be found in animal fats, but it is mostly present in processed foods and can be read on a label as "partially hydrogenated oil."

Trans fats are so harmful to human health that the CDC estimates somewhere between three thousand and seven thousand deaths in the U.S could be prevented each year if partially hydrogenated oils were removed from our food,[45] and your risk of cardiovascular disease may increase by as much as twenty-three percent from just a two percent increase in energy intake from trans fats.[46]

If a partially hydrogenated oil is one of the first few ingredients on a label, it may be best to swap that food out with a healthier alternative. Food items high in trans fats include shortening, margarine, fried potatoes, potato chips, packaged cakes, cookies, and crackers, and certain animal products,[47] so it's important to read labels when filling your pantry or grabbing a snack on the go.

DIETARY FAT AND REPRODUCTIVE HEALTH

Remember, menstruating bodies *need* fat, but not all fats are created equal.

While many steer away from products that are higher in fat, a study in 2017 found lower risk of infertility in individuals who consumed high-fat dairy, while low-fat dairy was associated with increased risk of infertility.[48] This may relate to the sugar content in low-fat dairy products and is an example of why reading labels is important. Foods marketed as low-fat, including yogurts, tend to be loaded with sugar, and high sugar content is not ideal for hormone balance.

Another consideration if you're struggling with infertility is the types of fats you're consuming. A 2016 study found that consuming more omega-3s may improve chances of healthy ovulation and increase progesterone during the luteal phase,[49] positively influencing your chances of getting pregnant.

FASCINATING FACT

If you have specific conditions like PCOS and endometriosis, decreasing trans fat may help with symptoms!

If you have endometriosis, it might be worth decreasing trans fats and increasing your intake of omega-3 fatty acids. According to a 2010 study, individuals in the highest fifth of trans fat consumption had a forty-eight percent higher chance of being diagnosed with endometriosis,[50] and another study from the same year found an association between higher omega-3 intake and lower risk of endometriosis.[51]

For individuals with PCOS, a 2017 study found that increasing fiber intake and decreasing trans fat may positively influence health.[52] This is one of the reasons we emphasize cooking at home—chances are, you're not going to consume as much saturated and trans fats, and it's much easier to increase healthy fats!

CHOLESTEROL

Of course, we can't talk about dietary fat without also talking about cholesterol.

Cholesterol is a molecule that is built from the same building blocks as fats (known as lipids). Because it repels water, it is attached to a protein to be carried throughout the body.[53]

While many of us associate cholesterol with cardiovascular risk, it has several important roles in the body. Cholesterol can be found in cell membranes, where it influences cell membrane function and signaling, and is one of the major building blocks for vitamin D, steroid hormones such as estrogen and progesterone, and bile acid, which helps with digestion.[54]

There are two types of cholesterol, often referred to as "good" and "bad"—here is why they're classified that way:

- **Low-density lipoprotein,** known as LDL, is referred to as "bad" cholesterol because, historically, research has correlated LDL levels with cardiovascular disease. However, this theory has recently come under scrutiny due to the methodology in some of the original studies.[55] It's important to stay open-minded as new scientific discoveries become available.

- **High-density lipoprotein,** also known as HDL, is referred to as "good" cholesterol. HDL has historically been associated with decreased cardiovascular risk and is thought to have antioxidant and anti-inflammatory properties.[56] However, a 2017 review found that HDL may not be an accurate marker of cardiovascular health in all populations.[57]

While new science is always emerging, your cholesterol levels can still help you determine if there are lifestyle changes that you can make to improve your overall health and are a valuable marker of health to discuss with your healthcare team.

LIFESTYLE FACTORS AND CHOLESTEROL

To improve your cholesterol levels (increasing HDL and decreasing LDL), stress management is key![58]

As we just discussed, cholesterol levels are often equated with cardiovascular risk, but stress may be a factor in this association as cholesterol levels have been seen to rise during times of stress.[59] Chronic stress has been linked to coronary heart disease, so even if your cholesterol levels are typically in the normal range, addressing stress might not be a bad idea![60]

Other ways to naturally improve HDL levels include quitting smoking and incorporating physical activity into your routine.[61]

SATURATED FATS, TRANS FATS, AND CHOLESTEROL

While you can consume cholesterol directly from food, other dietary fats may also influence your cholesterol levels.

The highest dietary sources of cholesterol consumed in the U.S. are meat, milk, eggs, and grains,[62] however, these may not be the culprit behind your high cholesterol levels. A 2017 review found that diets high in saturated and trans fats elevate LDL, our "bad" cholesterol, while trans fat may also lower our HDL, or "good" cholesterol levels.

If you want to improve heart health, be mindful of reducing your saturated and trans fat intake and replacing them with unsaturated fats, like olive oil, when possible.[63]

FASCINATING FACT

While reducing saturated fats may be beneficial, it would be nearly impossible to remove all saturated fats from your diet and may not be completely necessary.

In contrast to trans fats, which are *not* health-promoting in any way, not all saturated fats have undesirable effects in the body.

Coconut oil, although high in saturated fatty acids, was found to have similar effects to olive oil in regards to LDL, or "bad" cholesterol levels, and increased HDL, or "good" cholesterol levels, in a randomized controlled trial.[64]

Stearic acid, a saturated fat found in lard and cocoa butter, may have more of a positive effect on LDL, or "bad" cholesterol levels, than other saturated fats.[65]

These studies give us a glimpse into the complexity of fatty acids and their effect on the human body. We have so much to learn and explore, and making broad statements about saturated fats and cholesterol is neither correct nor helpful.

Based on the information above, sources of saturated fatty acids that may be more beneficial for cholesterol levels and overall health include coconut oil, cocoa butter, and lard. Fats that may be better in moderation include butter and processed foods high in trans fats.

LABEL READING AND DIETARY FAT

Remember, it's okay to eat fat. In fact, it's *good* to eat fat! Balance, as always, is key.

Generally speaking, here is a simple, helpful list to keep in mind when reading labels.

Friends

- Unsaturated fats: extra virgin olive oil, fatty fish, nuts, seeds, avocados, and avocado oil.
- Saturated fats: cocoa butter, beef tallow, lard, and coconut oil.

Foes

- Partially hydrogenated oils: and other refined oils such as corn, cottonseed, sunflower, soybean, wheat germ, safflower, canola,[66] and refined palm oil.

PRO TIP

We're pro-butter! If you look at the ingredients on most margarine spreads, they're loaded with different types of processed oils. Real butter is always better than the fake stuff.

Simple ways to improve your fat intake are cooking at home and monitoring what goes into your food—it may be better to roast potatoes with olive oil and salt than to open a bag of chips fried or baked in refined oils.

MACRONUTRIENT TAKEAWAYS

Carbs are not the enemy, not all proteins are alike, and fat isn't going to make you fat.

Ultimately, we want you to understand the importance of *balance* and the true necessity of including each macronutrient in your diet. If you're struggling with the enticing tug of some of the popular fad diets in the media, we encourage you to read our chapter Fad Diets, Sugar, and Your Cycle and speak with a nutritionist.

MICRONUTRIENTS

Micronutrients are the vitamins and minerals essential for basic processes in our bodies.[67] Micronutrients cannot be produced in the body, making a balanced diet important for obtaining all the necessary micronutrients.

In the next few pages, we will look at some of the micronutrients most relevant to your cycle.

FASCINATING FACT

Before you reach for a bottle of supplements, it's important to talk with a healthcare provider or pharmacist.

Even herbs and over-the-counter supplements can negatively influence the body when used incorrectly or in excess. In fact, in 2017, liver toxicity due to over-the-counter herbal remedies was estimated to be responsible for around twenty percent of liver toxicity cases,[68] and a 2022 article reports that drug-induced liver injury (from natural or manufactured compounds) has become the leading cause of acute liver failure in the United States.[69]

This is one of the reasons we emphasize talking to your healthcare team prior to supplementing. It's best to get lab work done to figure out what you actually need rather than assume your symptoms are from a micronutrient deficiency. And remember, how your body absorbs and uses micronutrients depends on gut health, making addressing the basics even more important!

A NOTE ON HORMONAL CONTRACEPTIVES AND NUTRIENT ABSORPTION

Hormonal contraceptives are one of the most commonly prescribed classes of medications, and unfortunately most people aren't aware that hormonal contraceptives have been linked with changes in nutritional status.[70]

Hormonal contraceptive use has been correlated with deficiencies in folate, B2, B6, B12, vitamin C, vitamin E, zinc, selenium, and magnesium.[71] B vitamins play a crucial role in maintaining healthy energy levels and vitamin C, vitamin E, zinc, selenium, and magnesium all have antioxidant properties. If you're on the pill or have a hormonal IUD or arm implant and are struggling with your health, it may be worth talking to your provider about getting lab work done to see if micronutrient deficiencies may be contributing to your symptoms.

To learn more about hormonal and non-hormonal contraceptives, check out pages 225 and 237.

VITAMINS: FAT-SOLUBLE VS WATER-SOLUBLE

It's important to understand there are two different types of vitamins, and they are processed differently in the body.

Water-soluble vitamins dissolve in water and can be easily absorbed into the bloodstream.[72] When the body reaches its threshold of a water-soluble vitamin, it will excrete the excess through urine. Because of this, Because of this, they typically cannot be stored in the body for long periods of time, making it difficult to reach a toxic level of these vitamins.[73]

Examples of water-soluble vitamins include B1, B2, B3, B6, B9, B12, and C.

Fat-soluble vitamins require fat to be absorbed and transported throughout the body, and unlike water-soluble vitamins, fat-soluble vitamins can be stored in body fat for extended periods of time.[74] It is important to consider the toxic thresholds of these vitamins since the excess isn't excreted in urine.

Examples of fat-soluble vitamins include A, D, E, and K.

MINERALS

Minerals are inorganic compounds, including sodium, potassium, chloride, calcium, phosphorus, magnesium, iron, copper, zinc, selenium, and iodine.[75]

It's important to note that popular fad diet plans may contribute to mineral deficiencies and imbalances.[76] We'll talk about this in our chapter Fad Diets, Sugar, and Your Cycle.

MICRONUTRIENTS ESSENTIAL FOR HORMONE HEALTH

VITAMIN B6

Vitamin B6 (also known as P5P) is a water-soluble vitamin involved in over one hundred enzymatic reactions in the body. Most of these chemical reactions are centered around protein metabolism and the creation of neurotransmitters such as serotonin.[77]

In regards to hormone health, B6 supports the production of progesterone and metabolism of estrogen,[78] making it relevant if you struggle with symptoms related to hormone imbalance.

> **FASCINATING FACT**
>
> The effectiveness of B6 in reducing PMS symptoms may be boosted when combined with calcium. In a randomized clinical trial, the combination of 40 mg of B6 with 500 mg of calcium had a greater impact on reducing PMS symptoms than vitamin B6 alone.[79]

Dietary sources of B6 include chickpeas, beef liver, tuna, salmon, chicken, potatoes, turkey, and bananas.

Recommended Dietary Allowance (RDA) for menstruating people:
1.3 mg per day.

FOLATE (B9)

Folate is most often associated with prenatal nutrition due to its positive impact on neural tube formation. While having healthy levels of folate *is* critical in the development of a fetus, it is also very important for the health of our cycles.[80]

If you've been reading labels, folate can be a little bit confusing.

Folate is a natural form of B9.

Folic acid is a synthetic form of B9.

> **FASCINATING FACT**
>
> For sixty to seventy percent of the population,[81] it may be difficult to break down the synthetic version, folic acid, into its more usable form in the body. If supplementing with B9, try to look for a supplement with a bioactive form of folate such as 5-methyltetrahydrofolate (5-Me-THF).[82]

Folate plays a critical role in menstrual health due to its positive influence on egg development,[83] progesterone levels, and ovulation. Folate may help improve luteal phase progesterone levels,[84] helping to balance the ratio of estrogen to progesterone during this time. We'll talk later in the book about how having a balanced ratio of estrogen to progesterone may help with your period problems!

Dietary sources of folate include dark green leafy vegetables, liver, bread, yeasts, and fruits.

Recommended Dietary Allowance (RDA) for menstruating people:
400 micrograms (mcg) per day.

VITAMIN B12

Vitamin B12, also called cobalamin, was the most recent vitamin to be discovered.[85] B12 plays a role in DNA synthesis, red blood cell formation, neurological health and helps maintain healthy energy levels.[86]

B12's involvement in red blood cell formation is critical for menstruating people since they lose 20-80 mL of blood each cycle. Heavy bleeders usually lose more than 80 mL of blood, so if you have a heavy period this may be a micronutrient worth paying attention to.

B12 deficiency can manifest as anemia, degeneration of peripheral nerves, neuropathy, mental confusion, depression, numbness, and tingling. B12 deficiency can develop slowly for years without notice until symptoms begin showing up, and it may take three to five years for symptoms to become evident.[87]

It is even more vital to pay attention to the above symptoms if you are vegetarian or vegan, as B12 is primarily found in animal products. Because of this, many processed grain products are fortified with B12 and other vitamins and minerals. This means that vitamins and minerals are added to the foods as a part of their processing. Although it may look like they have high amounts of nutrients on the labels, processed foods aren't always the most bioavailable sources of nutrients. When it's an option, we always recommend getting nutrients from whole food sources. If you're vegetarian or vegan, it might be worth talking with a nutritionist or other healthcare provider about the best ways to ensure you're getting enough B12 in your diet.

FASCINATING FACT

A small study from 2012 found that women with bladder leakage associated with coughing or sneezing, known as stress incontinence, tended to have lower levels of vitamin B12.[88] It may be worth getting your levels tested if you have incontinence, especially if you're not getting symptom relief with other treatment strategies.

Many people assume that because B12 is a water-soluble vitamin, you can't overdo supplementation. However, B12 is a water-soluble vitamin that can be stored in the body for longer periods of time (maybe even years!).[89]

A case study from 2020 found that after an individual had a total of 12 mg of B12 in one day, she started having symptoms like anxiety, acne, redness of her skin, palpitations, difficulty staying still, headaches, and insomnia.[90] The individual in this study was taking 5000 times the recommended daily amount, so if you're getting your B12 through food sources, you should be ok! If you are taking a higher dose supplement, make sure it's under the direction of a healthcare provider and that they are aware of the above symptoms.

Dietary sources of vitamin B12 include animal products such as beef, pork, poultry, fish, shellfish, eggs, and small amounts in dairy products.[91]

Recommended Dietary Allowance (RDA) for menstruating people:
2.4 micrograms (mcg) per day.

VITAMIN D

Did you know vitamin D is not a true vitamin? It's actually a steroid hormone created when sunlight touches bare skin. Once vitamin D has been made in the body, it travels to different tissues and organs where there are receptors ready to utilize it.[92]

Vitamin D receptors are highly prevalent in our reproductive organs, hypothalamus, and pituitary gland, making it a crucial player in reproductive health.[93]

A 2018 review found there may be a relationship between low vitamin D levels and the likelihood of developing a menstrual disorder,[94] and a 2020 clinical highlight lists vitamin D as having anti-inflammatory properties,[95] making vitamin D one to watch if you suffer from period problems!

FASCINATING FACT

Vitamin D levels have also been linked to the development of uterine fibroids. A 2013 study found lower rates of uterine fibroids in individuals with sufficient vitamin D levels compared to those with insufficient levels. This same study from 2013 discovered that only ten percent of the Black menstruating people and fifty percent of the white menstruating people who participated in the study had adequate vitamin D levels (>20ng/mL),[96] making it vital to advocate for yourself and make sure to get your vitamin D levels checked if you have fibroids!

While Western medicine standards categorize adequate vitamin D levels between 20-80 ng/mL,[97] you may feel your best at levels closer to 80 ng/mL. If you've had labs done, it's important to evaluate your levels in relation to how you feel even if your value comes back within a normal range.

It's also worth noting that iron and vitamin D have a symbiotic relationship,[98] so if you have problems with iron deficiency or anemia, you may also want to have your vitamin D levels checked!

Dietary sources of vitamin D: Although we get vitamin D primarily through sunlight, dietary sources of vitamin D include fortified dairy products, fish such as salmon, herring, sardines, and tuna, egg yolks, mushrooms, fortified orange juice, and cod liver oil, which has the added benefit of being a great source of omega-3.

Recommended Dietary Allowance (RDA) for menstruating people:
15 micrograms (mcg) or 600 IUs per day.

VITAMIN E

Vitamin E is a fat-soluble vitamin and antioxidant.[99]

While vitamin E naturally occurs in eight different forms, alpha-tocopherol is the only form human bodies are able to use.[100]

Because vitamin E is considered an antioxidant with anti-inflammatory properties, it may be beneficial for individuals suffering from menstrual disorders, menstrual pain, and migraines.[101]

> **PRO TIP**
>
> It may be beneficial to get your vitamin E from foods rather than supplements due to the high concentrations of vitamin E in some supplements.[102]

Dietary sources of vitamin E include nuts, egg yolks, cheese, oatmeal, avocados, olives, green leafy vegetables, and plant-based oils such as olive oil.[103]

Recommended Dietary Allowance (RDA) for menstruating people:
15 mg per day.

MAGNESIUM

Magnesium is a mineral necessary for menstrual and overall health. It plays a role in nervous system and cardiovascular function, metabolism, DNA synthesis, blood sugar regulation, bone formation, and may even relate to thyroid function.[104]

In regards to menstrual health, magnesium has been proposed to have anti-inflammatory properties and promote muscular relaxation,[105] which may explain its suggested benefits for cramps, period pain, and PMS.

While a 2019 review on magnesium and PMS symptoms found the current studies on the topic don't provide enough evidence to support the use of magnesium to treat PMS,[106] the benefits may depend on magnesium status prior to supplementation. A small 2015 study analyzing college students with PMS found individuals with PMS tended to have lower blood levels of magnesium compared to controls, and about one-third of them had magnesium deficiency.[107]

There is no standard lab test to accurately determine magnesium deficiency, making it very challenging for clinicians to diagnose. Until a good testing strategy emerges, it may be worth considering risk factors such as high consumption of coffee, soda and processed foods, use of medications such as diuretics, antacids, and oral contraceptives, which may influence magnesium status. Magnesium status may also be influenced by disease states such as diabetes, heart disease and osteoporosis and symptoms of low magnesium include leg cramps, sleep disorders and chronic fatigue. If any of the above symptoms are present, it may be beneficial to order a serum magnesium test and/or twenty-four-hour urine test to confirm suspicions based on symptom presentation.[108] Sometimes serum magnesium can be normal even in the presence of deficiency, so it's important to work with a provider who you trust and who will look at the whole picture.[109] Remember, like all supplements and medications, magnesium can have adverse effects with improper use. Some common side effects include low blood pressure, flushing, vasodilation, diarrhea, abdominal pain, gas, nausea/vomiting, and problems balancing electrolytes. Factors to consider prior to supplementation include neuromuscular conditions, pregnancy, and kidney function.[110]

For individuals with menstrual disorders, magnesium supplementation may be beneficial if you have a known deficiency or tend to be on the lower end of the spectrum. As always, starting with the whole food sources below is never a bad idea!

Dietary sources of magnesium include nuts, seeds, dark leafy greens, seaweed, legumes, dairy products, and whole grains.

Recommended Dietary Allowance (RDA) for menstruating people:
310–360 mg per day.

CALCIUM

Calcium is a mineral necessary for bone mineralization, muscle contractions and cardiovascular function.[111]

In relationship to menstrual health, 500 mg of calcium carbonate per day for two to three months has been seen to help with PMS symptoms like fatigue, appetite changes, cyclical depression, and mood disruption.[112]

However, don't reach for the supplements just yet! Minerals have symbiotic relationships, so too much of one can influence levels of another.[113] As always, it's best to talk with a provider before supplementing.

Dietary sources of calcium include dairy, green leafy vegetables, soy, sardines, and fortified grain products.

Recommended Dietary Allowance (RDA) for menstruating people:

1,000 mg of calcium per day.

IRON

Iron is a micronutrient necessary for cellular respiration, DNA repair and synthesis, and oxygen transfer throughout the body.[114]

The reason iron is such a critical micronutrient for menstruating people is because most of the iron found in the body is attached to hemoglobin in red blood cells. During menstruation, most individuals lose between 20-80 mL of blood and 10-40 mg of iron.[115] If you have a heavy cycle, you are likely to lose even more blood and iron, which is one of the reasons it's important to monitor for heavy bleeding.

When we talk about reproductive health, we cannot leave iron out of the equation. Iron plays a role in energy levels and may also influence ovulation and fertility! A 2006 study found low iron levels were correlated with increased risk of not ovulating,[116] which is important to consider if you're trying to conceive.

Low iron can manifest as weakness, fatigue, and may even contribute to hair loss and a feeling of restlessness in your legs.[117] If you suffer from chronic fatigue or tend to have low energy levels, check out our chapter on iron deficiency later in the book!

Diet plays an important role in iron status, with vegetarians and vegans being at a higher risk for iron deficiency.

There are two types of iron:

Heme iron is found in animal proteins and is very bioavailable, meaning that it can easily be absorbed and used in the body. Consuming heme iron is one of the best ways to boost iron levels and replenish nutrients lost during your bleed.

Non-heme iron is found in plants and is much less bioavailable than heme iron. Because non-heme iron is less easily used by the body, it is important for vegetarians and vegans to notice any symptoms that may be related to iron deficiency and keep in good communication with their healthcare team.[118]

PRO TIP

Vitamin C interacts with non-heme iron to make it more easily absorbed in the body.[119] A quick culinary trick for increasing the bioavailability of non-heme iron is to sprinkle citrus juice over a non-heme iron-rich plant, such as spinach.

If you're vegetarian or vegan, knowing that you're at risk for iron deficiency might make you want to reach for an iron supplement, but it's important to get lab work done before supplementing with iron. Iron is not easily excreted through urine and bowel movements,[120] meaning that it's possible to overdo supplementation.

Even if you have the symptoms of iron deficiency listed above, it's best to rule out any other health conditions that could be contributing to these symptoms. This is why we recommend having a healthcare team following your case; your specific lab reports may help figure out the root cause of your symptoms.

Sources of heme iron include beef, poultry, pork, and fish.

Sources of non-heme iron include dark leafy greens such as spinach, kale, and collard greens.

Recommended Dietary Allowance (RDA) for menstruating people:
15-18 mg of iron per day.

ZINC

Zinc is a mineral with known antioxidant and anti-inflammatory properties[121] that plays a role in cell growth, cognition, immune system function, and reproductive health.[122]

Preliminary research has found potential benefits for zinc supplementation in individuals with period pain and polycystic ovary syndrome (PCOS), and it *may* be beneficial for individuals with endometriosis due to its antioxidant status, but more research needs to be done.[123]

Although peer-reviewed research in regard to zinc and menstrual health is limited, a very small study in 1975 revealed some interesting results in terms of zinc and reproductive health. This study analyzed two women of reproductive age with dwarfism who had physical symptoms such as lack of breast tissue and pubic hair, under-development of external genitalia, and lack of menstruation. These individuals also had low levels of zinc, and once they were placed on a supplement regimen of zinc sulfate, both women received their first period and began growing pubic hair and breast tissue.[124]

Though the daily recommendation for zinc is 8 mg, a 2007 study found that 31 mg of zinc per day positively influenced premenstrual symptoms, whereas amounts closer to the daily recommendation did not. The study findings suggest that the current recommendation of 8 mg per day may not be adequate for individuals with a menstrual cycle.[125] Based on these findings, we believe more research needs to be done on zinc and reproductive health in menstruating people.

Although 8 mg per day *may* not be enough for menstruating people, don't reach for the high-dose supplements just yet! It is important not to over-supplement with zinc, which has an upper limit of 40 mg per day for adults.

Symptoms of dangerously high levels of zinc, known as zinc toxicity, include nausea, vomiting, stomach pain, lethargy, and fatigue. Although these symptoms usually occur at levels much higher than the recommended daily amount, high or low levels of zinc can influence levels of copper, cholesterol, and iron in the body,[126] potentially contributing to other health problems, including anemia.[127] With all of this in mind, it's important to get labs done prior to supplementation.

Dietary sources of zinc include oysters, beef, crab, lobster, pork, chicken, pumpkin seeds, cashews, chickpeas, and other legumes such as lentils and beans.

Recommended Dietary Allowance (RDA) for menstruating people:
at least 8–9 mg of zinc per day.

SELENIUM

Selenium is an essential trace mineral that plays a role in our body's antioxidant defense system.[128]

Selenium supports the menstrual cycle by defending against oxidative stress in the uterus and promoting the growth and maturation of follicles, which is necessary for ovulation.[129] Both are vital processes when it comes to fertility!

Dietary sources of selenium include sunflower seeds, Brazil nuts, chicken liver, beef liver, oysters, clams, fish roe, sardines, salmon, eggs, and beef.

Recommended Dietary Allowance (RDA) for menstruating people:
55 micrograms (mcg) per day.

IODINE

Iodine is a micronutrient that plays a role in thyroid function and metabolism.[130]

While there aren't many studies on iodine and reproductive health, low iodine may influence fertility and fibrocystic breast disease, so if you're having difficulty conceiving, or have painful, lumpy breast tissue, it may be worth talking to your provider about getting your iodine levels checked.[131]

In regards to PCOS, in small sample sizes with a lack of control for other treatments, some physicians have found iodine supplementation to help with period regularity, type II diabetes and ovarian cysts.[132]

It's important to note that iodine plays a critical role in thyroid function.[133] So, if you think you might have thyroid issues, have a history of thyroid disease, or have abnormal levels of thyroid hormones T3, T4, or TSH (thyroid-stimulating hormone), it's important to follow up with a healthcare provider before supplementing.

Dietary sources of iodine include seaweed, seafood, iodized salt, dairy, and eggs.

Recommended Dietary Allowance (RDA) for menstruating people:
150 micrograms (mcg) per day.

GLUTATHIONE

Glutathione is one of the most important antioxidants in our body.[134] It is found in most cells[135] and helps support our mitochondria, which are vital for maintaining healthy energy levels.[136] Glutathione aids the liver in the detoxification process[137] and may even play a protective role in the reproductive system due to its antioxidant properties.[138]

FASCINATING FACT

Did you know that your liver has a three-part detoxification process?

1. The first phase of detoxification is focused on bioactivation, which helps to make a toxin water-soluble. The water-soluble toxin is less stable and actually even *more toxic* than it originally was, however, it can be more easily excreted at the end of the detoxification process.

2. The second phase is where enzymes, such as glutathione, attach themselves to the toxin. Think of this phase as the neutralization phase that helps the molecule become less toxic to the body and more easily excreted in phase three.

3. The third phase is elimination of toxins attached to enzymes like glutathione through urine and bile.[139]

If detoxification started and stopped at phase one, you can imagine the havoc that would follow—our body would hold on to toxic substances, causing more harm than good.

While glutathione cannot be obtained directly through food, there are foods that support maintenance of healthy glutathione levels. These include fish, which are high in omega-3 fatty acids, foods rich in B vitamins, vitamin C, and vitamin E,[140] and whey protein, which is high in N-acetylcysteine.[141]

Other ways to increase glutathione levels include meditation and prayer, decreasing alcohol and sugar intake, and limiting exposure to environmental chemicals and toxins.[142]

MICRONUTRIENT TAKEAWAYS

Maintaining healthy levels of vitamins and minerals is crucial for menstrual health. We believe that, for most people, this is possible through consuming adequate nutrients in the foods we eat. Remember, if you want to supplement with specific vitamins and minerals, it's best to talk to your provider before starting a supplement regimen.

FOOD ALLERGIES AND INTOLERANCES

We would be remiss not to mention how each one of us processes food and medication differently. Reports of unfavorable physiological reactions to food have been on the rise in recent years,[143] and both food allergies and food intolerances can wreak havoc on your health.

So, what is the difference between food allergies and intolerances?

Food allergies are relatively immediate immune reactions to specific foods and involve an IgE antibody response to compounds in these foods.[144]

Food intolerances, also referred to as food sensitivities, are harder to identify because they involve a delayed immune reaction, which may be why they are under-diagnosed.[145] Food intolerances involve IgG, IgA, and IgM antibody responses, and symptoms may take several days to manifest after exposure to food triggers,[146] making it hard to identify which foods are causing your symptoms. Symptoms of food intolerance are wide-ranged and vary from person to person.[147]

So how do you know if you have food allergies or intolerances?

Skin prick tests help to identify allergies related to IgE mediated responses. Although they are commonly used, these tests may not be as helpful in identifying food intolerances due to the delayed response associated with IgG, IgM, and IgA mediated responses.[148]

When it comes to testing for food sensitivities and intolerances, there is debate in the medical field about the reliability of testing. A 2004 study found there are a number of tests that may be beneficial in identifying food intolerances and sensitivities, but the different tests may not catch *all* of the foods someone is reacting to.[149] A 2009 study suggests it may be beneficial to test antibodies in the blood against both raw and processed food particles, as how food is processed may influence reactions related to food sensitivities and intolerances.[150]

PRO TIP

AGEs, also known as advanced glycation end products, are chemicals that may be contributing to the rise in food allergies, due to their influence on the immune system.[151] How you cook your food can influence the number of AGEs present in your foods, with broiling and frying leading to higher amounts of AGEs.[152] If you're trying to decrease AGEs, start with the basics by decreasing highly processed and fried foods.

LOW FODMAP AND ELIMINATION DIETS

Because there is a lack of consensus in the medical field about how to test for food sensitivities and intolerances, it is common to use a trial-and-error approach to figure out what foods are causing symptoms.[153] Low FODMAP and elimination diets are two of the most popular approaches.

FODMAP is an acronym for "fermentable oligo-, di-, mono- and polysaccharides," which are short-chain carbohydrates that are not easily digested in the body. FODMAP sensitivity is one of the proposed mechanisms for the symptoms associated with food intolerances.[154] Because of the association between FODMAPs and GI symptoms, a low FODMAP diet, which involves eliminating foods high in FODMAPs from your diet, is often proposed to manage gastrointestinal problems.[155]

Some of the most common foods high in FODMAPs are foods high in fructose, including honey and fruits like pears, watermelon, mango, and fruits with pits, dairy, due to its lactose content, grains including wheat and rye, nuts, and vegetables like artichokes, onion, garlic, cauliflower, mushrooms, sugar snap peas, and snow peas.[156]

The **elimination diet** involves taking out certain foods over a specific period of time, usually two to three weeks. After the elimination period, symptoms are reviewed to see if eliminating the selected food(s) has helped with symptom management. If symptoms improve, the eliminated foods can be reintroduced, one by one, monitoring symptoms closely to ensure the problem foods are identified. It's important to note that if you have severe reactions to certain foods, reintroducing them might not be a good idea.[157]

FASCINATING FACT

Kola nut, often added to energy drinks due to its caffeine content, is used in the manufacturing of Coca-Cola and Pepsi and has been associated with food intolerances.[158] If you're having unexplained symptoms, it might be worth eliminating soft drinks and energy drinks!

Some of the foods most commonly removed in the elimination diet include gluten and dairy products.

Celiac disease is an autoimmune disease, in which ingestion of gluten triggers the body to attack the small intestine, leading to intestinal damage and inflammation. It's estimated that 1 in 100 individuals have celiac disease, and common symptoms include fatigue, loose bowel movements or constipation, vomiting and abdominal pain or discomfort.[159]

Even if you don't have celiac disease, you may still have symptoms related to gluten sensitivity.[160] Whether you have celiac disease or gluten sensitivity, some common symptoms associated with gluten intake include brain fog, fatigue, and GI irritation; this is why gluten is often one of the first items eliminated in the elimination diet.[161]

Dairy is another food that may be responsible for some of your digestive problems. There are two different types of proteins in animal milk: A1 casein and A2 casein. If you are part of the one in four Americans who cannot digest dairy, A1 casein may be the culprit of your digestive issues.[162] Sheep, goat and buffalo dairy are relatively accessible options containing minimal, if any, A1 proteins.[163]

We all process and metabolize foods differently, and the elimination and low FODMAP diets are meant to be tools to help you figure out which foods do, and do not, support your overall health. If you are following a low FODMAP or elimination diet it is wise to work closely with a nutritionist to ensure you are getting enough micro and macronutrients to support your overall health. It is not recommended that a low FODMAP diet be adopted for longer than four to eight weeks,[164] and it's important to gradually add foods back in if you're on an elimination diet.

ALLERGIES: HISTAMINE, HORMONES, AND GUT HEALTH

If you've ever experienced vague GI symptoms, dizziness, headaches or migraines, an unexplained runny nose, menstrual cramps, or skin problems like itchy skin, hives, or flushing, it might be related to histamine.[165]

Histamine is a chemical messenger found in the skin, gut, and immune system. It plays a large role in allergy and inflammatory responses,[166] and problems regulating histamine can lead to various non-specific symptoms in the body.[167]

High levels of histamine can be caused by ingestion of foods high in histamines, high production of histamine in the body, and problems with how our body processes histamine.[168]

FASCINATING FACT

Making matters more complicated, histamine levels can also be related to our physical environment. Exposure to environmental mold or extended time in a dry environment may influence symptoms related to histamine, and more recently, it has been proposed that electromagnetic fields (EMF) may influence histamine levels.[169] You may also experience symptoms related to high histamine if you have had prolonged activation of your immune system in response to an infection.[170]

Gut-related issues due to histamine may be difficult to isolate and reproduce, which can be frustrating if you're trying to figure out where your GI symptoms are coming from. This is where it's important to keep track of ALL your symptoms—your skin and gut issues just may be linked!

Histamine intolerance is a type of food intolerance related to the accumulation of histamine in the body, whether it's from our bodies' production of histamine, ingestion of histamine, or a combination of both, making it difficult to track.[171]

Like other food intolerances, symptoms of histamine intolerance can be vague and vary from person to person. The low-histamine diet is the gold standard for determining if your symptoms may relate to histamine; if you notice decreased symptoms on a low-histamine diet, this may indicate histamine is playing a role in your symptoms.[172]

Foods high in histamine include fish, wheat, cheese, wine, beer, eggplant, spinach, tomato, and avocado.[173]

This is where working with a functional nutritionist or healthcare provider is vital; in order to get better, it's important to figure out the root cause of your symptoms.

So how do hormones relate to histamine?

Estrogen receptors can be found on the immune cells responsible for the production and release of histamine,[174] and estrogen may slow down the activity of some of the enzymes that break down histamine, allowing histamine to stay in the body for longer periods of time.[175]

Progesterone may help decrease the release of histamine,[176] so if you suffer from low progesterone in relation to estrogen, you might also experience physical symptoms related to excess histamine.

This is one of the reasons tracking *all* of your symptoms is vital. If you experience vague GI and allergy symptoms, these may be influenced by histamine and hormone levels. Luckily, we have a whole chapter on how to balance the ratio of estrogen to progesterone; check out page 136 to learn more!

STRESS AND YOUR GUT

Did you know gut health and stress may go hand in hand?

Stress can create physiological changes in the gastrointestinal system.[177]

Stress can alter the gut microbiome, increase intestinal permeability (think "leaky gut" here), and impact how quickly food moves through your GI tract. It might even influence how you perceive pain and discomfort in your gut.[178]

This is important to understand because if stress is the root cause of your digestive issues, your symptoms might not resolve if you don't incorporate stress management into your routine.

The good news is, there are techniques to help us tap into our relaxation or "rest-and-digest" response. One of the simplest strategies is to slow down your breathing, focusing on breathing in and out for a count of five.

FASCINATING FACT

There's actually research directly connecting the diaphragm, our primary breathing muscle, with bowel problems like IBS. The diaphragm functions like a pump, aiding in digestion, and also has ties to our vagus nerve, promoting a relaxation response.[179]

To incorporate diaphragmatic breathing into your routine, bring one hand to your chest and one hand to your abdomen. Keeping the hand on your chest still, inhale and allow your abdomen to expand into your opposite hand. As you exhale, feel the abdomen gently draw up and in.

If you have a difficult time with diaphragmatic breathing or think stress may be influencing your GI symptoms, pelvic health physical therapy is a great resource to help with breathing, GI function and stress management.

GUT HEALTH TAKEAWAYS

If you're having unexplained GI symptoms, it's best to work with a healthcare provider to find the best plan for you. We're big fans of functional nutritionists because they can order blood work and stool samples to help get to the root cause of your issues.

Consider tracking how what you eat makes you feel—you may be able to fill in some of the mystery yourself through careful observation of your food choices and how they affect your body. Chances are you will notice almost immediate symptom reduction if you cut out packaged and fast foods high in processed sugar and fats for two to three weeks.

If you choose to do a low FODMAP or elimination diet, it's important to remember these diets are not meant to be followed for more than four to eight weeks. Without the supervision of a provider, these diets may lead to lack of adequate calories and nutrients and can have negative effects on the gut microbiome.

It's important to have open conversations with your providers if they recommend following a low FODMAP or elimination diet, especially if you have a history of disordered eating. These diets may trigger a relapse in the unhealthy behaviors you've worked so hard to overcome.

While some of your gut symptoms may be related to the foods you're eating, stress may also influence your gut, so it may be worthwhile to incorporate some stress management techniques into your routine.

MOVEMENT OVERVIEW

USING YOUR CYCLE TO OPTIMIZE ATHLETIC PERFORMANCE

Did you know that many world-class athletes view their menstrual cycle as a tool to enhance their athletic performance rather than something that inhibits it?

The U.S. women's soccer team is a prime example! Their players vary training based on where they are in their cycles and look at how successful they are. Some of their stats include most Women's World Cup titles won, most consecutive World Cup Finals, most times in the top four at the Women's World Cup, and most goals scored in the World Cup.[1]

Regardless of your athletic background, understanding how hormones influence your body's performance is crucial to optimizing how you move throughout your cycle. We will get into tips for each phase of your cycle later in this chapter, so stay tuned!

PRO TIP

Dr. George Bruinvels is a leading researcher in the field of menstruation and athletic performance. His team created an app called FitR Woman to help menstruating people track their cycles. This app provides relevant information about nutrition, activity, and general health throughout your cycle, so if you're not already using a period tracking app, it might be worth checking it out! As always, remember that when you use apps, there's no guarantee that your data will be secure. Old-school pen and paper might be the best way to keep track if you're concerned about security.

EXERCISE RESEARCH AND YOUR CYCLE

While there is compelling evidence for the benefits of exercise, a large portion of this evidence may not take into account individuals with a menstrual cycle.

This is especially true in sports medicine research. A 2014 article in the *European Journal of Sports Medicine* discovered that over a three-year period in articles from three major sports medicine journals, menstruating people only accounted for thirty-nine percent of the individuals studied.[2]

FASCINATING FACT

Exercise may not be the only field where menstruating people are not properly represented in research. In a 2001 review analyzing articles on adverse drug reactions, one of the top factors found to increase the likelihood of having an adverse drug reaction was *being a menstruating person!*

This review found that menstruating people were 1.5–1.7x more likely to have an adverse drug reaction compared to their non-menstruating counterparts. The reasoning behind this could be multifactorial,[3] which is why we believe there is no "one-size-fits-all" approach when it comes to health. Even drugs with the same purpose may affect each unique body differently.

The other problem with research regarding exercise, even if it does include menstruating individuals, is that there are many different types of exercise and varying protocols used in the literature. Because of this, some results may be more or less relevant to your goals or preferred exercise routine.

What we *do* know is that movement is good for the body, so choosing ways to stay active that you can be consistent with is what matters.

Before we talk about general exercise recommendations, let's talk about specific nutrition hacks if you are a menstruating person with high activity levels.

MACRONUTRIENTS, EXERCISE, AND THE MENSTRUAL CYCLE

Nutritional needs may vary from person to person, affecting athletic performance. But did you know menstruating endurance athletes may have different nutritional needs than their non-menstruating counterparts?

Two studies, one from 1985 and one from 1995, found menstruating endurance athletes tend to rely more heavily on fats for fuel than carbohydrates and proteins like their non-menstruating counterparts.[4]

PRO TIP

While this is good information to know, it's also important to remember that these studies specifically looked at individuals performing high-intensity activity lasting more than half an hour; if you're a recreational athlete, your energy needs may be a little bit different.

With this information in mind, you might be wondering—*should I be carbo-loading?*

If you've been told to carbo-load or eat more carbohydrates the day before an athletic event, it's important to note that carbo-loading may be more effective in non-menstruating people. The goal of carbo-loading is to increase carbohydrate storage in the body, which may be more efficiently done in individuals without a menstrual cycle.[5]

Though carbo-loading may not demonstrate identical results between individuals with and without a menstrual cycle, it shouldn't be completely written off for menstruating people.

In a 2000 study analyzing a high-carbohydrate diet in six endurance athletes during their luteal phase, increasing carbohydrate intake to about seventy-eight percent of their diet was seen to improve carbohydrate stores and athletic performance, even if at a smaller magnitude than in their non-menstruating counterparts.[6] While this study found benefits for carbo-loading in the second half of your cycle, it's important to remember that this research focuses on a group doing long, intense workouts; individual energy needs may vary by activity levels. Your baseline energy needs may also be higher in the luteal phase, making carbs more beneficial for athletes during this time. We'll talk about this in the next chapter!

The research we've highlighted shows there may be differences in what macronutrients are most effective for menstruating athletes, and this might shift throughout our cycles. The above studies had very small sample sizes, and future research looking at how menstruating individuals use specific macronutrients like carbs, fats, and proteins for fuel during exercise is warranted, especially across different stages of our cycle.

Carbohydrates are essential, but it's also important to recognize that fat may play a critical role in sports performance for menstruating people. As always, balance is key!

EXERCISE RECOMMENDATIONS

Our bodies thrive with movement and physical activity! Exercise can support your mental well-being, mood, sleep, and immune function.[7]

Unfortunately, with the online world expanding, most aspects of our lives, including work, school, and recreational activities, are now available on a screen. In general, we're spending more time sitting and less time moving, which can be detrimental to both our physical and mental health.

Both the American Heart Association and the World Health Organization have similar recommendations for physical activity.

Their recommendations include:

- **Aerobic activity:** at least 150 minutes per week of moderate-intensity aerobic activity or 75 minutes per week of vigorous aerobic activity.

  - **Moderate aerobic activity:** brisk walking at least 2.5 miles per hour, water aerobics, ballroom or social dancing, gardening, tennis doubles, and biking slower than 10 miles per hour.

  - **Vigorous aerobic activity:** hiking uphill or with a heavy backpack, running, swimming laps, aerobic dancing, heavy yard work, tennis singles, cycling 10 miles per hour or faster, and jumping rope.

- **Strength training:** two days per week of moderate to high-intensity strength training with use of resistance or weights.

On a happy note, you can get your minimum aerobic requirement by combining moderate and vigorous activity, and even short exercise sessions count!

FASCINATING FACT

Before 2018, the World Health Organization recommended the duration of physical activity sessions be longer than ten minutes, but new research suggests you may get benefits from even just a few minutes of exercise! Short bursts of exercise, often referred to as "exercise snacks," can be more manageable schedule-wise, and may still positively impact cardiovascular health.[8]

Keep in mind these are the *minimum* recommendations to reduce the risk of preventable disease and premature death. If your goal is to decrease your risk of conditions like type II diabetes and cardiovascular disease, aim for at least 150 minutes of physical activity per week.

If you have slightly more ambitious goals, you'll need to increase your time commitment closer to 300 minutes of aerobic activity per week to maximize health benefits. Make sure to mix in some strength training, too.

Remember, it's never too late to get moving, regardless of your exercise background or athletic ability!

Simple ideas for increasing physical activity include getting outside for a walk or hike, doing yard work, doing arm exercises or squats while watching TV, or practicing chair yoga and stretches.

Adding short bits of exercise throughout the day can help, too! If you're a student or primarily sit at a desk for work, we love the Pomodoro timer because it encourages you to get up from your work and move around every twenty-five minutes. Bonus points if you can get your movement in while outdoors, as the sun is a great source of vitamin D!

AEROBIC VERSUS ANAEROBIC EXERCISE: WHAT'S THE DIF-FERENCE?

Aerobic exercise is what we think of when we hear "cardio." Some of the most common forms include cycling, swimming, walking, and running. Aerobic activity relies on oxygen to create energy. Because of this, aerobic activities are usually lower or moderate-intensity and can be performed over longer periods of time.

Anaerobic exercise does not rely on oxygen for the creation of energy and tends to be high intensity over short periods of time.[9] Anaerobic activity consists of quick bursts of activity, as is common during High-Intensity Interval Training workouts, also known as HIIT. Anaerobic exercises are much harder to sustain over a long period of time.

FASCINATING FACT

Carbohydrates are the only macronutrient that can be used for energy without utilizing oxygen, which makes carbohydrates essential for high-intensity activity or training that relies on the anaerobic system.[10]

A well-rounded routine will include both aerobic and anaerobic training to maximize health benefits.

A NOTE ON STRENGTH TRAINING

If you're not doing any strength training, now is the time to start!

Resistance training, also referred to as strength training, is exercise using resistance, most commonly in the form of bands or weights. Resistance training may help athletes optimize performance by reducing muscular imbalances and decreasing the likelihood of overuse injuries. It can also help untrained individuals gain strength and confidence with daily activities.

FASCINATING FACT

In untrained individuals, almost any type of resistance training program will result in improvements in strength, regardless of the number of sets and repetitions. In individuals who already have a program and are trying to gain muscle bulk, or hypertrophy, doing three or more different exercises per muscle group is the most effective strategy.[11]

Strength training is crucial for optimizing bone health and preventing injuries. By having a consistent strengthening routine, you make sure that you're able to do daily tasks without worrying about tweaking your back, hips, or knees.

For those of you who love cardio and don't do anything else, we're talking to you, too!

Think about it this way: if you do the same motions over and over without strengthening other muscles, you're more likely to become injured. We all know that injuries can put a damper on your daily life and training routine, so it's definitely worth adding some strength training into the mix!

PRO TIP

It's important to remember that strength training creates long-term changes in the body. You may not notice results until you're six to eight weeks into your program, so don't get frustrated if you're not seeing immediate changes. This is why we stress the importance of creating sustainable habits to establish greater health over time.

The most important thing to take away from this chapter is to get moving! We encourage you to get out of your comfort zone by trying different fitness activities throughout the week. "Exercise snacks" are a great way to get some exercise in if you're in a time crunch, and those short bouts of exercise really add up!

MUSCLE SORENESS – IS IT A NECESSARY PART OF WORKING OUT?

If you've ever been sore after a workout, you most likely experienced delayed onset muscle soreness, also known as DOMS.

DOMS is common after intense exercise and is usually highest twenty-four to forty-eight hours post-exercise.[12]

FASCINATING FACT

While it was previously thought that DOMS may be due to lactic acid production, more recent theories suggest that it is related to microtrauma in the muscles and connective tissue and the associated inflammatory response.[13]

A little bit of soreness can be a normal byproduct of working out, especially if you're trying something new, but excessive soreness may be a sign that you overdid it. If you're still sore for up to five days after your exercise session, it may be a sign that you worked out too hard!

While the "go-hard or go-home" mentality is common, if you're not experiencing soreness, that doesn't mean you're *not* building strength! A 2017 study found strength gains in both a group with soreness and muscular damage and a group who reported minimal soreness.[14] These findings indicate that a consistent routine starting at a low or moderate intensity and gradually increasing in difficulty may be a sustainable approach to improving strength.

PRO TIP

Massage and foam rolling may help ease some of the symptoms associated with DOMS.[15] If you don't have access to a massage therapist post- workout, a foam roller is a great alternative! A foam roller is a tube made of compressed foam, often used as a tool for muscular recovery. A 2014 study found foam rolling immediately after and at twenty-four and forty-eight hours post-exercise may help reduce symptoms of DOMS and improve recovery.[16]

THE BENEFITS OF EXERCISE: LOOKING AT THE WHOLE BODY

We all know exercise is good for us, but sometimes, it's easier to commit to a routine when you understand why it's beneficial. When you can connect exercise with improved mental health, sleep, and immune function, you may be more likely to set aside some time for it in your busy schedule.

The next few sections discuss how exercise can positively influence the whole body. While there is a ton of research out there about the benefits of exercise, we wanted to include a few examples in this section to get you thinking about how adding movement into your routine can positively influence your body and mind.

EXERCISE, MOOD, AND MENTAL HEALTH

Did you know depression is the most common cause of health-related disability in menstruating people? Individuals with a menstrual cycle are almost two times more likely to experience a major depressive episode compared to their non-menstruating counterparts.[17]

Medical management of mental health disorders like anxiety and depression often includes prescription medication. However, medication alone doesn't necessarily address the root cause of your symptoms and may lead to less than desirable side effects.

This is one of the reasons we are passionate about this book; before we reach for medications to address health problems, it's important to start with the basics.

While we are not against the use of medications, we encourage you to start with the health pyramid on page 8 to see if there are any basic aspects of health that can be improved. Pay attention to your mental health symptoms; sometimes, they can have a cyclical component without us even realizing it!

Whether you have anxiety or depression, it's important to honestly assess your exercise patterns. Are you getting any exercise on a daily basis? Or are you exercising too much as a coping mechanism?

Remember, everything, including exercise, should be practiced in moderation. Some people suffering from anxiety or depression may use excessive exercise as a coping strategy. If you feel like you have to exercise for multiple hours per day to "burn off" something you consumed or to deal with minor everyday stressors, it might be beneficial to add a mental health professional to your team.

Though we do not think exercise is a "cure-all" for mental health issues, research has shown that exercise may be beneficial for individuals with depression,[18] and it can be a great addition to your treatment plan for moderate or severe depression, whether or not you are using medications to manage symptoms.[19]

What about exercise and anxiety?

For individuals with anxiety, exercise alone may not be enough to manage symptoms at the same levels achieved by prescription drugs.[20] However, if you have anxiety and you're not currently active, it may be worth adopting a consistent movement routine. A 2011 review found that low activity levels were linked to a higher likelihood of developing psychiatric disorders, including anxiety and depression, and a 2017 review found anxiety to be more prevalent among individuals with low activity levels.[21] If you're not moving your body regularly, we encourage you to start with the activity recommendations mentioned earlier in this chapter!

If you are seeing a mental health provider and exercise is not currently a part of your treatment plan, talk to your provider about adding exercise into your routine. While we are not against the use of medication by any means, there is plenty of research indicating that, in some cases, physical activity may be an effective treatment option, and you can add it into your routine whether or not you are on medications or in therapy.

PRO TIP

Sometimes, mental health problems can interfere with your desire to exercise,[22] even if you know you'll feel better after working out.

If you're having a low-energy day, we suggest the three-minute test—set a timer for three minutes and walk briskly until the timer goes off. If you feel better or more energized after this test, exercise may be a great idea! If you feel worse or more fatigued, this may be a sign that your body needs to rest.

EXERCISE AND THE IMMUNE SYSTEM

Did you know exercise helps support our immune system?

The lymphatic system is part of our immune system. You can think of the lymphatic system as our bodies' natural filter, clearing out cellular waste and toxins that build up in our tissues. It also helps transport fats and fat-soluble vitamins from the GI tract to other parts of the body.[23]

The lymphatic vessels pick up fluid from the body. This fluid, referred to as lymph, is then filtered by specific organs and returned back into the cardiovascular system.[24]

How does exercise relate to this process?

Capillaries pick up fluid from the body, bringing it into the lymphatic vessels. Both smooth and skeletal muscle contractions help move fluid forward through the lymphatic vessels, helping it move towards the lymph nodes to be filtered.[25]

This is where exercise is key! Skeletal muscle contractions are estimated to contribute to about a third of the forward movement of lymph in the lower body. If you're not moving regularly, you may be missing out on the benefits of your body's natural filtering system![26]

EXERCISE AND SLEEP

Sleep is *vital* to health and well-being, and exercise may help with sleep!

The age-old theory of "go hard or go home" may not apply when it comes to the benefits of exercise on sleep. According to a 2019 review, moderate-intensity activity was associated with better sleep outcomes than vigorous activity.[27]

You might think of cardio as the best way to tire yourself out and improve sleep, but a 2019 review of thirteen studies found consistent resistance exercise improved quality and quantity of sleep, with the biggest impact on quality.[28] So, whether you choose to run, cycle, or lift, moderate-intensity exercise may help you get better sleep and feel well-rested throughout your cycle!

EXERCISE TIPS AND THE IMPORTANCE OF COMMUNITY

The hardest step is always the first one. Knowledge is both power and motivation, and we want you to feel empowered as you understand how the choices you make regarding movement influence the whole body.

Simple Ways to Get Started:

- **Start where you are and do what you can:** Chair exercises are better than no exercises, and walking is a great way to promote whole-body health. Find ways to incorporate little bursts of exercise into your day.

- **Create more time in your schedule:** It's easy to binge-watch our favorite shows for hours, especially when we're tired.

If you know you have this habit, stream your favorite show and do some cleaning, meal prep, laundry, or even lift some weights while you're watching. If you combine something you enjoy such as music, podcasts, or binge-watching a series with daily activities that you need to get done, not only will you enjoy these activities more, but you'll have more time to add some exercise into your routine and enjoy other aspects of your life.

- **Spend less time sitting:** Even light activity can offset some of the health issues associated with being sedentary. If you're sitting at a desk for work all day, try sitting on a large exercise ball. This small change can help improve your posture and engage your core while you're working. If your job allows you the option, moving throughout the day may be more beneficial than spending your full day in one position, whether that's sitting or standing. You might even ask your employer if they're willing to reimburse you for a standing or convertible workstation. If you're sitting for most of the day and are interested in learning more about how to transition into better biomechanics, check out the book *Deskbound* by Juliet and Kelly Starrett.

- **Set a timer:** We love the Pomodoro timer for those who spend most of their day at a desk! One of our favorite websites for this is pomofocus.io/app. The Pomodoro timer encourages you to get up from your work every twenty-five minutes for a five-minute break. Some ideas of ways to incorporate more physical activity into your day include using this break for walking, pushups, planking, or jumping jacks. It might be just the brain break you need to be more productive with whatever you're working on!

- **Put it on your calendar:** If you have specific days and times scheduled for exercise, you'll be more likely to make sure it happens.

- **Set a fitness goal:** Setting a fitness goal can look like "I'll walk with friends three times per week," "I'll add one strength training session a week," or "I'll start prepping for a race or triathlon." Having a goal can motivate you to consistently stay active. If you're new to activity and are craving a structured routine, the CouchTo5K app is a really great place to start. It provides a sustainable routine to help motivate individuals to get moving and provides gradual walking/jogging progressions week to week, easing you from a sedentary lifestyle all the way to completing a 5k (3.1 miles).

- **Create a community:** Sometimes, it can be difficult to feel motivated to move our bodies. One tip we love is to make working out social. Ask friends to join you or work out with a trainer in a small group setting or one-on-one. When you create a culture that supports physical activity, it's much easier and more fun to get moving!

PRO TIP

It's important to remember that pain is not a necessary part of working out. We encourage you to take care of any aches and pains before they develop into injuries that interfere with your daily life. If you need exercise guidance, working with a trainer is a great place to start! If you can't figure out where your pain is coming from, physical therapy is an awesome place to learn more about injury prevention and work on pain management without surgeries, medications, or injections. In most states, you can see a physical therapist without a physician referral.

EXERCISE TAKEAWAYS

With any exercise program, it's important to find what's right for you. In later chapters, we explore some examples of how to exercise throughout your cycle, and we encourage you to build a routine you can stick with.

If you love tennis, play tennis! If you love strengthening, keep strengthening! We want to remind you that it's also good to keep a well-rounded routine in order to maximize health benefits and avoid injury, and we encourage you to try activities outside of your comfort zone. While it's easy to think *I can't* when it comes to exercise and fitness, you'd be surprised at how much you can accomplish when you consistently show up! If you feel limited by your schedule, remember that doing ten minutes of exercise on a busy day is *way* better than doing nothing, and those ten minutes really add up over a year.

And if you're not an "athlete," no sweat (pun intended)! Athletes in our society are often glorified with that "go-hard-or-go-home, push-through-the-pain" mentality, but it's important to note that athletes aren't always optimally healthy. If your goal is overall health, it's key to find a routine that works and feels good for you, and that might look different for each of us reading this book.

EATING AND MOVING FOR YOUR CYCLE

A NOTE ON EATING AND MOVING FOR YOUR CYCLE

This chapter will focus on exercise and nutrition hacks for each stage of your cycle, including options for vegetarians, vegans, and meat-eaters alike. We're not here to judge your dietary decisions or how you choose to move your body but to give you an idea of healthy options to fit your lifestyle.

Each body is unique and may function best with different approaches to nutrition and fitness. What works for you may not only look different from what someone else is doing but may also vary day to day depending on where you are in your cycle and what's happening in your life.

Contrary to what pop culture may tell you, food holds no morality, and you are *not* a "better" person if you exercise more.

We want to strip away any feelings of judgment or shame around your food choices and how you choose to move your body. There is no such thing as "bad" food or "good" food. Food is just food, and your decisions around both food and movement do not make you any more or less of a human being worthy of love and acceptance. The foods you eat, the amount you exercise, or the way your body looks does not determine your character and the beautiful things only you can bring into this world.

With that being said, food and exercise *do* influence how you feel and function, so using both as a way to nourish and love your body is a great place to start!

ENERGY NEEDS THROUGHOUT YOUR CYCLE

Do you feel hungrier in the second half of your cycle? Or completely drained when you do the same activities you did earlier in your cycle, even when eating the same amount of food?

This may be due to higher baseline energy expenditure during the second half of your cycle; you may use more energy at rest during the luteal phase, making it vital to properly fuel your body during this time.[1]

FASCINATING FACT

A 2020 study analyzing nine individuals found an increase in body temperature at night and a 6.9% increase in energy expenditure, with higher use of carbs as an energy source during the luteal phase.[2]

These physiological changes may relate to progesterone levels, so if you're tracking basal body temperature and your temperature isn't rising during the second half of your cycle, this may signify low progesterone levels and lack of ovulation.[3]

Once you understand your energy needs vary throughout your cycle, you can start to recognize your hunger cues and increase your food intake without being self-critical or depriving yourself of much-needed energy.

Now let's talk about each distinct part of the menstrual cycle.

Disclaimer: We are using the textbook length of a menstrual cycle as an example in this book. Not everyone has a fourteen-day follicular phase, ovulates on day fourteen, and gets their period on day twenty-eight. This is why we encourage you to track your monthly rhythms—they might be slightly different for each of us reading this book and may vary month to month.

MENSTRUATION: DAY 1 – END OF BLEEDING

Menstruation, also known as your period or menses, is when the inner wall of the uterus is shed.

Estrogen and progesterone are at their lowest levels during menstruation. Bleeding is triggered by the drop in progesterone just before your period, causing the inner wall of the uterus to disintegrate. Towards the end of menstruation, a rise in estrogen promotes clotting and the regrowth of the uterine lining.[4]

During menstruation, you may feel more tired and need extra rest due to the low levels of estrogen and progesterone. Not only are estrogen and progesterone at the bottom of the bell curve making you feel "bleh," your uterus is also contracting due to an increase in prostaglandins,[5] which may contribute to the cramping sensation during your period.

> If you are following the Fertility Awareness Method, known as FAM, your basal body temperature, also known as BBT, usually drops significantly at the onset of your period ranging from 97.00-97.70.[6]

EATING DURING MENSTRUATION

While some fatigue is normal, if you suffer from significant fatigue during your period, it may be related to the loss of iron and other micronutrients. Remember, you lose an average of 10-40 mg of iron per bleed,[7] which may result in decreased energy and increased need for rest. Knowing this, it's important to get adequate nutrition during this time.

During this time, the dietary focus should be on three things: warming foods, energy- and mineral-rich foods, and foods that fight inflammation.

Warming foods are exactly what they sound like: foods that are warm and soothing. Warming foods are not only comforting to the soul but also bring comfort to your cooler-than-normal body since your basal body temperature (BBT) is low during menstruation.[8]

Mineral-rich foods are also critical to help replace the minerals lost via bleeding, and it's important to maintain adequate fat and protein intake during menstruation. Incorporating both fat and protein at every meal can help regulate blood sugar levels and sustain energy throughout the day, which is especially important to combat period-related fatigue.[9]

Rich stews with energy and mineral-dense ingredients such as beets, kale, animal protein such as beef or chicken, kidney beans, and miso are a great place to start. Not only are soups and stews warming foods, but they also are high in micro and macronutrients, making them a wonderful option!

Anti-inflammatory foods help to combat inflammation, which may contribute to period problems such as headaches, cramps, and period pain. Check out the list on the next page for some examples!

FASCINATING FACT

You may also experience GI changes during your period! Have you ever started your period and then seemingly out of nowhere you're urgently running to the bathroom? This is actually common and may be related to hormonal shifts. Progesterone is associated with gut motility,[10] or how quickly food moves through the GI tract. This means when progesterone levels change throughout the cycle, gut motility may also change. For example, as progesterone rises in the luteal phase, you may be more prone to constipation, and as progesterone drops during menstruation and prostaglandins increase GI contractions, your bowel movements might be looser. As always, if you suffer from severe GI dysfunction (whether or not it is related to your cycle), it never hurts to follow up with a healthcare provider.

WHAT TO EAT DURING MENSTRUATION

- **Ten Iron-Rich Foods:** beef, chicken, pork, venison, fish, shellfish, dark leafy greens, dried apricots, lentils, and grains.
  - When using leafy greens as an iron source, remember to pair them with a source of vitamin C to make the iron more available for use in the body. Citrus fruits such as lemon and lime are great options!
- **Ten Anti-Inflammatory Foods:** salmon, blueberries, raspberries, blackberries, walnuts, ginger, broccoli, avocado, mushrooms (specifically lion's mane), and extra virgin olive oil (EVOO).

MEAL IDEAS FOR MENSTRUATION

Vegetarian & Vegan

Breakfast: Chickpea Scramble	Lunch: Spinach Berry Salad	Dinner: Lentil and Mushroom Stew

Non-Vegetarian/Vegan

Breakfast: Avocado and Smoked Salmon Toast	Lunch: Chicken, Broccoli, and Mushroom Stir-fry	Dinner: Jazzy Chickpea Pasta

Note: See the back of the book for full recipes!

MOVING DURING MENSTRUATION

During menstruation, you may crave slow, gentle movement. Listen to your body by doing more or less depending on what you need, and don't hesitate to add in a few rest days. This is a great time to focus on activities like walking, stretching and gentle yoga. It may also be beneficial to incorporate deep breathing into whatever movement routine you choose!

> **PRO TIP**
>
> If you're not feeling up for moving, you can still get health benefits from adding some deep breathing into your routine! An easy place to start is setting a timer for a few minutes and focusing on breathing in and out through your nose, counting to five for each inhale and exhale. There are also some YouTube videos that cue for deep breathing; an example of one that we like is "Guided Meditation of HRV Resonate Breathing at 6 BPM" by Forrest Knutson.

If you feel up for higher-intensity exercise, go for it! Studies have shown that you may be less likely to injure yourself during this time due to the low estrogen levels.[11]

Examples of physical activity during menstruation include walking, hiking, gentle biking, and restorative or gentle yoga.

THE FOLLICULAR PHASE: DAYS 1 - 14

Did you know your period is actually a part of the follicular phase?

During your period, estrogen begins to rise, which prompts the end of your menstrual bleed.[12] Along with the rise in estrogen, there is also a rise in follicle-stimulating hormone (FSH). FSH is secreted by the pituitary gland to help prepare our bodies for ovulation, which is the next stage of our cycle.

FASCINATING FACT

While most of us think of ovulation as our most fertile time, did you know your fertile window actually starts at the end of the follicular phase, about five days prior to ovulation?

The follicular phase has two stages: the early follicular phase, characterized by low levels of both estrogen and progesterone, and the late follicular phase, characterized by low progesterone and the highest amount of estrogen throughout your cycle.[13]

If you are following the Fertility Awareness Method, known as FAM, you may notice that your cervical mucus is absent or sticky, like the residue from a sticker, and your basal body temperature, also known as BBT, remains in the 97.00-97.70 range during the follicular phase.[14]

EATING DURING THE FOLLICULAR PHASE

The dietary focus in this phase should be replenishing nutrients lost during menstruation and increasing foods that energize you.

With this in mind, it is important to include foods rich in micronutrients, such as vitamin B12 and iron, which can be found in animal proteins and dark leafy greens.

WHAT TO EAT DURING THE FOLLICULAR PHASE

- **Ten Iron-Rich Foods:** beef, liver, venison, chicken, salmon, shellfish, eggs, dark leafy greens, legumes, and molasses.

  - When using leafy greens as an iron source, remember to pair them with a source of vitamin C to make the iron more available for use in the body. Citrus fruits such as lemon and lime are great options!

- **Ten B12-Rich Foods:** beef, liver, venison, chicken, salmon, shellfish, eggs, dark leafy greens, legumes, and whole milk dairy products.

MEAL IDEAS FOR THE FOLLICULAR PHASE

Vegetarian & Vegan

Breakfast: Fueled-Up Oatmeal and Broiled Grapefruit	Lunch: Roasted Broccoli and Black-Eyed Pea Salad	Dinner: Grilled Portobello Collard Wraps

Non-Vegetarian/Vegan

Breakfast: Veggie 'N Cheese Omelet	Lunch: Roasted Broccoli and Chicken Salad	Dinner: Simple Baked Salmon Dinner

Note: See the back of the book for full recipes!

MOVING DURING THE FOLLICULAR PHASE

With your period occurring at the beginning of this phase and estrogen and progesterone levels remaining relatively low, you might notice increased fatigue. Most individuals can benefit from easing into activity in the early follicular phase and gradually increasing intensity as they get closer to ovulation.

A small 2014 study found strength training may reveal the most gains during the late follicular phase as you approach ovulation.[15] This may be a great time to incorporate more strength training into your routine!

> **PRO TIP**
>
> There is some conflicting evidence and not all studies have found differences in strength gains in different phases of your cycle.[16] However, there is still benefit to strength training, so we encourage you to add strength training into your routine, not only during this phase, but throughout your cycle!

You may be more prone to injury in the late follicular phase if you participate in contact sports or high-impact activities.[17] But don't let this stop you from doing what you love!

Injury risk can be prevented by improving *how* you're moving. This is one of the reasons we emphasize adding whole-body strength training, core work, and balance work into your routine. We'll talk more about ways to reduce risk of injury in our section Injury Prevention and Your Cycle—check it out to learn more.

Examples of physical activity during the follicular phase include running, high-intensity interval training (HIIT), and strength training.

OVULATION: DAYS 12 – 14

Ovulation, the time when you're most fertile, is when you may feel more energetic and social. As your sex hormones signal that it's time to make a baby, you might notice a stabilized mood and increased libido or sex drive.

Ovulation occurs when luteinizing hormone (LH) and estrogen signal the mature follicle to release an egg from one ovary into the fallopian tube to travel to the uterus[18] and potentially be fertilized if it comes in contact with healthy sperm. If it has been fertilized, it will implant into the uterine lining...hello, pregnancy! If it has not been fertilized, it will disintegrate.

When possible, ovulation is a great time to schedule important presentations or meetings at work, focus on creative projects, and engage in big events and social gatherings.

> If you are following the Fertility Awareness Method, known as FAM, you may notice that your cervical mucus becomes clear, resembling egg whites, and your basal body temperature, also known as BBT, increases just after ovulation. Remember, the increase in temperature can differ between individuals and from cycle to cycle.[19]

EATING DURING OVULATION

The dietary focus during ovulation should be centered on "cooling foods," due to the increase in basal body temperature right after ovulation, and foods that support your liver.

Chinese medicine teaches that "cooling foods" can work to slightly cool your warmer-than-usual body. Some examples of cooling foods include green veggies and green tea.[20]

Cruciferous veggies, such as broccoli, cauliflower, kale, and collard greens, are a great option during this time as they are considered cooling foods and are high in fiber which helps with bowel movements. They also contain phytochemicals which support liver health and the breakdown of estrogen![21]

By incorporating these vegetables into your diet during ovulation, you can begin preparing your body to help manage PMS symptoms in the second half of your cycle.

Hunger may start to rise during ovulation, continuing to increase into the luteal phase. This may be due to the higher energy requirements at rest, so it's important to listen to and honor your hunger cues!

WHAT TO EAT DURING OVULATION

- **Ten Cooling Foods:** mushrooms, cauliflower, cabbage, zucchini, cucumber, tofu, pear, snow peas, cherries, and strawberries.

- **Ten Liver-Supporting Foods:** Brussels sprouts, cabbage, garlic, leeks, grapefruit, avocados, kale, spinach, walnuts, and dandelion greens (and dandelion root tea).

MEAL IDEAS FOR OVULATION

Vegetarian & Vegan

Breakfast: Baked Pear Breakfast	Lunch: Ovulatory Support Salad	Dinner: Grilled Veggies with Lentils and Wild Rice

Non-Vegetarian/Vegan

Breakfast: Mushroom and Cabbage Breakfast Sauté	Lunch: Chicken Salad Sammie	Dinner: Zoodle Pad Thai

Note: See the back of the book for full recipes!

MOVING DURING OVULATION

Because you may feel more energetic and social during ovulation, it is the perfect stage in your cycle to consider running with a friend, hitting up a group power yoga class, or attending a cardio dance class. Accountability and growing your community are major benefits of this approach to fitness!

Injury risk may be slightly higher with contact sports or high-impact activities during the late follicular phase and into ovulation,[22] but don't be afraid to build some heat!

Injury risk can be prevented by improving *how* you're moving. It's vital to include whole body strength training, core work and balance work into your routine, especially if you're an athlete. We'll talk all about ways to reduce your risk of injury in our section Injury Prevention and Your Cycle—check it out to learn more.

Examples of physical activity during ovulation include cardio dance class, running, cycling, or power yoga.

THE LUTEAL PHASE: DAYS 15 – 28

The luteal phase is the final stage in our cycle. This phase preps our bodies for menstruation if an egg doesn't get fertilized.

After ovulation, luteinizing hormone (LH) drops back to its baseline, and the early luteal phase is characterized by high estrogen and progesterone.[23] Estrogen and progesterone both decline towards the end of the luteal phase, right before menstruation.

This is the stage often associated with the dreaded premenstrual syndrome, also known as PMS. We have a whole chapter diving into PMS and ways to naturally improve your symptoms later in the book.

> If you are following the Fertility Awareness Method, known as FAM, you may notice that your cervical mucus is absent or you may have sporadic days of lotion-like mucus, and your basal body temperature, known as BBT, will be elevated, usually greater than 97.80 during the luteal phase.[24]

EATING DURING THE LUTEAL PHASE

You may feel hungrier during the luteal phase—honor this hunger! Your energy needs change throughout your cycle, and because of this, your hunger patterns will change, too. During the second half of the menstrual cycle, increased progesterone results in increased body temperature and basal metabolic rate,[25] meaning you will likely need more energy at baseline.

Honoring your hunger cues may mean increasing energy intake in the second half of your cycle.

This may include changes like having a bigger breakfast and packing more hearty, whole-food snacks during the day to hold you over until dinner.

While you may crave sugar during this time, complex carbs are going to be more beneficial for your body. Try to reduce your intake of refined sugars and carbs, and instead focus on increasing proteins, healthy fats, and fiber-rich complex carbs to help stabilize blood sugar.[26] Some examples of complex carbs include quinoa, millet, oats, sweet potatoes, lentils, kidney beans, squash, cabbage, Brussels sprouts, and plantains.

PRO TIP

In addition to decreasing sugar and increasing complex carbs, when you're packing extra food during the luteal phase, make sure to add sources of tryptophan, which can be found in meats, milk, bread, chocolate, peanuts, oats, bananas, prunes, and apples.[27] We'll talk all about the benefits of tryptophan in our chapters on PMS and PMDD!

B vitamins, which play an important role in energy levels, are especially important during this phase as they promote the breakdown of estrogen and production of progesterone.[28] Liver-supporting foods are also beneficial since the liver is responsible for processing excess estrogen.

Incorporating whole foods high in dietary fiber, such as the complex carbs listed above, and drinking plenty of water are key in this phase to promote healthy bowel movements. Remember, constipation is not normal, and if you're struggling with constipation or don't usually have daily bowel movements, estrogen and other waste byproducts may be getting recirculated back into your body,[29] contributing to PMS and other hormonal issues.

FASCINATING FACT

If you get "period poops" right before you start your period, this may be related to the quick drop of progesterone at the end of the luteal phase. As your period approaches, it may be helpful to avoid caffeine, foods that you are sensitive to, and high-fiber smoothies, which may speed up food transit in your digestive tract and result in loose stools.

WHAT TO EAT DURING THE LUTEAL PHASE

- **Ten Foods High In B6:** chickpeas, beef liver, tuna, salmon, chicken, potatoes, turkey, bananas, acorn squash, and butternut squash.

- **Ten Liver-Supporting Foods:** Brussels sprouts, cabbage, garlic, leeks, grapefruit, avocados, kale, spinach, walnuts, and dandelion greens (and dandelion root tea).

MEAL IDEAS FOR THE LUTEAL PHASE

Vegetarian & Vegan

Breakfast: Sweet Potato Chickpea Hash	Lunch: Warm Lentil Quinoa Veggie Salad	Dinner: Veggie Stir Fry

Non-Vegetarian/Vegan

Breakfast: Sweet Potato Brussels Sprout Hash	Lunch: Chicken Quinoa Bowl	Dinner: Simple Shrimp Stew

Note: See the back of the book for the full recipes!

MOVING DURING THE LUTEAL PHASE

With the increase in energy demands at rest, it's vital to monitor how you're feeling and make sure you're eating enough to support your activity levels during the luteal phase.

PRO TIP

Do you feel like you're not sleeping well in the second half of your cycle? If you're not eating enough to fuel your activity levels during the late luteal phase, this may interrupt your sleep.[30] While exercise may help with hormonal issues including PMS symptoms like painful periods,[31] it's important to consume enough healthy, energizing food to get you through your workouts and promote restful sleep. If you're experiencing sleep issues, consider how much you ate the previous day—chances are, you may need more fuel. Try adding in a snack high in protein and complex carbs in your day and notice how your sleep. Our general rule of thumb is, if you're hungry, eat!

Higher levels of activity may feel good right after ovulation, but as you approach menstruation, you may feel more fatigued. Whether you are an endurance athlete or enjoy less strenuous exercise, we encourage you to honor these cyclical shifts in energy. This may not be the time to set personal records, and that's okay!

FASCINATING FACT

While you can definitely still be successful in your sport throughout your cycle, if you're an endurance athlete, it may be beneficial to plan your longer workouts for the beginning or middle of your cycle when possible.

A small study looking at elite soccer players found that endurance performance tends to be lower during the mid-luteal phase, but no significant changes were observed for jumping or sprints between the mid-luteal phase and the early follicular phase.[32]

Remember, anything in excess is not good for the body. Think about a bell curve; you want to be somewhere in the middle, not overdoing exercise on one end or being completely sedentary on the other end. If you tend to maintain high activity levels throughout your cycle, make sure to fuel your body well.

Examples of physical activity during the luteal phase include doubles tennis, gentle yoga, swing dancing, and hiking.

PROBLEMS WITH YOUR CYCLE

By now, you are probably aware that hormone balance, general health, and the health of your cycle are intricately linked. But how do you know if your hormones are out of sync?

This section will go through common signs of hormonal imbalance, possible causes, and ways to help manage any symptoms you're experiencing. You may have symptoms of hormone disruption and not even realize it!

Disclaimer: The following section is intended for informational purposes only, not as a way to diagnose specific medical issues. While this section includes helpful tips, it's important to follow up with a medical provider if you resonate with any of the symptoms discussed. Remember, with any health concern, a team approach is the best approach, so don't be afraid to get opinions from multiple providers.

EMOTIONAL FLUCTUATIONS AND YOUR CYCLE

Do you ever feel like you experience changes in your ability to think critically or respond to emotional stress during different stages of your cycle? Well, you're not alone!

When we think about emotional changes during our cycle, we usually think of PMS. However, minor changes in your ability to respond to emotional stressors and social situations throughout your cycle may be normal, even if you don't have PMS!

We're here to tell you it's okay if you don't feel the same every day of your cycle.

A small 2013 pilot study suggests slight emotional fluctuations may be a normal part of your cycle. This study discovered the time required to solve problems involving emotional conflict was higher in the luteal phase compared to the follicular phase in both those *with and without PMS.* While individuals who had PMS demonstrated higher markers of stress and depression, this study's findings indicate that some fluctuation in mood and response to stress throughout your cycle may be normal.[1] Taking this into consideration, try to be gracious with yourself when dealing with high-stress situations in the second half of your cycle.

If you are feeling "off" or are experiencing anxiety or depression, track these symptoms. By doing so, you may realize some symptoms are more prevalent during certain phases of your cycle.

When you are aware that certain symptoms may be related to cyclical hormone changes, it may be easier to understand your feelings and be less critical of yourself. Not only that, but you will be better able to communicate with your team so they can ultimately find the root cause of your symptoms. And remember, it's okay to seek help if you are struggling with anxiety, depression, or other mental health issues. We consider it a sign of strength to ask for help!

PMS - IS IT JUST SOMETHING WE HAVE TO SUFFER THROUGH?

If you suffer from significant mood swings, fatigue, pain, or feelings of depression in the second half of your cycle, *this is not normal.*

Historically, it has been assumed that having PMS is just part of having a menstrual cycle, but this simply isn't true! Just because something is common doesn't make it normal. You shouldn't have to call out from work, cancel plans with friends, or be stuck in bed because of symptoms related to your cycle. What is to be expected is mild discomfort or twinges in the pelvis, slight breast tenderness, and an increase in desire for comforting affection.

THE SYMPTOMS OF PMS

If you're one of the three out of four menstruating people who report symptoms of PMS,[2] you might recognize some of the following symptoms. According to the American College of Obstetricians and Gynecologists (ACOG), symptoms of PMS include:

- food cravings, thirst and appetite changes
- breast tenderness
- headaches
- aches and pains
- fatigue
- skin problems
- GI symptoms

- abdominal pain
- depression
- anger and irritability
- crying spells
- anxiety
- confusion
- social withdrawal
- poor concentration

- sleep problems including difficulty sleeping at night and feeling like you need a nap midday
- changes in sexual desire
- bloating and weight gain
- swelling of the hands or feet[3]

Usually, these symptoms are at their worst five days before your period and end four days after your period starts. ACOG recommends keeping track of your symptoms and talking with a healthcare provider if you struggle with any of the symptoms listed above. For a true diagnosis, a healthcare provider should confirm that there is a pattern of symptoms consistent with PMS.[4]

Even if you haven't been officially diagnosed with PMS, any symptoms you experience are valid, and we believe that once you understand your body, you can start making positive changes that will benefit you throughout your cycle. There are ways you can naturally manage hormonal fluctuations to improve your mood, energy levels, and even relationships. Using a cycle-tracking app is a great place to start!

PRO TIP

Apps we like include Clue, Flow, Ovia, Eve by Glow, MagicGirl, Kindara, and Natural Cycles. Remember, not all apps are secure and private, so if that's a top concern for you, old-school pen and paper might be your best bet!

So, why do some of us experience PMS?

As with all issues related to hormones, the answer is complex and may vary individual to individual. Before we talk about general tips on eating and moving for PMS, we want to address some of the key players that may be influencing your symptoms. These include an imbalance of estrogen to progesterone, diet culture, sugar, inflammation, and environmental toxins.

HORMONE BALANCE AND PMS

Too much estrogen in relation to progesterone, also called estrogen dominance, may be contributing to some of those less-than-ideal symptoms in the second half of your cycle. This is one of the reasons we dedicated a whole section to it! Check out page 136 for more information on estrogen dominance.

In regard to PMS specifically, excess estrogen in the second half of your cycle has been linked to heightened PMS symptoms, especially those involving mood and emotion.[5]

FASCINATING FACT

Hormones may also influence bloating. Estrogen encourages sodium retention, increasing water retention and potentially affecting bloat. Progesterone may help to counteract the effects of estrogen on sodium and fluid retention.[6] This is good news for those who have healthy, balanced hormones; a normal ratio of estrogen to progesterone may help prevent bloating.

DIET CULTURE AND PMS

While "dieting" is common in Western culture, it may be contributing to your period problems.

Both high consumption of processed foods *and dieting* have been linked to PMS.

A 2013 study found PMS symptoms were most common in adolescents who were not physically active, those who were "overweight," those who ate processed foods, and those who were dieting or decreasing food intake in order to lose weight. On top of PMS, painful periods and clots were more common in the individuals who were dieting.[7]

These findings emphasize the importance of a bell curve. Health lies somewhere in the middle of the extremes, whether that's with diet or exercise.[8] Too much or too little of either is going to wreak havoc on your hormone health and overall well-being.

SUGAR AND PMS

Now, let's talk about sugar and PMS.

Do you notice an increase in desire for sugar in the second half of your cycle? Do you find yourself reaching for sweet treats between meals more often? You're not alone!

Did you know individuals with PMS tend to increase carbohydrate intake during the second half of their cycle? A small study in 1989 found a twenty-four percent increase in carbohydrate intake during meals and a forty-three percent increase in carbohydrate consumption during snacking in those suffering from PMS.[9]

This is where it's important to pay attention to the *types* of carbohydrates you're consuming. Nutrient-dense complex carbs (think fruits, vegetables, grains) are going to be much better for managing PMS symptoms than processed carbs (think bagged or boxed foods).

FASCINATING FACT

It's been proposed that some of the reason for this increased desire for sweets is to promote improved serotonin levels. There are other health-promoting ways to increase serotonin levels rather than focusing solely on carbs. Increasing your intake of foods high in tryptophan like lean chicken, turkey, beef, pork, salmon, eggs, edamame, tofu, oatmeal, quinoa, whole-wheat pasta, brown rice, and regular and soy milk may help improve serotonin levels.[10] We'll talk more about serotonin in our next section on PMDD.

Other natural ways to improve serotonin levels include exercise, sunshine or light therapy, and positive affirmations.[11] We'll talk more about positive affirmations in the chapter Restoring Your Cycle—check it out for more details!

Regardless of the specific period problems you have, remember that you use more energy during the luteal phase, so we encourage you to reach for the most nourishing, health-promoting foods to fuel your body during this time. Pack extra whole food snacks, including those high in tryptophan, to help prevent yourself from reaching for high-sugar and processed foods that will only make your symptoms worse!

INFLAMMATION AND PMS

Remember prostaglandins? Prostaglandins are a key player in our inflammatory response and may play a role in some of those less-than-ideal period symptoms. In addition to influencing uterine contractions or "cramps," prostaglandins may also influence menstrual-related migraines, painful periods,[12] and GI issues in the second half of your cycle.

> ### FASCINATING FACT
>
> Speaking of inflammation, if you're looking for another reason to quit smoking, look no further. Individuals who smoke have been found to be more than twice as likely to develop PMS within the next two to four years compared to those who have never smoked. This risk increases if you've been smoking longer and consuming more packs of cigarettes.[13] And remember, while vaping and e-cigarettes have gained popularity, they are still not good for your health, especially if you're having period problems!

ENVIRONMENTAL CHEMICALS AND PMS

We would be remiss to not mention environmental toxins and how they can influence hormone health and PMS symptoms.

Chemicals commonly found in cleaning products and personal hygiene products can affect hormone function and communication in our bodies. These chemicals, known as "endocrine-disrupting chemicals" or "endocrine disruptors," have gained attention recently due to the increasing prevalence of health problems related to our hormone system.[14]

There is a specific subset of endocrine disrupting chemicals, known as xenoestrogens, that can mimic estrogen in the body, wreaking havoc on hormone regulation.[15] We'll have an in-depth discussion about these environmental chemicals as they relate to your cycle in our chapter on estrogen dominance.

MICRONUTRIENTS AND PMS

While we usually think about taking over-the-counter medications such as Ibuprofen or Midol to manage period symptoms, certain micronutrients may also be beneficial.

Micronutrients that may be beneficial for PMS include calcium, vitamin D, magnesium, curcumin, omega-3, vitamin B6, DIM complex (diindolylmethane), and calcium-D-glucarate.

While supplementing can be useful, we believe that sourcing nutrients from whole foods is the best way to promote optimal health, and it's best to get lab work done to understand your body's specific needs.

Remember, even herbs and over-the-counter supplements can negatively influence the body when used in combination or in excess.[16]

Now let's talk about some of the micronutrients relevant to PMS!

Calcium may positively influence PMS symptoms like fatigue, appetite changes, depressive symptoms, and irritability.[17]

FASCINATING FACT

A 2019 review looking specifically at the evidence on calcium and vitamin D in relationship to PMS found that low levels of these micronutrients during the second half of your cycle may influence the onset and severity of PMS symptoms.[18]

Dietary sources of calcium include milk, cheese, other dairy products, leafy greens like collard greens, broccoli rabe, and kale, seafood, and foods that are fortified with calcium, meaning that they have calcium added to them.[19]

Vitamin D may be beneficial for PMS.

As you might recall, vitamin D is not a true vitamin but a steroid hormone that is mostly synthesized by sunlight touching bare skin.[20] A 2019 meta-analysis found that vitamin D is beneficial for optimal wellness and may have a positive effect on PMS symptoms.[21] Who would have thought getting out in the sun could help with PMS?

Although we get vitamin D primarily through sunlight, dietary sources of vitamin D include fortified dairy products, fish such as salmon, herring, sardines, and tuna, egg yolks, mushrooms, fortified orange juice, and cod liver oil, which has the added benefit of being a great source of omega-3.

Magnesium is another micronutrient that may be beneficial for PMS.

While a 2019 review on magnesium and PMS symptoms found the current studies on the topic don't provide enough evidence to support the use of magnesium to treat PMS,[22] magnesium supplementation may be beneficial if you have a known deficiency or tend to be on the lower end of the spectrum.

In a small 2015 study, only about one-third of the individuals with PMS had a magnesium deficiency, although those with PMS tended to have lower levels compared to the control group.[23] Older results from a 1989 study found that magnesium might be beneficial for those with period pain, due to increased inhibition of a specific prostaglandin (PGF2 alpha) and because of its positive effects on blood flow and muscular relaxation.[24]

Working with a professional can help you figure out if supplementing with magnesium might be helpful. When in doubt, start by adding some whole foods high in magnesium into your diet.

Dietary sources of magnesium include nuts, seeds, dark leafy greens, seaweed, legumes, dairy products, and whole grains.

Curcumin is a plant compound with known antioxidant and anti-inflammatory properties.[25] A small double-blind study in 2015 found a significant decrease in PMS symptoms when individuals took curcumin a week prior to menstruation and three days into their period for three cycles.[26]

Dietary sources of curcumin include turmeric, which is why it's one of our favorite spices for cooking!

PRO TIP

In order to make the most out of cooking with turmeric, add some black pepper and healthy fats into your recipe to aid in the absorption of curcumin.[27]

Omega-3 fatty acids are another nutrient that may help ease the severity of cramps and PMS symptoms.

A 2011 study found that fish oil, which is high in omega-3 fatty acids, was more beneficial than Ibuprofen for decreasing period pain without an underlying medical cause.[28] While supplementation with fish oil is great, you may also be able to alleviate some of your PMS symptoms through whole food sources of omega-3, including the ones listed below!

FASCINATING FACT

A study in 1995 found that individuals with premenstrual symptoms tended to have lower intake of omega-3 and B12 and a lower ratio of omega-3 to omega-6.[29] To keep the omega-3 and omega-6 ratio in a health-promoting balance, eat plenty of the healthy fats listed below and avoid processed oils.

Dietary sources of omega-3 include fish and marine animals,[30] such as salmon, tuna, and herring, as well as flaxseeds, chia seeds, and walnuts.

Vitamin B6 (also known as P5P) is a water-soluble vitamin involved in many chemical reactions in the body, including the creation of neurotransmitters such as serotonin.[31]

While there is preliminary research about vitamin B6 and PMS, a literature review from 2000 found the quality of the existing research is low.[32] The benefit may depend on your baseline, which is another reason lab work can be beneficial!

FASCINATING FACT

Despite the limitations in the current research, B6 may be more beneficial when combined with calcium! In a 2016 randomized controlled trial, it was discovered that the combination of 40 mg of B6 and 500 mg of calcium had a greater impact on reducing PMS symptoms than vitamin B6 alone.[33] It may be beneficial to add whole food sources of both vitamin B6 and calcium into your diet, especially in the second half of your cycle.

Dietary sources of B6 include chickpeas, beef liver, tuna, salmon, chicken, potatoes, turkey, bananas, acorn squash, and butternut squash.

Other compounds to consider are **DIM complex (diindolylmethane)** and **calcium-D-glucarate.** Don't worry; they're not as scary as they sound!

DIM is a derivative of indole 3-carbinol, which is created from a compound called glucobrassicin, found in cruciferous vegetables. DIM may help the body metabolize steroid hormones, including estrogen.[34] Calcium-D-glucarate also supports healthy estrogen metabolism.[35]

Dietary sources of glucobrassin, which is necessary for the synthesis of DIM, include the cruciferous vegetables listed on the next page.

Dietary sources of glucaric acid, which calcium-D-glucarate is derived from, include cruciferous veggies, apples, grapefruits, and oranges.[36]

Cruciferous vegetables:

- Cauliflower
- Brussels sprouts
- Cabbage
- Bok Choy
- Arugula

- Radish
- Turnip
- Kohlrabi
- Watercress
- Rutabaga

- Maca
- Broccoli
- Kale
- Horseradish
- Daiko

EXERCISE AND PMS

Along with the nutritional hacks for PMS, there's evidence supporting exercise as another tool for managing PMS symptoms.

Note: While we are all for improving health through exercise, it is important to remember research regarding exercise is difficult to analyze due to variations in protocols and outcome measures. A 2020 review of randomized controlled trials found that exercise *may* be a beneficial treatment strategy for PMS, but there is still a high risk of bias in the current studies and some uncertainty about the reliability of the outcomes.[37]

Taking that into consideration, exercise is still a low-risk strategy that may also positively influence other markers of health, so let's get moving!

If you're overwhelmed at the thought of the exercise recommendations previously mentioned, remember, you don't have to do it all at once! While the recommendations are helpful, you'll still reap the benefits at smaller doses of exercise, especially if you have PMS or period problems.

FASCINATING FACT

A small 2019 study found an eight-week, whole-body exercise program decreased PMS symptoms, including headaches, nausea, and bowel problems like constipation and diarrhea. Even better? The program was only thirty minutes three times per week![38]

While we encourage you to move in ways that feel good throughout your cycle, don't be afraid to work up a sweat! A 2011 study analyzing sixty-one individuals who menstruate found that those who performed moderate or high-intensity workouts over a six-week period had decreased PMS symptoms and improved markers of general health.[39]

With these findings in mind, aiming for a few sessions per week of moderate- or high-intensity exercise may be a great option to help alleviate some of your PMS symptoms and improve overall health.

For our athlete friends, if you're experiencing period pain and irregular periods, this may be a sign of overtraining. A 2009 study analyzing thirty-one menstruating athletes found seventy-one percent of the athletes studied experienced symptoms of PMS. The most common symptoms included irritability, fluctuations in mood, and menstrual cramps among other complaints.[40] Remember, our bodies change throughout the month, so there will be times when your body needs more rest. Learn to listen to your body, and if you feel like you need more rest and recovery, honor your body's cues. Rest is not a sign of weakness or a reward for your hard work—it's something we all need and deserve.

PMS TAKEAWAYS

PMS isn't something you have to suffer through!

There are multiple factors that may influence PMS symptoms. Some of the most common include an imbalance of estrogen to progesterone, diet, inflammation, environmental toxins, and getting too much or too little exercise.

What can you do if you have PMS?

- Add foods like cruciferous veggies into your diet
- Consume plenty of water and fiber
- Decrease alcohol and sugar consumption
- Quit smoking
- Get adequate sleep
- Manage stress levels
- Avoid environmental toxins (we'll discuss strategies for this in our chapter on estrogen dominance)
- Exercise regularly, at least three times per week for thirty minutes, as a baseline

If you're having significant and debilitating PMS symptoms, it's important to follow up with a medical provider. While the tips we've provided may be helpful, sometimes your PMS and painful periods may be due to underlying medical conditions.[41] We encourage you to track your PMS symptoms and share your findings openly with a medical provider.

PMDD – HOW IS IT DIFFERENT FROM PMS?

Premenstrual dysphoric disorder, referred to as PMDD, is similar to PMS, but PMDD symptoms significantly disrupt daily life. A 2005 review on menstrual disorders found PMDD symptoms may negatively impact work productivity, relationships, and social interactions. Many people with PMDD have high medical costs from the number of doctor visits and lab tests they undergo due to their symptoms.[42]

Similar to PMS, PMDD symptoms usually start a week prior to your period and last a few days into menstruation, but PMDD also includes diagnosable psychiatric symptoms. Common symptoms associated with PMDD include:

- significant mood swings or changes in emotion, including being tearful, sudden onset of sadness, or heightened sensitivity to rejection
- anger, irritability, and increased conflicts with the people around you
- self-deprecating thoughts
- feelings of hopelessness or depression
- anxiety, tension, or feeling on edge
- lack of interest in normal activities
- difficulty concentrating
- fatigue, decreased energy
- changes in appetite and overeating
- feeling tired during the day or unable to sleep at night
- feeling overwhelmed or like you're lacking control
- physical problems, including pain, breast tenderness, "bloating," and increased weight[43]

If you feel like we're describing you in this section, *track your symptoms.* This way, you can tell your healthcare provider exactly what's going on, and they can create a care plan specific to your needs. If you feel like your concerns are being dismissed, we recommend finding a new provider.

TRAUMA, PTSD, AND PMDD

If you have a history of trauma, whether physical or emotional, it is especially important to let your healthcare team know what's going on.

According to a 2013 cross-sectional study, having PTSD and a history of trauma may put you at a higher risk for developing PMDD.[44] A small study in 2003 analyzing twenty-eight individuals with PMS and PMDD in two separate groups of individuals found that twenty in the PMDD group and ten in the PMS group reported a history of sexual or physical abuse.[45]

We want you to know if you are suffering, you are not alone, and it's not your fault. We are firm believers in seeking the care you need, and there should be no stigma around including mental health providers on your team. In fact, a 2016 review in *American Family Physician* suggested medications and cognitive behavioral therapy may be the best treatment options for PMDD.[46] We love our counterparts in the mental health field, and working with a mental health provider may be just what you need to help alleviate your period problems!

FASCINATING FACT

Did you know if you have ADHD, you might have a higher chance of developing PMDD and postpartum depression with your first child? As always, keep track of all of your symptoms so that you and your healthcare provider can find the plan that's best for you![47]

SEROTONIN AND PMDD

Serotonin, one of our "feel-good" neurotransmitters, regulates many aspects of human physiology and behavior. Some of the processes modulated by serotonin include mood, anger, attention, aggression, sexuality, memory, and appetite.[48]

Serotonin may be especially relevant if you have PMDD, as the mood symptoms associated with PMDD may be related to an altered serotonin response, among other changes in brain activity, according to a 2019 review.[49]

Mood symptoms are a prevalent and disruptive aspect of PMDD, but many people don't realize the foods we eat can positively influence our bodies' ability to produce serotonin!

Your diet is the source of tryptophan, which is one of the building blocks for serotonin. This means if you're not getting enough tryptophan, your ability to synthesize serotonin may be disrupted.[50]

Dietary tryptophan may be beneficial for mood regulation. A 2015 study analyzing a group of college students without diagnosed anxiety or depression found those who consumed a high tryptophan diet reported improved mood, decreased anxiety, and decreased symptoms of depression.[51]

With the cyclical mood changes associated with PMS and PMDD, tryptophan intake may be even more important to monitor! In a study analyzing sixteen individuals diagnosed with PMS, depleting tryptophan increased premenstrual symptoms, especially irritability, which is consistent with other research associating serotonin with the severity of premenstrual symptoms.[52]

FASCINATING FACT

Increased sugar cravings and consumption are common in individuals with PMS and PMDD. One reason for this may be due to the positive influence having a high-carbohydrate, low protein meal can have on serotonin levels.[53] While this may temporarily help with symptoms like depression, sadness, anger, and fatigue,[54] high sugar intake can wreak havoc on the body and may make your PMS symptoms worse in the long-term. The good news is, there are other ways to help with serotonin levels, including increasing dietary tryptophan and the following strategies!

Dietary sources of tryptophan include lean chicken, turkey, beef, pork, and salmon. Vegetarian sources of tryptophan include eggs, edamame, tofu, oatmeal, quinoa, whole-wheat pasta, brown rice, and soy milk.[55]

According to a review in *The Journal of Psychiatry and Neuroscience,* some other natural ways to improve serotonin include:

- Exercise
- Sunshine or light therapy
- Positive affirmations (we'll talk more about positive affirmations in the chapter Restoring Your Cycle—check it out for more details!)[56]

If you have PMDD, track your symptoms and give yourself grace. Our physical bodies and mental health are intricately linked, so therapy or counseling and medication may be key in reducing some of the symptoms associated with your cycle.

Since serotonin may influence some of the mood and emotional disturbances associated with PMDD, if you're craving sugar, try adding in some sources of dietary tryptophan, such as those listed above. Other options for improving serotonin levels include exercise, sunshine, and positive affirmations, so be sure to incorporate some of each into your routine!

HORMONES AND PMDD

While PMDD symptoms may be influenced by estrogen and progesterone, the levels of these hormones may be similar to individuals without PMDD; new research is suggesting that it is not the levels of estrogen and progesterone, but altered response to the fluctuations of these hormones that may influence PMDD symptoms.[57]

There may also be other nervous system changes influencing symptoms. Along with low serotonin availability, PMS and PMDD may be influenced by the effects of inflammation on our nervous system, and there may also be changes in progesterone receptors in the brain and conversion of progesterone into metabolites, influencing nervous system function.[58]

PAIN RELIEF MEDICATIONS FOR PMS AND PERIOD PAIN: NSAIDS, CRAMPS, AND FERTILITY ISSUES

NSAIDs, short for non-steroidal anti-inflammatory drugs, are commonly used for aches and pains, including cramps and premenstrual symptoms.

Some popular NSAIDs are:

- Aspirin (acetylsalicylic acid)
- Advil (ibuprofen)
- Aleve (naproxen)
- Voltaren (diclofenac)

FASCINATING FACT

Tylenol, also known as acetaminophen, is actually *not* an NSAID, although it is another commonly used over-the-counter pain relief medication.

The reason non-steroidal anti-inflammatory drugs like Advil (ibuprofen) and Aleve (naproxen) are frequently used for menstrual symptoms is that they inhibit the formation of prostaglandins, which play a large role in period problems.[59]

While they may help with premenstrual symptoms and cramps, long-term use of NSAIDs may have negative implications for reproductive health.

As a quick review, ovulation is when the follicle surrounding the egg in the ovary bursts and releases the egg into the fallopian tube for potential fertilization.

It's important to consider timing if you're using NSAIDs on a regular basis for aches and pains, especially if you're having difficulty conceiving. Taking NSAIDs during menstruation may not influence ovulation (an observational cohort study actually found a possible protective mechanism),[60] but if you're taking them daily for other aches and pains, it may be best to get to the root cause of your pain.

There is preliminary evidence that taking NSAIDs frequently, especially in the middle of your cycle, may influence follicular rupture and ovulation. A 2005 review suggests avoiding them if you have known fertility issues,[61] and a small 2015 study found when taken ten days in a row, starting on the tenth day of your cycle, there were negative effects on ovulation and progesterone levels. Functional cysts were also common, which may be related to issues with the follicle rupturing.[62]

So, NSAIDs are likely okay for cramps and menstrual-related pain every once in a while, but if you use them every day (especially in the middle of your cycle), it's best to figure out the true source of your pain so you don't have to rely on them.

ESTROGEN DOMINANCE: THE GREAT BALANCING ACT

Estrogen dominance has become a popular term over the past few years, but what does it actually mean?

Estrogen dominance refers to an imbalance between estrogen and progesterone. While estrogen dominance can mean you have high levels of estrogen, it is technically the ratio of estrogen to progesterone, which can also be influenced by low levels of progesterone.

Some cycle-related issues that might point to estrogen dominance include heavy menstrual bleeding, mood swings, irritability, poor sleep quality, cysts in your breasts, fibroids, and even problems with your gallbladder and thyroid![63] Estrogen dominance can also influence conditions like polycystic ovary syndrome (PCOS), endometriosis, autoimmune diseases, and cancer.[64]

And *no,* hormonal contraception isn't the only option for treating hormonal imbalances such as estrogen dominance. We'll talk more about this in our section on hormonal contraception.

So what causes estrogen dominance?

Some of the major culprits include stress, gut issues, liver problems, and exposure to chemicals in foods, cleaning supplies, and beauty products.

STRESS AND ESTROGEN DOMINANCE

We're talking about stress again?

Yes, we are! And in this case, it may be directly related to the hormonal imbalances associated with estrogen dominance.

Chronic stress may negatively impact progesterone levels.[65]

One of the major building blocks of progesterone is also one of the main building blocks of our stress hormone, cortisol. This building block can be "stolen" from progesterone in order to make more cortisol, causing decreased progesterone levels while we build cortisol during times of stress.[66] This can lead to a skewed ratio of estrogen to progesterone, potentially leading to estrogen dominance.

Check out our section Restoring Your Cycle for tips and tools to manage everyday stress!

ESTROGEN AND THE GUT

Did you know the gut has specific bacteria for metabolizing estrogen? These bacteria, collectively known as the estrobolome, are particularly important for maintaining proper metabolism of estrogen in the GI tract.[67] This is why problems with the gut may lead to larger problems such as hormone imbalances and, in particular, symptoms of estrogen dominance.

And while for some, constipation is "normal," constipation can be another GI factor affecting hormone balance!

When you aren't having bowel movements daily, estrogen found in your waste may be absorbed from your colon back into your body,[68] increasing circulating estrogen and influencing symptoms related to estrogen dominance.

FASCINATING FACT

An older study from 1987 comparing individuals consuming a normal Western diet, consisting of about forty percent fat and low-fiber intake, and those consuming a vegetarian diet, with about thirty percent fat and high fiber, found the vegetarians excreted three times more estrogen than their Western diet counterparts in bowel movements and had a fifteen to twenty percent decrease in plasma estrogen levels. Remember, you don't need to be vegetarian or vegan to get these benefits; simply work on increasing dietary fiber and decreasing processed fats and oils!

If you can't figure out why you're struggling with constipation, start with the basics. Are you drinking half your body weight in ounces of water? Are you eating five servings of fruits and veggies a day? Are you getting some sort of movement each day? If not, start there! If you're still struggling after incorporating the basics, we recommend working with a pelvic health physical therapist or functional nutritionist to get to the root cause of your digestive issues.

YOUR LIVER AND HORMONE BALANCE

While the liver has multiple functions in the body,[69] it plays a vital role in hormone balance since it is where estrogen is broken down to be sent to the colon.[70]

There are three pathways for estrogen metabolism in the liver, each having very different effects in the body.

Estrogen Metabolism Pathways:

- 2-hydroxy metabolic pathway
- 4-hydroxy metabolic pathway
- 16-hydroxy metabolic pathway[71]

The pathway resulting in the most beneficial metabolites for the body to use is 2-hydroxy. Even though the 4- and 16-hydroxy break down estrogen, they actually promote an estrogenic effect in the body,[72] which may amplify problems associated with high estrogen.

Put simply, we want our body to use the 2-hydroxy pathway as opposed to the 4-hydroxy and 16-hydroxy pathways because estrogen is more favorably and efficiently metabolized down the 2-hydroxy.

The good news is that we can influence how estrogen is metabolized in the body and which pathway it takes!

A 2011 study found that supplementation with DIM (diindolylmethane) increased the ratio of 2-hydroxy metabolites to 16-hydroxy metabolites.[73] This means that DIM helps to redirect estrogen metabolism toward the more health-promoting pathway (2-hydroxy) and away from those promoting estrogen dominance (4-hydroxy and 16-hydroxy).

While the study above looked at supplementation with DIM, you can also get DIM from your diet! DIM is synthesized from indole 3-carbinol, which is made from glucobrassicin commonly found in cruciferous and brassica veggies. Check out page 128 for a full list of cruciferous and brassica veggies.

FASCINATING FACT

Since we're talking about estrogen dominance, it's interesting to know that indole 3-carbinol may help stop the growth of tumors in estrogen-dependent cancers such as breast cancer, endometrial cancer, and cervical cancer.[74] This makes cruciferous veggies even more of a win!

To improve liver health, it's important to decrease exposure to chemicals that get processed in the liver, such as pesticides, herbicides, and environmental toxins in household cleaning and personal hygiene products.[75] Medications may also influence liver health, so it's never a bad idea to do a medication check with a pharmacist. We'll talk more about this in the next section.

Alcohol and high sugar consumption are also environmental factors to watch!

Alcohol and excess sugar get processed in the liver,[76] making them very relevant if you suffer from period problems related to estrogen dominance. We'll take a deeper look at sugar and the liver in our section Fad Diets, Sugar, and Your Cycle.

Besides decreasing exposure to substances that negatively impact the liver, you can improve liver health by increasing antioxidants that aid in the detoxification process.

One antioxidant that plays a vital role in liver health is glutathione. While you cannot directly consume glutathione by way of diet, there are multiple ways to improve levels of this health-promoting antioxidant.

WAYS TO IMPROVE GLUTATHIONE LEVELS

- **Meditation and prayer:** Meditation is a wonderful, free tool for improving glutathione levels. A pilot study in 2008 found that individuals who had practiced a specific type of meditation regularly for more than a year had higher glutathione levels compared to controls.[77] While the study looked at a type of meditation known as Sudarshan Kriya, we believe there are benefits in finding a meditation practice that works for you!

- **Consuming whey protein:** Whey protein contains a form of cysteine, known as N-acetylcysteine, which is easily absorbed by the body,[78] and cysteine may be beneficial for replenishment of glutathione stores.[79] This is especially important when we are in immune-deficient states like being ill or participating in extreme exercise. If you're sick or have a big athletic event coming up, it may be beneficial to add some whey protein into your diet![80]

    - **Note:** If you have trouble with dairy, there are also N-acetylcysteine supplements. We always recommend following up with a nutritionist or healthcare professional prior to starting any supplements in order to figure out what's right for you.

- **Decreasing alcohol intake:** Chronic alcohol consumption can negatively impact glutathione levels.[81] While we're all for moderation and balance, it might be better to put that second or third drink down, especially if you're in the second half of your cycle.

- **Decreasing sugar intake:** Too much sugar may deplete the body of glutathione,[82] which is why it's vital to check labels and avoid added sugars, especially high-fructose corn syrup.

- **Decreasing exposure to environmental toxins:** One of the ways certain pesticides and herbicides may negatively influence liver and hormone health is through their influence on glutathione levels. Decreasing exposure to persistent organic pollutants (POPs), environmental toxins primarily found in conventionally grown foods, can help maintain our bodies' levels of glutathione.[83] While we will never be able to get rid of all of the environmental toxins we are exposed to, incremental, health-promoting changes in the food we eat and the products we put on our skin and use in our homes can go a long way in reducing risk and maintaining healthy glutathione levels.

ENVIRONMENTAL CHEMICALS AND ESTROGEN DOMINANCE

If you suffer from symptoms of estrogen dominance or other period problems, it might be worth doing an environmental check. Household cleaners and personal hygiene products often contain chemicals that have the ability to disrupt our hormones.

As you might recall from earlier, our hormones are part of our endocrine system. Chemicals known to disrupt our hormones are called "endocrine-disrupting chemicals" or "endocrine disruptors."[84]

Some common sources of endocrine disruptors are:

- Cosmetics: especially those containing parabens
- Plastic bottles: specifically, those containing BPA
- Food cans: which often contain BPA[85]
- Pesticides and herbicides: used commonly on non-organic foods to keep them free of bugs[86]

- Dish soaps and laundry detergents: often contain perfumes and other endocrine disruptors[87]

- Medical devices: which often contain phthalates

- Toys: specifically, those containing phthalates

- Flame retardants: often contain polybrominated diphenyl ethers and are commonly found in furniture, mattresses, curtains, carpets, electronics, household appliances, building and construction materials, and transportation materials in cars, planes, and trains[88]

XENOESTROGENS AND HORMONE BALANCE

There is a specific subclass of endocrine disruptors, known as xenoestrogens, which can mimic estrogen in the body and influence your menstrual cycle as well as other hormones and systems.[89] Because of their similarities to estrogen, these chemicals may be detrimental to the natural functioning of estrogen in the body.[90]

Unfortunately, xenoestrogens are common in our modern environment. This is why it's important to read labels—many of these ingredients are hidden in plain sight.

Common xenoestrogens include:

- Parabens[91]

- DDT (Dichlorodiphenyltrichloroethane), which is an insecticide

- BPA and other bisphenols

- Alkylphenols

- Dichlorophenols

- Methoxychlor

- Chlordecone

- PCBs (polychlorinated benzol derivatives)
- Dioxins[92]

FASCINATING FACT

Dioxin is a persistent organic pollutant (POP) particularly dangerous for menstruating people. According to a fact sheet by the EPA, dioxins are extremely toxic and have been linked to conditions like cancer, hormonal imbalance, problems with the immune and reproductive systems, and developmental issues.[93] A mouse study in 2010 showed that exposure to dioxin influenced the development of characteristics associated with progesterone resistance, potentially leading to estrogen dominance. These changes in progesterone responses in mice persisted over several generations.[94]

Even if we've been previously exposed to dioxin or other endocrine disruptors, being mindful of our environment can help decrease future risk. The food sources with the highest amount of dioxin include meat, dairy products, fish, and shellfish. Dioxin can also be found in smaller amounts in herbicides, pesticides, and water.[95] Dioxin accumulates in the fat stores of animals, but you don't have to give up meat to avoid this toxin, just try to make sure you're choosing grass-fed and organic options when possible!

FRAGRANCES

If you've been told to avoid fragrances for hormone health, this is good advice.

Fragrances often contain chemicals that disrupt our hormones, including parabens, phthalates, hydroperoxides, glutaraldehyde, and metals.

FASCINATING FACT

Even essential oils, in high amounts may be able to interact with estrogen receptors.[96]

We suggest avoiding anything that states "fragrance" on its label without saying exactly what that fragrance is made from.

AVOIDING ENVIRONMENTAL TOXINS

While we will never be able to get rid of all of our exposure to environmental toxins, the following resources may be helpful as you work to eliminate what exposure you can.

- Environmental Working Group's "Dirty Dozen" List: Updated yearly, the EWG's list contains the top twelve produce items likely to have large amounts of herbicides and pesticides in their non-organic state.

- Environmental Working Group's "Clean Fifteen" List: Also updated yearly, the EWG has a list called "The Clean Fifteen," which contains produce items safest to eat non-organically.

- The Environmental Working Group's Skin Deep Cosmetic Database: Allows you to search common personal and beauty products to screen for toxic load. Find these helpful resources on www.ewg.org, or download EWGs app, which is helpful when you're on the go!

- The Think Dirty App: Helps identify toxins in common beauty and household products.

MANAGING ESTROGEN DOMINANCE

While managing your hormones can seem overwhelming, there are simple, daily actions you can take to help alleviate symptoms related to your cycle and improve your overall health.

Basic strategies to improve hormone balance include keeping a healthy diet full of whole foods high in micronutrients and fiber, managing gut and liver health, moving daily, and maintaining healthy relationships.

FASCINATING FACT

Did you know positive social interactions may influence hormone balance? A 2009 study analyzing progesterone levels after tasks with and without social closeness found increased progesterone levels in individuals who participated in the task involving close social interactions.[97] If a person is estrogen dominant due to low progesterone, social support and a sense of community may help regulate the ratio of these two hormones.

If you feel like you're lacking social support, we highly recommend investing time doing what you're interested in—this can help you find your people and grow your community organically. And if you're feeling especially lonely, it never hurts to add a mental health provider to your team.

If you're struggling with estrogen dominance, your diet and having regular bowel movements are imperative! High fat intake and low fiber intake have been associated with higher plasma estrogen, or levels of estrogen in the blood, making it vital to consume whole foods naturally high in fiber and avoid packaged and fast foods high in processed fats and oils.[98]

As we've mentioned, a healthy liver is important for hormone balance.

Ways to decrease stress on the liver include reducing alcohol and excess sugar consumption and trying to decrease exposure to environmental toxins. It may even be worth doing a medication check with your pharmacist to see if any of the medications or supplements you're taking may be negatively impacting your liver.

Along with decreasing substances that put extra stress on the liver, you can positively influence the liver by increasing antioxidants like glutathione that aid in the detoxification process.

Some ways to improve glutathione levels include meditation, prayer, and consuming whey protein, which is high in N-acetylcysteine. Glutathione levels are also positively influenced by decreasing alcohol, sugar, and exposure to environmental toxins, making these steps a great place to start when addressing liver and hormone health!

NATURALLY IMPROVING PROGESTERONE

After reading this chapter, you now know that estrogen dominance doesn't always mean high estrogen, it can also mean low progesterone. So, what can we do to improve progesterone levels?

Besides maintaining healthy social connections, certain micronutrients, including folate, vitamin C, vitamin E, and L-arginine may help improve progesterone levels.

Make sure you check with a healthcare provider before supplementing, and remember, whole foods high in these micronutrients are a great place to start if you think you're deficient.

Folate (B9) is an antioxidant that plays a critical role in hormone balance. A 2012 study found that menstruating people with higher folate intake tended to have higher progesterone levels than those with low folate intake.[99]

Dietary sources of folate include dark green leafy vegetables, liver, bread, yeasts, and fruits.

Vitamin C is another micronutrient that may help with progesterone levels. A 2003 article found higher progesterone levels in the mid-luteal phase in individuals who supplemented with 750 mg of vitamin C compared to a control group.[100]

FASCINATING FACT

Vitamin C may also positively influence glutathione levels, making it a win-win when it comes to hormone balance![101]

Dietary sources of vitamin C include citrus fruits, strawberries, tomatoes, hibiscus tea, broccoli, spinach, bell peppers, and kiwi fruit.

Vitamin E and L-arginine, which act as antioxidants, have both been found to promote improved progesterone levels in the mid-luteal phase according to a 2009 study.[102]

It may be beneficial to get your vitamin E from foods rather than supplements due to the high concentrations of vitamin E in some supplements.[103]

Dietary sources of vitamin E include nuts, egg yolks, cheese, oatmeal, avocados, olives, green leafy vegetables, and plant-based oils such as olive oil.[104]

Dietary sources of L-arginine include red meat, poultry, fish, and dairy products.

ESTROGEN DOMINANCE TAKEAWAYS

Managing estrogen dominance is all about keeping a healthy ratio of estrogen to progesterone.

Some common symptoms of estrogen dominance include:

- heavy menstrual bleeding
- mood swings

- irritability

- poor sleep quality

- cysts in your breasts

- fibroids

- endometriosis

- PCOS

- gallbladder and thyroid issues[105]

If you struggle with estrogen dominance, it is a good idea to talk to a healthcare practitioner who can help you troubleshoot the specifics of your case. Every body is unique, therefore, it is unlikely that your hormone issues are stemming from the same cause as your friend who also has estrogen dominance. It's important to get individualized care in order to get to the root cause of your symptoms.

Basic lifestyle hacks can be a great place to start. Here are a few daily steps to help with hormone balance and overall health:

- Getting regular exercise, including "exercise snacks," and aiming for at least three thirty-minute sweat sessions per week

- Eating more dietary fiber and less processed foods high in sugar and refined oils

- Increasing your consumption of cruciferous veggies like cabbage, broccoli, cauliflower, and Brussels sprouts

- Working on stress management with strategies like therapy and meditation/prayer

- Getting adequate sleep and having a good bedtime routine

- Establishing healthy relationship boundaries and spending time with your favorite people, remembering positive social interactions may support healthy progesterone levels

- Choosing organic foods when possible and using the Dirty Dozen and Clean Fifteen lists on EWG.org to prioritize which produce to try to purchase in organic form

- Using the EWG Skin Deep Cosmetic Database and the Think Dirty app to check personal hygiene and household products for toxin exposure

POLYCYSTIC OVARY SYNDROME (PCOS)

Polycystic ovary syndrome, also known as PCOS, is one of the most common hormone-related disorders in menstruating people, affecting an estimated five to fifteen percent of individuals who cycle.[106]

FASCINATING FACT

Just because you have ovarian cysts doesn't necessarily mean you have PCOS.

An ovarian cyst is a fluid-filled sac on your ovary. Functional ovarian cysts are the most common type and can be a normal byproduct of the menstrual cycle. Because they are generally harmless and tend to resolve on their own without treatment, your provider might suggest the wait-and-see approach.[107]

PCOS is characterized by not only ovarian cysts but also hormonal imbalance and menstrual dysfunction.[108]

So, how do you know if you have PCOS?

Some tell-tale signs include growth of hair on your face, chest, and back, thinning hair on your head, difficulty with weight management, acne, skin tags, darkening of your skin, and irregular menstrual cycles.[109]

The most recent criteria for the diagnosis of PCOS is the Androgen Excess Society's criteria, which includes:

- Hyperandrogenism, which is high levels of sex hormones called androgens. Hyperandrogenism plays a role in some of the most common physical characteristics of PCOS,[110] including excess facial or body hair (known as hirsutism), hair loss or balding (known as androgenic alopecia), insulin resistance, persistent acne, oily skin, darkly pigmented areas of skin, and more.[111] Signs of hyperandrogenism can be found based on physical characteristics or lab findings.[112]

- Ovarian dysfunction, which can include multiple cysts on your ovaries, irregular ovulation, lack of ovulation, or infrequent periods.[113]

- Exclusion of other medical diagnoses that may cause similar symptoms.[114]

Note: It's important to understand that some of the same symptoms that characterize PCOS are common during adolescence. A 2015 review found characteristics such as lack of ovulation, irregular menstrual cycles, and acne frequently occur during puberty. Because of this, it is challenging to diagnose PCOS in adolescents.[115] If you're a teen who has been diagnosed with PCOS, we highly recommend making some of the lifestyle changes in this section and monitoring your symptoms.

If you relate to any of the symptoms above, it's important to follow up with your provider and bring a list of your symptoms and questions to review with them.

Even though PCOS is very common, it can take a year or more to get a diagnosis. This sometimes requires going to multiple providers and getting second opinions. The time it takes to get a diagnosis of PCOS can lead to the progression of symptoms and can be very frustrating for patients.[116]

In good news, environmental factors, which in general can be easily changed, can heavily influence PCOS symptoms in most cases. While addressing symptoms related to PCOS may seem overwhelming, making lifestyle changes including good nutrition, regular exercise, and decreasing exposure to environmental chemicals can be a great place to start.

FASCINATING FACT

Although your environment does play a role in the symptoms associated with PCOS, it's important to be patient as you make changes. A 2019 review found it may take significant time to show improvement in the physical symptoms associated with PCOS, even if you're doing all the right things. For example, while acne tends to respond relatively quickly to treatments, decreasing excess hair on your face, back, and chest may take more than three months. Improving thinning hair and balding may take even longer than that, sometimes taking twelve to eighteen months.[117]

The slow healing process can be discouraging, and over the course of time that it takes to see positive change, other health issues may arise. A 2019 review found individuals with PCOS may have a higher risk of developing binge eating disorder, which may be related to sugar management[118] as well as the often frustratingly slow healing process of PCOS.

The negative emotions associated with poor body image and the slow healing process may also influence quality of sleep, making almost everything more challenging! A 2020 cross-sectional study found individuals with PCOS tended to report poorer sleep quality, worse daytime functioning, and higher use of sleep medication than controls. Sadly, the strongest psychological variable negatively influencing sleep patterns was body image.[119]

Friends, this is where the hard work comes in. If you're having negative thoughts about your body, try this. Think of your three favorite people. What are your favorite characteristics about them? Nine times out of ten, physical appearance doesn't make the list! Some of the qualities that come to mind when we think of our favorite people include being kind, trustworthy, genuine, funny, goofy, and ultimately, being okay with being themselves.

Who you are on the inside is so much more valuable than how you look on the outside!

If you are working through PCOS and the healing process is affecting your mental well-being, there is no shame in seeking help and adding a mental health provider to your team.

If you feel a lack of progress no matter how hard you try, *it's not your fault and is not a reflection of poor effort or lack of hard work. It's just the biology of healing.* This is one of the reasons we emphasize giving yourself a year; sometimes, these changes just take time.

LIFESTYLE TIPS FOR PCOS

On a happy note, lifestyle modifications including nutrition and exercise may positively influence your PCOS symptoms!

Let's talk about some specific lifestyle hacks for PCOS.

NUTRITION AND PCOS: MACRONUTRIENTS

For those of you who have PCOS, some of your symptoms may be related to the *types* of macronutrients you're eating!

Remember, macronutrients include carbs, proteins, and fats, and balancing macronutrients is vital for those with PCOS.

In individuals with PCOS, fiber and protein intake tend to be low, while sugar, saturated fat, and cholesterol intake tend to be high.[120]

A small 2016 study analyzing individuals with PCOS found protein intake was low in almost thirty-seven percent of participants, and over eighty-three percent were not getting enough fiber in their diet.[121]

If you struggle with weight management, low dietary fiber may be playing a role in your symptoms. A 2019 cohort study found weight management problems and obesity in individuals with PCOS may not be due to overeating and inactivity, but instead may relate more to low fiber and magnesium levels.[122] Menstruating friends, this gives you even more of a reason to get those whole foods in, especially ones high in magnesium such as nuts, seeds, dark leafy greens, seaweed, legumes, and whole grains!

And remember, not all fats are created equally. A 2017 study found that on top of increasing fiber intake, decreasing trans fat intake may positively influence health in individuals with PCOS.[123]

A great place to start is reading labels and decreasing heavily processed foods from your diet. Remember, fat is not "bad" for you, and the quality of fat matters! If you are getting your fats from whole foods and healthy sources, you are more likely to feel full and satisfied versus getting fats from highly processed foods. A grass-fed or black bean burger with potatoes roasted in olive oil and salt is going to be a much better option than a fast-food burger and fries.

FASCINATING FACT

To put into perspective why we emphasize eating at home when possible, here is the ingredients list for McDonald's fries: Potatoes, Vegetable Oil (Canola Oil, Corn Oil, Soybean Oil, Hydrogenated Soybean Oil), Natural Beef Flavor [Wheat And Milk Derivatives]*, Dextrose, Sodium Acid Pyrophosphate (maintain Color), Salt. *Natural Beef Flavor Contains Hydrolyzed Wheat And Hydrolyzed Milk.[124]

Potatoes cooked at home in olive oil and salt are sounding much better now, huh?

NUTRITION AND PCOS: MICRONUTRIENTS

Before we talk about micronutrients and PCOS, it's important to understand that gut health plays a role in how our body processes and absorbs nutrients.

If you have PCOS, we highly recommend starting with the basics. The easiest way to start is by increasing fiber and protein, decreasing packaged and fast foods high in processed sugars and oils, and making sure you have bowel movements daily!

If you've been making those changes consistently and still feel "off," it may be worth getting lab work done. There are specific micronutrients that tend to be low in individuals with PCOS, and increasing some of these nutrients may be beneficial for the healing process.

Individuals with PCOS commonly have low levels of calcium, magnesium, potassium, folic acid, vitamin C, and vitamin B12,[125] and research has found potential benefits of zinc, iodine, vitamin D, calcium, and magnesium.

PRO TIP

Especially if you haven't had lab work, we recommend whole food sources of nutrients whenever possible. Whole foods may be especially beneficial if you have PCOS due to their high fiber content. Before adding supplements into your routine, make sure to talk to a healthcare provider, especially if you are taking medications.

Zinc may be beneficial for individuals with PCOS and period pain.[126] In a study analyzing individuals with PCOS, those who supplemented with 50 mg per day of elemental zinc over an eight-week period demonstrated decreased hair loss, known as alopecia, and decreased hair growth on the face, chest, and back, known as hirsutism. While there were no significant changes in hormonal profiles, inflammatory markers, or other markers of oxidative stress,[127] this is promising news for addressing some of the most common physical symptoms associated with PCOS.

Disclaimer: The study above had subjects taking 50 mg of zinc per day, which is above the upper limit for adults of 40 mg per day. Always consult with a healthcare professional before adding supplements into your routine. Refer to page 71 to refresh your memory on the common symptoms of zinc toxicity.

Dietary sources of zinc include oysters, beef, crab, lobster, pork, chicken, pumpkin seeds, cashews, chickpeas, and other legumes (lentils, beans, etc.).

Iodine levels may play a role in PCOS and the development of ovarian cysts. Unfortunately, research is lacking in regards to iodine supplementation, and we could not find any randomized controlled studies on the topic. On a hopeful note, in small sample sizes, some physicians have found iodine supplementation to positively impact period regularity, cyst growth, and the management of type II diabetes in those with PCOS.[128] Getting your iodine levels checked may help you determine whether an iodine deficiency is contributing to your symptoms.

Dietary sources of iodine include seaweed, seafood, iodized salt, dairy, and eggs.

Vitamin D and **calcium** may help with hormone balance and blood pressure in individuals with PCOS. A small study of twelve overweight and vitamin D deficient people with PCOS found that taking 3533-8533 IU of vitamin D and 530 mg of calcium daily decreased levels of certain sex hormones known as androgens and improved blood pressure in those starting with blood pressure higher than 120/80.[129]

Although we get vitamin D primarily through sunlight, dietary sources of vitamin D include fortified dairy products, fish such as salmon, herring, sardines, and tuna, egg yolks, mushrooms, fortified orange juice, and cod liver oil, which has the added benefit of being a great source of omega-3.

Dietary sources of calcium include dairy, green leafy vegetables, soy, sardines, and fortified grain products.

Magnesium, zinc, calcium, and **vitamin D,** when taken in combination over a twelve-week period, were seen to improve hormonal profiles, hirsutism, and some biomarkers of inflammation and oxidative stress in individuals with PCOS.[130]

Dietary sources of magnesium include nuts, seeds, dark leafy greens, seaweed, legumes, dairy products, and whole grains.

Remember, it's important to follow up with a health care provider before starting supplements, especially if you are on medications. You can get vitamin D from sunlight and fortified foods, and the rest of these micronutrients can be found in the whole food sources listed above. Even better, getting your micronutrients from whole food sources will naturally increase your fiber intake, making it a win-win!

EXERCISE AND PCOS

The thought of exercise may seem overwhelming, but if you're not currently active, we encourage you to add some movement into your routine. Exercise can positively impact health, especially if you have PCOS!

FASCINATING FACT

According to a 2015 study, low activity levels may increase your risk of developing PCOS.[131] Another study from 2012 found adolescents with PCOS tended to have lower physical activity levels than those without PCOS. All individuals in the 2012 study were sedentary for more than four hours per day, which is in excess of the current public health recommendations.[132]

Many folks aren't aware of the positive effects exercise can have on PCOS symptoms and their overall health.

So, if you have PCOS, try adding social workouts into your routine such as walking, biking, or dancing with a friend.

Exercising for physical and mental well-being has benefits that don't always translate to changes on the scale, so it's important to think of all of the ways you're building a healthy body when you move regularly.[133]

Exercise may positively influence cardiovascular health, decrease inflammation, improve insulin sensitivity, and improve your chances of ovulating,[134] which are all changes you can't see externally. So before you get frustrated and give up, remember...

Your health is not determined by your weight!

Both strength training and aerobic exercise, when performed at a moderate intensity consistently over the course of three to six months, can help increase your chances of ovulating and improve insulin sensitivity.[135]

If you don't already have an exercise routine, today is a great day to start! There are no scientific findings suggesting people with PCOS should avoid exercise because of their diagnosis,[136] and regular movement may be a great tool for symptom management! Remember, exercise can be in the form of little bursts of exercise throughout the day, and you can also get benefits from doing three thirty-minute exercise sessions throughout the week. Both aerobic exercise and strength training can be useful tools to improve health, especially if you're consistent with them for three to six months. If you're looking for a little motivation, find a friend and make a plan together!

ENVIRONMENTAL CHEMICALS AND PCOS

We know from previous chapters that environmental chemicals can affect our hormones, and there are specific chemicals that may be especially relevant for individuals with PCOS.

BPA, also known as bisphenol A, has gotten a lot of attention over the past few years due to its negative impact on human health.[137] BPA levels tend to be higher in individuals with PCOS, and high levels of BPA have been associated with increased levels of androgens,[138] which is a common problem among individuals with PCOS.

- BPA is commonly found in plastics, including disposable water bottles. It may be worth trying to fill up your reusable bottle (preferably stainless steel) at home prior to going out.

AGEs, also known as advanced glycation end products, are another environmental chemical relevant if you have PCOS. Multiple studies have found the concentration of AGEs to be higher in individuals with PCOS compared to controls.[139]

- AGEs can be produced in the body when breaking down food, or they can be absorbed directly from your diet.[140] Broiling and frying foods leads to the highest AGEs content.[141] The Standard American Diet, which is high in processed meats, meat substitutes, fats, oils, and foods full of fat and sugar cooked at high heats, is full of AGEs.[142]

- Some easy ways to decrease dietary exposure to AGEs include decreasing your intake of processed meats, meat substitutes, and packaged foods high in fats and sugar, and increasing whole foods, which tend to be naturally higher in fiber and lower in AGEs. Smoking cigarettes may also increase AGEs in the body, adding to your list of reasons to quit smoking.[143]

FASCINATING FACT

Along with BPA and AGES, a 2014 study in China found other specific environmental factors associated with the development of PCOS include alcohol consumption, eating foods packaged in plastic, high pesticide exposure, and eating fruits with skins, which may have higher exposure to pesticides.[144]

If you have PCOS, it may be worthwhile to try to limit exposure to certain plastics, including those with endocrine-disrupting compounds like BPA. Decreasing the intake of fast foods and highly processed animal products will help decrease exposure to AGEs. Remember to look at the Dirty Dozen List to see which fruits might be most highly contaminated in their non-organic forms. Last but not least, smoking increases your toxic load and exposure to AGEs, giving you another reason to quit!

MEDICATIONS AND MANAGEMENT OF PCOS

If you have PCOS, you may be taking multiple medications for symptom management. But do you know why these medications have been prescribed to you?

We believe if you are taking medications, it's important to understand why you are taking them and what symptoms they are treating.

Two of the most commonly prescribed medications for PCOS include hormonal contraceptives and Metformin.

According to a 2017 review, hormonal contraceptives are often the first choice for treating individuals with PCOS. While current practice guidelines for prescribing hormonal contraceptives are based on research, much of this research has not specifically looked at the use of hormonal contraceptives in individuals with PCOS. Hormonal contraceptives may help with some of the symptoms associated with PCOS, including hyperandrogenism and cancer risk, but might *not* help with underlying metabolic disorders.[145]

This is important to understand because insulin and metabolic problems play a large role in the symptoms associated with PCOS. When addressing hormone imbalance, we want to heal the *root cause* and not just put a Band-Aid over the symptoms, which is why it's vital to look at lifestyle factors like movement and nutrition if you suffer from PCOS.

FASCINATING FACT

As far as hormonal contraception and ovarian cysts go, a systematic review of the literature in 2009 analyzing findings from seven studies found no decrease in the healing time for functional ovarian cysts in individuals taking hormonal contraceptives. Most cysts, especially functional ovarian cysts, resolved on their own in a few cycles without any treatment. If a cyst was persistent, this was usually a sign that it was pathological (a cyst due to abnormal cell growth).[146]

Metformin is also commonly prescribed, but did you know it actually hasn't been FDA approved specifically for PCOS? Metformin addresses the metabolic problems such as high blood sugar and insulin resistance common in patients with PCOS.[147]

While we are not anti-medication, the problem, in this case, is often a lack of education. The prescribing providers won't always ask about the lifestyle factors that may be contributing to insulin resistance... nutrition and exercise! We are all for medications when they are necessary, but if you are trying to treat problems related to blood sugar and insulin management, decreasing sugar and processed or fast foods should most definitely be included in your plan.

We encourage you to ask thorough questions about side effects, efficacy, and long-term use of any medications you are prescribed. If you can't get a hold of your physician, pharmacists are a great resource for these sorts of questions! While there is a time and place for medications, it is wise to gather all the facts before adding anything new into your routine. Besides medications when appropriate, lifestyle factors such as nutrition and exercise should also be addressed.

Remember, eating well does not have to be boring! There are lots of delicious low-sugar recipes that can fuel your body and help you manage your PCOS symptoms. Check out our recipes at the back of the book for some inspiration.

PCOS TAKEAWAYS

If you have PCOS, your daily habits matter! Lifestyle changes like increasing dietary fiber intake, decreasing sugar and processed fats, and exercising regularly can play key roles in symptom management.

While the thought of these changes can seem overwhelming, it doesn't have to be! Try starting with the basics—cook at home using whole food sources, read labels when you're on the go, and try to get at least thirty minutes of exercise three times per week as a baseline. Remember, "exercise snacks" really add up, so make sure to take some breaks throughout your day if your job is sedentary. The Pomodoro timer (pomodoro.io/app) is a great resource for this!

We want to remind you: you are so much more than your physical appearance!

Sometimes, addressing PCOS can be mentally taxing. We encourage a team approach when it comes to your health, and mental health providers can often help bring your healing full circle!

If you feel frustrated trying to address the physical symptoms associated with PCOS, remember that change takes time. This is one of the reasons we emphasize giving yourself a year; we want you to create a sustainable plan to promote overall health and well-being. Small daily steps over the course of a year will help you continue to grow in your physical and mental health. While the healing process takes its course, remember that who you are on the inside is so much more valuable than how you look on the outside.

ENDOMETRIOSIS

Did you know an estimated ten to fifteen percent of individuals with a menstrual cycle have endometriosis?[148]

But what is endometriosis?

As you might recall, the endometrium is the inner lining of the uterus that is shed during menstruation. Endometriosis occurs when tissue sharing similar properties to the endometrium is found in other areas of the reproductive system, and in rare cases, other areas of the body, including the GI tract, lungs, brain, and skin.[149]

Endometrial-like tissue outside of the uterus has the same qualities as the lining of the uterus, causing cyclical swelling and bleeding in areas of the body where these byproducts may not easily be shed.[150]

Endometriosis is classified as both an estrogen-dependent condition and a chronic inflammatory condition, meaning that addressing both hormonal imbalances and inflammation are vital!

The heightened inflammatory response may contribute to the formation of scar tissue adhesions, influencing some of the most common physical symptoms of endometriosis such as pelvic pain, painful periods, and pain with sex.[151] Symptoms may also be influenced by hormone imbalances such as estrogen dominance and progesterone resistance,[152] which both contribute to a high ratio of estrogen to progesterone and the not-so-fun associated symptoms, which we talk about in our chapter on estrogen dominance.

Some of the verbiage related to endometriosis can be difficult to navigate, so here are a few definitions that might be helpful:

- **Ectopic** is defined as being in an abnormal place or position; in regard to endometriosis, ectopic lesions or ectopic endometrium refer to endometrial-like tissue found outside of the uterus in other areas of the reproductive system or body.

- **Eutopic** means in a normal position; in this case, it is referring to endometrial tissue found in the uterus.

- **Eumenorrhea** means normal or regular menstruation.

THE SYMPTOMS OF ENDOMETRIOSIS

While pain is the most common symptom of endometriosis, it is not the only symptom. Other common symptoms include fertility issues,[153] heavy menstrual bleeding, long menstrual cycles,[154] and digestive problems.[155]

It's important to let your team know all of your symptoms to help them figure out if you have endometriosis and to give them a better idea of where the lesions may be located.

For example:

- In relation to GI symptoms, different types of digestive issues, including constipation, difficulty with bowel movements, or diarrhea, may be associated with endometriosis in different parts of the GI tract.[156]

- There have also been multiple case studies examining endometriosis in the colon as a cause of rectal bleeding.[157] If you have persistent rectal bleeds or rectal bleeding requiring hospitalization, it's important to see if your bleeding follows a cyclical pattern. If this is the case, it may be worth adding a specialist well-versed in endometriosis to your team to see if there is a possibility that you have endometrial-like tissue contributing to your symptoms.

- In regard to fertility, a 2014 retrospective cohort study analyzing a group of individuals with infertility found spotting for more than two days between cycles was a better indicator of whether or not someone had endometriosis than relying on patient reports of period pain or pain with intercourse.[158]

- It's estimated that between seventy-one to eighty-seven percent of individuals with chronic pelvic pain have endometriosis, so if you have chronic pelvic pain, make sure to keep track of your symptoms.[159]

PRO TIP

Although pelvic pain and pain with intercourse are common, it's not always a comfortable subject to talk about; sometimes, there can be hesitation from both patients and healthcare providers to address this issue.[160] We want to remind you that you are not alone and encourage you to have open conversations with both your providers and partners. The book *Come as You Are* by Emily Nagowski is a great read if you're struggling in this area, and it's never a bad idea to follow up with a mental health provider or pelvic health physical therapist to address the emotional and physical components of your pain.

So, how do you know if you have endometriosis?

One of the most challenging aspects of endometriosis is that the symptoms can be vague and mimic other conditions, making it difficult to diagnose.

A 2008 case-control study found individuals with endometriosis spend more time at the doctor's office and are twice as likely to take time off from work than controls.[161] Many individuals with endometriosis feel like they lack support from healthcare professionals,[162] which is one of the reasons we encourage you to understand your body and find a team that you feel supports *you*.

If you have symptoms consistent with endometriosis, talk to your doctor about the various ways to diagnose endometriosis. Surgery, although the gold standard and the only way to truly confirm endometrial lesions, is an invasive technique. Because of this, providers in recent years are relying more heavily on patient history and imaging to assist in the diagnosis of endometriosis.[163]

Unfortunately, surgery is the only way to truly get rid of endometrial lesions. If you are having surgery for endometriosis, we highly recommend finding a specialist who is well-versed in these surgeries; if any of the endometrial-like tissue gets left behind, the cells can divide and create new lesions.[164]

FASCINATING FACT

Although surgery is the only way to get rid of lesions, it may not necessarily decrease pain.[165]

When it comes to the pain associated with endometriosis, it is commonly assumed that it is caused directly by the lesions, but the size and location of the lesion don't always correlate with pain.[166] Recent research has shown that some of the primary factors contributing to pain include nerve growth to the lesion, inflammation, and hormonal imbalance.[167] Estrogen may influence both inflammation and nerve growth to the lesions, making estrogen management vital.[168] If you're interested in learning more about strategies to help manage estrogen levels, check out our chapter on estrogen dominance on page 136.

The good news is that adjunct therapies like physical therapy, massage therapy, acupuncture, exercise, and dietary changes may help decrease some of the symptoms of endometriosis. We'll go over the details later in this chapter!

ENDOMETRIOSIS: MAINTAINING HORMONAL BALANCE

Endometriosis is characterized by estrogen dominance and progesterone resistance.[169]

Estrogen dominance is the term for high estrogen in relation to progesterone. In the case of endometriosis, this promotes the growth of the endometrial-like tissues. Besides promoting the growth of lesions,[170] estrogen and changes in estrogen receptors may increase inflammation as well as neural and vascular stimulation to the area, contributing to pain.[171]

FASCINATING FACT

The goal of hormonal therapies, including hormonal contraception, for individuals with endometriosis is to decrease the production of estrogen in the ovaries.[172] We hope that you will feel more educated on your options for managing estrogen levels through lifestyle modifications, including nutrition and movement, after reading this book.

Along with the changes in the lesions due to high estrogen and changes in estrogen receptors, the tissue in endometrial lesions may be *less* responsive to progesterone, known as progesterone resistance. This can be caused by both a lack of progesterone *and* changes in how the tissues respond to progesterone. Progesterone resistance allows the growth of the endometrial tissues caused by estrogen to go unchecked.[173]

ENVIRONMENTAL CHEMICALS AND ENDOMETRIOSIS

We've previously mentioned how environmental chemicals in commonly used cleaning and personal hygiene items can influence hormone balance. Dioxin is one to pay particular attention to if you have endometriosis.

As you might recall from our chapter on estrogen dominance, dioxin is a persistent organic pollutant and is considered to be one of the most toxic chemicals in its class. A 2010 study found menstruating people with high plasma concentrations of dioxin-like compounds were at a higher risk of developing endometriosis than individuals whose plasma concentrations were within the normal environmental exposure range.[174] A mouse study from 2010 found dioxin may influence the development of characteristics related to progesterone resistance. Even scarier, these changes in the mice persisted over several generations.[175] This is important information to consider if you have endometriosis, as one of the common characteristics of endometrial lesions is progesterone resistance.

Although you can't control previous exposures, you can take daily steps to reduce your risk moving forward. While most dioxin comes from fat in animal products, such as meat, fish, and dairy, it can also be found in pesticides, herbicides, and drinking water.[176] Easy ways to decrease dioxin exposure include choosing lean cuts of meat, limiting high intake of animal fats, and decreasing pesticide and herbicide exposure when possible. To make sure your water is free from unhealthy contaminants, we recommend finding a good water filter to help decrease unnecessary exposure to the chemicals often found in tap water. You can check tap water quality in your local area at EWG.org.

PRO TIP

Because one of the characteristics of endometriosis is estrogen dominance, it may be worth decreasing your exposure to xenoestrogens, or chemicals that can mimic estrogen in the body. Check out page 143 for a list of xenoestrogens commonly found in everyday items, and read the full section for other tips and tricks to reduce exposure.

While we may not be able to avoid all the environmental toxins we are exposed to, small and incremental changes in the products we use and the food we eat can go a long way in reducing risk and minimizing exposure.

LIFESTYLE FACTORS AND ENDOMETRIOSIS

Endometriosis can be a scary diagnosis, and although surgery is the only option to completely remove endometrial lesions, small daily decisions can make a big difference in your symptoms!

Embracing bodily autonomy and self-efficacy, the right to your own body and the knowledge that you can make decisions to positively influence your health, can help you create sustainable lifestyle changes. Having a good support team, including friends and family, is also vital in helping you stay consistent with dietary and lifestyle changes.[177]

From a medical standpoint, do your research and find providers well-versed in endometriosis, and know that pelvic health physical therapists can help with the physical symptoms and mental health providers can help with any overwhelm due to your diagnosis.

Massage therapy and acupuncture may also be beneficial as they both can help alleviate some of the physical symptoms, such as painful periods, associated with endometriosis.[178]

If you're feeling overwhelmed and have appointment fatigue associated with your diagnosis, start with little daily actions. Keep reading to learn more about nutrition and movement tips for endometriosis and ways to incorporate these tips into your life!

DIET AND ENDOMETRIOSIS

If you're feeling discouraged trying to find the "perfect" endometriosis diet, we get it! There is a lot of information out there, and some of it is contradictory.

This is where an individualized approach is vital. Using nutrition as a part of the healing process for endometriosis means finding a plan that makes you feel good, which may look different for each of us.[179]

If you're not sure where to start, it might be worthwhile to make some basic dietary changes like decreasing gluten, dairy products, and refined carbohydrates, and increasing fruits, veggies, fish, and lean meat.

A 2020 study found individualized diet changes, emphasizing decreased intake of processed foods, cooking at home from scratch, and making the dietary changes listed above, reduced pain, fatigue, and heavy menstrual bleeding, and improved sleep and energy levels in individuals with endometriosis. These nutritional changes proved to be instrumental in encouraging positive changes in other aspects of well-being, including activity levels, coping skills, stress management strategies, and the ability to manage conflict.[180]

FASCINATING FACT

You may be wondering about the effects of alcohol and coffee on endometriosis.

Alcohol consumption may have a negative impact on endometriosis.[181] With our knowledge of how estrogen is affected by alcohol, it might be good to replace your nightly wine with another antioxidant-rich beverage like tart cherry juice.

As for coffee, an analysis of current data in 2021 concluded no association between coffee or caffeine intake and your risk of developing endometriosis.[182] It's probably okay to have your morning coffee, just make sure not to load it with cream and sugar!

FRUITS, VEGGIES, AND ENDOMETRIOSIS

Different bodies may respond differently to foods that are generally considered healthy, which is why an individualized plan is so important.

PRO TIP

If you're confused about which foods you do well with, functional nutritionists are great resources to troubleshoot your specific dietary needs.

Although fruits are usually considered to be a healthy option, there is conflicting evidence about fruit intake and endometriosis. Some studies have found that certain fruits decrease the risk of developing endometriosis,[183] while other studies have found higher fruit consumption is related to an increased risk of developing endometriosis.[184]

This contradictory information may be partially due to different fruits having differing concentrations of pesticides and herbicides, influencing your environmental chemical exposure.

Taking this into consideration, with both fruits *and* veggies, it may be beneficial to look at the Dirty Dozen list on EWG.org to decrease unnecessary exposure to environmental chemicals.

As far as vegetables go, although we've previously discussed the health benefits of cruciferous vegetables, some studies have demonstrated an association between cruciferous vegetables and the risk of developing endometriosis.[185]

A 2018 study found an increased risk of developing endometriosis in individuals who ate more than one serving of cruciferous vegetables per day compared to less than one serving per week.[186] While this is not what the authors expected, this study found specific vegetables to be more related to endometriosis risk.

Some of the vegetables found to be most related to endometriosis risk included: Brussel sprouts, raw cabbage/coleslaw, and cauliflower. Corn, peas, and lima beans, although not cruciferous vegetables, were also correlated with increased risk.[187]

PRO TIP

A 2017 review found that individuals with endometriosis who also have GI symptoms may do best on a low FODMAP diet.[188]

This is where the importance of creating an individualized plan is so important. If you feel good eating cruciferous veggies, great! If you've been struggling and "doing the right things" and are still having symptoms, it may be worth eliminating the vegetables listed above and monitoring symptoms.

DIETARY FAT AND ENDOMETRIOSIS

If you have endometriosis, it may be beneficial to increase your intake of healthy fats!

The types of fats you're eating may influence your risk of developing endometriosis. A 2010 study found a *lower* risk of developing endometriosis in individuals who had a diet high in omega-3 fatty acids and a *forty-eight percent higher* chance of developing endometriosis in individuals who consumed high amounts of trans fat.[189]

Food items linked to an increased risk of developing endometriosis include packaged foods and processed meats, such as beef and ham.[190] These foods contain a high amount of saturated and trans fats and low amounts of omega-3 fatty acids.[191] Cooking at home with whole foods is a great way to improve the quality of your diet and decrease symptoms related to endometriosis.

MICRONUTRIENTS AND ENDOMETRIOSIS

Certain micronutrients may be beneficial if you have endometriosis. Ones worth monitoring include thiamine, folate, vitamin C, vitamin E, and L-arginine.

> **FASCINATING FACT**
>
> If you have endometriosis, it's important to get your nutrients from whole foods. A 2013 study found a decreased risk of developing endometriosis when thiamine, folate, vitamin C, and vitamin E were consumed in *whole food sources*. Supplements were not seen to reduce the risk of endometriosis in this study.[192]

Thiamine (also known as vitamin B1) has been found to be inversely related to endometriosis risk, meaning low thiamine intake may increase your risk of developing endometriosis.[193]

Dietary sources of thiamine include whole grains, meat, and fish.[194]

Folate (B9) is another micronutrient that is inversely related to endometriosis risk.[195] In fact, folate may improve luteal phase progesterone levels, helping to manage the balance of estrogen to progesterone in the second half of your cycle.[196]

Dietary sources of folate include dark green leafy vegetables, liver, bread, yeasts, and fruits.

Vitamin C and **Vitamin E** are both antioxidants that may help with pain related to endometriosis[197] and may protect the endometrium from damage due to oxidative stress, which can lead to chronic inflammation.[198]

Dietary sources of vitamin C include citrus fruits, strawberries, tomatoes, hibiscus tea, broccoli, spinach, bell peppers, and kiwi fruit.[199]

Dietary sources of vitamin E include nuts, egg yolks, cheese, oatmeal, avocados, olives, green leafy vegetables, and plant-based oils such as olive oil.[200]

It may be beneficial to get your vitamin E from foods rather than supplements due to the high concentrations of vitamin E in some supplements.[201]

L-arginine may influence the steroid hormone receptors that play a role in endometriosis[202] and has been inversely related to endometriosis risk.[203]

Dietary sources of L-arginine include walnuts, peanuts, soy protein, and fish.[204]

EXERCISE AND ENDOMETRIOSIS

Did you know that exercising regularly at a moderate to high intensity may reduce your chances of developing endometriosis? A 2003 study found individuals who exercised at a moderate to high intensity for more than thirty minutes three or more times per week for two years had a reduced risk of developing endometriosis.[205]

Some ideas for moderate- to high-intensity exercise include tennis singles, hiking, jogging at six miles per hour, shoveling, cycling at a speed of fourteen to sixteen miles per hour, basketball, and soccer.

If you've already been diagnosed with endometriosis, there are still benefits to staying active! A small 2017 study found that an eight-week exercise program may help improve posture and decrease pain in individuals with endometriosis.[206]

FASCINATING FACT

While we couldn't find any human studies analyzing the effect of exercise on endometrial lesion size, a 2019 study analyzing rats with endometriosis showed some promising results. All of the rats who participated in swimming demonstrated decreased lesion sizes, with the most improvement seen in those who exercised three or five times per week compared to once per week.[207] Although this was a study done on rats, this is good news for those of you getting out more than three times per week for a good sweat session!

ENDOMETRIOSIS TAKEAWAYS

If you think you might have endometriosis, we highly recommend finding a specialist that is well versed in treating endometriosis. Laparoscopic surgery is the only way to remove lesions, but lifestyle factors can positively influence pain levels and improve your quality of life.

Endometriosis can be a frustrating diagnosis, and while it's easy to feel discouraged, there are ways to manage symptoms that are within your control, including nutrition and exercise! If you know that you tend to reach for quick and easy foods that are processed, start with the basics: decrease dairy, gluten, and foods high in refined fats and carbohydrates, and increase fruits, veggies, and fish. As for exercise, aim for three thirty-minute sessions per week of moderate- to high-intensity activity.

It is vital to feel supported as you work through the healing process; this includes having a trustworthy medical team and the encouragement of friends and family. If you feel like you're lacking this support, mental healthcare professionals or community support groups can be beneficial. Check out myendometriosisteam.com or Nancy's Nook Endometriosis Education Facebook group for some great resources. And if you're struggling with pain, pelvic health physical therapy, massage therapy, and acupuncture are great adjunct therapies to add into the mix!

HEAVY MENSTRUAL BLEEDING

Needing to change your tampon or pad or having to empty your menstrual cup every hour is *not* normal!

Heavy menstrual bleeding, often referred to as menorrhagia, is a type of abnormal uterine bleeding in which a menstruating person loses more than eighty mL of blood per cycle.[208]

FASCINATING FACT

To put things into perspective, one tablespoon is a little less than fifteen mL. In a usual cycle you'll lose about two to three tablespoons of blood. If you're losing more than about five and one-third tablespoons of blood over the course of your period, which is roughly a third of a cup, chances are, you have heavy menstrual bleeding.[209]

According to the CDC, you may have an increased risk of heavy menstrual bleeding if you have the following symptoms:

- Your period lasts more than seven days
- You soak through one or more pads or tampons per hour for several hours in a row
- You're worried you will bleed through your tampon, so you wear a pad for extra coverage "just in case"
- You need to change your tampon or pad at night
- You have blood clots the size of a quarter (or larger)
- Your heavy bleeding keeps you from doing your normal activities

- You have lower abdominal pain during your bleed
- You have increased fatigue, lack of energy, or have shortness of breath during your period[210]

PRO TIP

Small amounts of clots, which resemble a jelly-like substance, can be a normal part of menstruation. If you're consistently getting clots that are larger than the size of a quarter, it's important to follow up with a healthcare provider.

If you resonate with any of the above symptoms, we recommend compiling a list of questions and concerns to bring to your next physical or annual appointment.

Heavy periods are an especially important talking point if you feel tired and fatigued.

A study from 1995 found about three-quarters of individuals who thought they had heavy menstrual bleeding had a specific type of anemia due to low iron levels, known as iron deficiency anemia, even if they didn't lose eighty mL or more of blood during their periods.[211] Iron deficiency anemia can affect energy and quality of life, which is why we have a whole section devoted to iron deficiency. If you have a menstrual cycle, it's important to know the signs and symptoms of iron deficiency so that you can bring all relevant information to your healthcare team.

MEDICAL MANAGEMENT OF HEAVY MENSTRUAL BLEEDING

It's important to have a healthcare team following your case if you have heavy cycles because you may have an underlying bleeding disorder or other problems like uterine fibroids contributing to your symptoms.[212]

According to a 2015 review, uterine fibroids occur in about one in ten patients with heavy menstrual cycles, and in those with severe heavy menstrual bleeding, this increases to about four in ten.[213] We'll talk all about uterine fibroids in the next section.

FASCINATING FACT

According to a 2022 review, about thirty percent of hysterectomies performed in the U.S., which is the surgical removal of the uterus, are due to heavy menstrual bleeding.[214] Unfortunately, it is common for the uterus to be removed only to find out after the surgery there was no pathology in the uterus contributing to the heavy bleeding.[215]

This is why we're passionate about providing education on how lifestyle factors such as nutrition and movement can influence your hormones and period. If you don't need to get surgery and can manage your symptoms by making daily changes, we're all for it! If you are considering surgery, it never hurts to get a second opinion prior to making your decision.

MANAGING HEAVY PERIODS

Surgery and medications are often the first treatment strategies offered for heavy menstrual bleeding, but what if you don't want to manage your symptoms with these interventions?

Heavy periods may be influenced by the overgrowth of the endometrium due to estrogen dominance.[216] Some easy tips for managing estrogen dominance include increasing your intake of cruciferous veggies like cabbage, broccoli, cauliflower, and Brussels sprouts, eating more fiber, eating less processed foods and refined oils, getting regular exercise to promote overall health, and using the tools in this book to help manage stress. And remember, positive social interactions have been linked with increased progesterone levels, favorably influencing the ratio of progesterone to estrogen, making it vital to keep a good community!

We have a whole chapter devoted to estrogen dominance and symptom management strategies—check out page 136 for more details!

> **PRO TIP**
>
> Managing inflammation is another key aspect in regulating heavy periods, as prostaglandins may play a role in heavy menstrual bleeding.[217] Easy tips for managing inflammation include decreasing processed and packaged foods, increasing fruit and veggie intake, and making sure to move daily.

NUTRITION AND HEAVY MENSTRUAL BLEEDING

Certain foods and nutrients may also be beneficial!

Ginger and vitamin E both have antioxidant and anti-inflammatory properties, and they've both been studied specifically in individuals with heavy menstrual bleeding![218] Vitamins A, K, C, B complex, and iron can also be beneficial for those with heavy periods.[219]

Ginger may have similar effects to NSAIDs on prostaglandins, making it a great, natural option for managing period pain.[220]

A small 2015 study analyzing individuals in high school with heavy menstrual bleeding found a significant decrease in blood loss with very few side effects in individuals receiving ginger compared to controls.[221]

Vitamin E is an antioxidant that may help with heavy periods. In a 2005 double-blind study analyzing high school students aged fifteen to seventeen, individuals who supplemented with vitamin E for four months reported lower pain levels and less blood loss compared to controls.[222]

It may be beneficial to get your vitamin E from foods rather than supplements, due to the high concentrations of vitamin E in some supplements.[223]

Dietary sources of vitamin E include nuts, egg yolks, cheese, oatmeal, avocados, olives, green leafy vegetables, and plant-based oils such as olive oil.[224]

Vitamin A plays a role in vision and immune function, and low vitamin A levels may influence heavy menstrual bleeding.[225]

Dietary sources of vitamin A include beef liver, sweet potato, spinach, pumpkin, carrots, Atlantic herring, milk, and cantaloupe.[226]

Vitamin K may be beneficial for heavy periods because of its effect on blood clotting. However, it may be best to get vitamin K from food sources rather than supplementing. If you want to supplement, it's important to speak with a healthcare provider because it may not be beneficial for everyone,[227] especially those with blood clotting disorders.

Dietary sources of vitamin K include collard greens, spinach, broccoli, cabbage, fermented soybeans (natto), and hard and soft cheeses.[228]

Vitamin C helps with iron absorption and may also help with heavy bleeding.[229]

Dietary sources of vitamin C include citrus fruits, strawberries, tomatoes, hibiscus tea, broccoli, spinach, bell peppers, and kiwi fruit.[230]

Vitamin B complex may help the liver break down estrogen, therefore decreasing overgrowth of the endometrium and reducing the risk of heavy menstrual bleeding.[231]

Dietary sources of B-complex (B1, B2, B3, B5, B6, folate, biotin, B12) include meat, organ meat, fish, eggs, dairy, whole grains, nuts, legumes, green leafy vegetables, potatoes, non-citrus fruit, and tomatoes.[232]

Iron is important to monitor if you have heavy menstrual bleeding because of the associated blood loss. It's imperative to consume enough iron in your diet,[233] so keep reading because we'll talk all about iron deficiency later in this chapter!

Check out page 69 for a full list of dietary sources of iron!

HEAVY MENSTRUAL BLEEDING TAKEAWAYS

If you lose more than one-third of a cup of blood per period, fill up multiple pads or tampons in less than a few hours, or have clots bigger than a quarter, you might have heavy menstrual bleeding!

If you have a heavy period, you have a greater loss of blood and nutrients during menstruation. It's important to focus on eating a well-rounded diet that incorporates a wide variety of foods to ensure you're getting all the nutrients you need. Incorporating whole foods full of the nutrients listed above and making sure to get enough iron is vital! We'll talk more about the importance of iron and food sources of iron later in this section.

While surgery for heavy periods is common, hormonal imbalances may also be contributing to your symptoms. High estrogen levels compared to progesterone, known as estrogen dominance, is common in individuals with heavy menstrual bleeding. We have a whole chapter on estrogen dominance, so check it out to learn more.

UTERINE FIBROIDS

Uterine fibroids, also known as uterine leiomyomas or myomas, are extremely common, affecting more than seventy percent of menstruating people.[234]

FASCINATING FACT

Did you know that uterine fibroids are considered to be estrogen-dependent, non-cancerous tumors? Uterine fibroids are a sign of abnormal tissue growth in the smooth muscle of the uterus, and estrogen may influence this uncontrolled cell growth.[235] Check our section on estrogen dominance for tips and tools for hormone management!

Some common symptoms of uterine fibroids include pelvic pain, bowel and bladder problems, back pain, and heavy periods, all of which can have a devastating impact on physical and mental well-being.

While asymptomatic uterine fibroids may not require medical treatment,[236] an estimated twenty-five percent of people with uterine fibroids suffer from clinically significant symptoms.[237]

Unfortunately, a 2017 review found that there are currently no treatment strategies that provide long-term symptom relief, are cost-effective, and don't negatively impact fertility.[238] If your symptoms are severe, the most common treatment options include surgery or medications.[239]

While this may sound discouraging, there is preliminary evidence that lifestyle modifications, such as dietary changes, exercising regularly, decreasing exposure to environmental toxins, and the alternative therapies listed listed on the next page, may help alleviate some of the symptoms related to uterine fibroids.[240]

PRO TIP

A small 2002 study found a combination of Chinese medicine, therapies focused on the mind-body connection, and guided meditation may be helpful for individuals suffering from symptoms related to fibroids. Over half of the individuals who participated in these treatments for six months demonstrated decreased fibroid size, and the alternative treatments were found to be as effective as pharmacological treatments.[241]

NUTRITION AND FIBROIDS

Nutrition may influence the development of uterine fibroids, with sugar and alcohol being major contributing factors.

A 2009 study found that alcohol intake tended to be higher in individuals with fibroids,[242] and another study in 2010 found that foods with a high glycemic index (high in refined carbohydrates and sugar) increased the likelihood of developing fibroids in individuals under thirty-five years of age.[243] Processed foods and sugary drinks tend to have a high glycemic index, so if you have uterine fibroids, it may be worth avoiding these!

Along with decreasing alcohol, sugar, and processed foods, it may be beneficial to increase your intake of fruits and veggies (which are high in micronutrients) and make sure you're getting enough vitamin D.[244] We'll talk about micronutrients and fibroids in the next section.

MICRONUTRIENTS AND FIBROIDS

Micronutrients that may be beneficial if you have fibroids include calcium, vitamin D, and green tea extract.

Calcium may help decrease the risk of developing uterine fibroids according to a 2020 study analyzing data from 1991-2009. This study found that consumption of foods high in calcium, like yogurt, had the greatest impact on decreasing fibroid risk.[245]

Dietary sources of calcium include milk, cheese, other dairy products, leafy greens like collard greens, broccoli rabe, and kale, seafood, and foods that are fortified with calcium, meaning that they have calcium added into them.[246]

Vitamin D is another micronutrient that may reduce your risk of developing fibroids. A 2013 study found lower rates of uterine fibroids in individuals with sufficient vitamin D levels compared to those with insufficient levels.

FASCINATING FACT

This same study from 2013 discovered that only ten percent of the Black menstruating people and fifty percent of the white menstruating people who participated in the study had adequate vitamin D levels (>20ng/mL),[247] making it vital to advocate for yourself and make sure to get your vitamin D levels checked if you have fibroids!

Although we get vitamin D primarily through sunlight, dietary sources of vitamin D include fortified dairy products, fish such as salmon, herring, sardines, and tuna, egg yolks, mushrooms, fortified orange juice, and cod liver oil, which has the added benefit of being a great source of omega-3.

Green tea extract, also known as epigallocatechin gallate or ECGC, may be beneficial for individuals who have been diagnosed with uterine fibroids. A small double-blind study from 2013 found that green tea extract may help decrease fibroid size and symptoms associated with fibroids, improve quality of life, and decrease the likelihood of being diagnosed with anemia. In this same study, the placebo group had a 24.3% increase in fibroid size![248]

It's important to talk with a healthcare provider before supplementing with green tea extract. There is evidence that it may lead to liver problems in some people,[249] so be mindful of reaching for high-dose supplements for problems that may be multifactorial in nature.

FASCINATING FACT

Heavy metals may influence fibroid development and the associated symptoms! A 2002 study found that individuals with fibroids tended to have low zinc levels and high copper and chromium levels.[250] If you have uterine fibroids, it may be worth asking your provider about testing for heavy metals to ensure heavy metals aren't contributing to your symptoms.

EXERCISE AND FIBROIDS

Exercise may have a protective effect in terms of fibroid development.

A 2007 study found individuals who reported the highest activity levels were less likely to have fibroids,[251] and having an active job may also help decrease risk, according to a 2013 study.[252]

We encourage you to keep moving, whether that's going to the gym or staying active at work or home!

ENVIRONMENTAL CHEMICALS AND FIBROIDS

A 2016 article proposed that exposure to endocrine-disrupting chemicals may be a risk factor for developing uterine fibroids.[253] This makes sense when we remember that some endocrine-disrupting chemicals can mimic estrogen in the body and fibroids are considered to be estrogen-dependent tumors.[254]

Easy daily practices to help decrease your exposure to endocrine-disrupting chemicals include using the Dirty Dozen list to decrease exposure from herbicides and pesticides, using the EWGs Skin Deep Cosmetic Database and Think Dirty App to screen beauty and household products, and limiting use of certain plastics, especially those containing compounds like BPA.

UTERINE FIBROID TAKEAWAYS

Uterine fibroids are classified as estrogen-dependent, non-cancerous tumors and are a sign of abnormal tissue growth in the smooth muscle of the uterus.[255]

Some common symptoms of uterine fibroids include pelvic pain, bowel and bladder problems, back pain, and heavy periods.[256]

While asymptomatic uterine fibroids may not require medical treatment,[257] if your symptoms are severe, the most common treatment options include surgery and medications.[258]

We want to remind you there are lifestyle modifications and daily decisions that you can make to positively influence symptoms, including decreasing sugar, alcohol and highly processed foods, getting regular exercise, and decreasing exposure to environmental chemicals.

IRON DEFICIENCY

Iron is a micronutrient involved in cellular respiration, DNA repair and synthesis, and oxygen transfer throughout the body.[259]

Sixty percent of iron is found in red blood cells, making it a critical micronutrient to monitor if you have a menstrual cycle. Even if you don't have heavy menstrual bleeding, you're still losing 20-80 mL of blood per cycle, which can deplete iron stores in the body.[260]

Lack of iron is the most common cause of anemia, known as iron deficiency anemia. This type of anemia is commonly found in individuals who experience heavy menstrual bleeding.[261] Symptoms of anemia include fatigue, weakness, restless legs, and shortness of breath.[262]

FASCINATING FACT

The rates of iron deficiency anemia among white menstruating people is likely between nine to twelve percent and may be closer to twenty in Black and Mexican American menstruating people.[263] It's important to monitor for symptoms of anemia and advocate to get labs, especially if you have a heavy period!

While most of the iron in the body is found attached to hemoglobin in red blood cells[264], iron can also be attached to a protein called ferritin. Serum ferritin, or the amount of ferritin in the blood, is used to determine how much iron is stored in the body,[265] making it a valuable biomarker for menstruating people.

Getting lab work, including ferritin, is crucial for menstruating people who have chronic fatigue and other vague symptoms to rule out iron deficiency, with or without anemia. Because hemoglobin and hematocrit are the traditional measurements for anemia,[266] if these lab values are normal, patients often receive other diagnoses, including Lyme disease, chronic fatigue syndrome, burnout, overtraining, and pain disorders like fibromyalgia prior to being diagnosed with low iron levels.[267] This is why ferritin can be such a useful lab value!

PRO TIP

Even if you've had lab work done, the "norms" for ferritin may not correlate with optimal wellness. While iron deficiency is typically classified as ferritin levels less than fifteen µg/L, if you're struggling with low energy levels, it's important to work with a provider and try to get your levels closer to 100 µg/L.[268] If your ferritin levels are less than fifty µg/L, supplements may be beneficial. A 2012 study found supplementing with eighty mg of ferrous sulfate daily for twelve weeks improved hemoglobin and ferritin levels and decreased fatigue in individuals with low ferritin.[269] This is why working with a provider is so important!

It's also crucial to note that if you have a chronic inflammatory disease, cancer, infection, or a collagen disease, ferritin may not be an accurate marker due to the fact that it may increase during times of inflammation.[270]

While you lose iron directly from blood loss, the root cause of your low iron levels may be poor nutrient absorption in the GI tract, which can be influenced by difficulty breaking down food or conditions like Celiac disease, Crohn's disease, cystic fibrosis, and parasitic infections.[271] Like all things health related, finding a good provider to help you solve the specifics of your case will help you find long term solutions to any health problems you're struggling with.

IRON DEFICIENCY IN ATHLETES

Did you know many menstruating athletes struggle with iron deficiency?[272]

Endurance athletes may be at a higher risk, with an estimated fifteen to thirty-five percent of menstruating athletes being affected by iron deficiency.[273]

Many active individuals aren't aware that iron status can influence athletic performance. A 2016 study found a large proportion of the athletes studied had not talked to their medical provider about their heavy periods or symptoms related to iron deficiency, but many of them had supplemented with iron without getting any lab work done.[274]

While supplementing might seem like the easy option, we recommend getting your iron levels checked before doing so, especially if you are increasing iron intake to combat fatigue, because other health conditions or micronutrient deficiencies can also make you feel tired. Excess iron is not removed through urine or bowel movements,[275] and supplementation may lead to GI distress and constipation,[276] making it even more important to follow up with a provider before supplementing.

Check out the section below to learn more about dietary sources of iron!

FOOD SOURCES OF IRON

Did you know iron cannot be produced in the body? This makes iron an essential part of our diets.

There are two types of iron found in food sources.

Heme iron is more easily absorbed by the body than non-heme iron.[277] Heme iron is found primarily in meat and seafood, and because of this, vegetarians are at a higher risk for iron deficiency.[278] Consuming sources of heme iron is one of the best ways to boost iron levels and has the added benefit of replenishing other micronutrients lost during your bleed.

Dietary sources of heme iron include beef, poultry, pork, and fish.

Non-heme iron is found primarily in plants and is not as easily absorbed and used by the body as heme iron. It is important for vegans and vegetarians to be mindful of their iron intake to avoid anemia and other health problems associated with low iron.[279]

Dietary sources of non-heme iron include dark leafy greens like spinach, kale, and collard greens.

FASCINATING FACT

Vitamin C and fermented foods rich in organic acids may improve the absorption of non-heme iron.[280] For this reason, sprinkle some lemon or lime juice on your green leafy vegetables to get the biggest nutrient "bang for your buck."

Calcium may decrease the absorption of both heme and non-heme iron,[281] which may be one of the reasons it is often recommended that iron supplements be taken on an empty stomach to help with absorption.

IRON DEFICIENCY TAKEAWAYS

Since menstruating people lose blood monthly, iron is a critical micronutrient to monitor if you have a menstrual cycle.[282]

Low iron levels are the most common cause of anemia, which frequently occurs in individuals with heavy menstrual cycles. Being a menstruating athlete may put you at a higher risk of developing iron deficiency.[283]

If you experience fatigue, weakness, restless legs, shortness of breath, or have been diagnosed with Lyme disease, chronic fatigue syndrome, fibromyalgia, burnout, or overtraining, it's important to work with a healthcare provider and make sure low iron isn't contributing to your symptoms. Remember, while hematocrit and hemoglobin are important lab values, it is also important to get your ferritin levels checked, as this gives a picture of your body's iron stores.[284]

If you're vegetarian or vegan, it's important to make sure you're consuming enough iron in order to avoid anemia and other health conditions associated with low iron.[285] Remember, iron is not easily excreted from the body, so it's best to work with a healthcare provider if you're considering supplementing.[286]

MISSING PERIODS

What if you're not getting your period regularly or at all?

Missing your period is a signal from your body that something isn't right.

Some of the verbiage can be difficult to navigate so here are a few definitions:

- **Amenorrhea:** not getting your period for more than three months.

- **Hypothalamic amenorrhea:** missing your period without a known medical cause.

- **Primary amenorrhea:** when someone has never had a bleed, even though they are of reproductive age.

- **Secondary amenorrhea:** when someone has previously had a period but stops cycling for several months in a row.

While we'll focus on tips and tools for hypothalamic amenorrhea in this section, it's important to follow up with a medical provider if you're not consistently getting your period to rule out any underlying medical conditions.

If you've been missing your period for several months, it is always a good idea to take a pregnancy test if you've been sexually active since your last bleed. If you aren't pregnant, it's wise to consult with a health professional to gain further insight into what is going on.

Some common causes of missing periods include caloric restriction, excessive exercise, and high stress.[287]

FASCINATING FACT

Eating disorders may increase your risk of problems with your cycle, including missing periods and low estrogen levels.[288]

Other causes of your missing period could be nutrient deficiencies, postpartum hormones, pituitary tumors,[289] and recently discontinuing the use of hormonal contraceptives.

Remember, hormonal contraceptives work by shutting down your body's normal production of sex hormones. Because your body's natural production of sex hormones ceases when taking hormonal contraceptives, it can take time for your hormones to return to normal after discontinuing use. Everyone's body is different, so we are wary of stating a time frame for when your body will return to "normal." If you recently stopped using hormonal contraceptives, we suggest you follow Dr. Jolene Brighten's post-pill protocol in her book *Beyond the Pill.*

A good plan for addressing your missing period may include eating more high-quality, nutrient-dense foods, exercising less and in a way that feels good in your body, and managing both physical and mental stress.

MISSING PERIODS TAKEAWAYS

Missing periods can be caused by multiple factors,[290] but unless you're pregnant, missing your period is a signal from your body that something isn't right. It's important to follow up with a medical provider if you don't consistently get your period to rule out any medical conditions that may influence your cycle.

Fueling your body well is key if you're not getting your period! You may feel better if you increase your caloric intake.

Remember, if you recently stopped using hormonal contraceptives, this may influence your hormones! Because your body's natural production of sex hormones is disrupted when taking hormonal contraceptives, it can take time for your hormones to return to normal. We highly recommend following the Post Pill Protocol from *Beyond the Pill* by Dr. Jolene Brighten if you are trying to get your period back after the use of hormonal contraceptives.

ATHLETES AND PERIOD PROBLEMS

UNDEREATING, OVEREXERCISING, AND YOUR CYCLE: RELATIVE ENERGY DEFICIENCY IN SPORT (RED-S)

Athletes, although often glorified in our society, are not always healthy and tend to have a higher rate of restrictive eating behaviors, especially if their sport favors a lean body type.[291]

Energy availability is an important concept for individuals with high activity levels to understand, and is defined as the amount of energy left for basic bodily functions after activity.[292]

It's important to properly fuel your body, especially if you're active! When you're undereating and continue to exercise at a high level, this can cause a whole host of health problems. A 2018 cross-sectional study analyzing 1,000 menstruating athletes found individuals with low energy availability had an increased risk of menstrual dysfunction, decreased bone density, metabolic problems, psychological problems, cardiovascular problems, and GI dysfunction. These changes may negatively impact things like coordination, concentration, training response, and endurance performance and may lead to higher instances of irritability and depression.[293] Let's face it, all of the problems listed above can affect your athletic performance and quality of life!

PRO TIP

It's important to remember that BMI may not be a reliable indicator of health. A 2015 study analyzing forty menstruating endurance athletes found that although technically these individuals were in a normal BMI range, sixty-three percent of these subjects had low energy availability, sixty percent had menstrual dysfunction, forty-five percent had poor bone health, and twenty-five percent demonstrated characteristics of disordered eating. These stats make it evident that you can't assume a person is healthy just because they're an athlete.[294]

The Female Athlete Triad was the original term for the low energy availability, menstrual dysfunction, and poor bone health commonly found in menstruating athletes. Relative Energy Deficiency in Sport, referred to as RED-S, is the term that was adopted in 2014 to replace the Female Athlete Triad. RED-S addresses a larger range of symptoms due to low energy availability and also acknowledges similar problems can occur in individuals who don't have a menstrual cycle.

Along with menstrual dysfunction and poor bone health, RED-S includes immune system dysfunction, changes in metabolic rate and cardiovascular health, and decreased protein synthesis. RED-S may also involve a psychological component, although whether the psychological aspect starts prior to or after its onset is difficult to know.[295]

FASCINATING FACT

Did you know high-level athletes may have a weakened immune response and a higher chance of illness? Among Olympic athletes surveyed in 2018, 100% reported one illness symptom in the previous month, with upper respiratory symptoms being especially common.[296]

Endurance athletes who don't have regular periods may also be at an increased risk of getting sick. Runners with irregular or missing periods tend to have higher instances of headaches, fevers, runny noses, and coughs when compared to individuals with a regular menstrual cycle.[297]

If you're an athlete with any of the characteristics of RED-S, a team approach to creating healthy behaviors pertaining to food and exercise is recommended. Key players on the healthcare team may include a physician, dietitian, mental health professional, physical therapist, certified athletic trainer, exercise physiologist, coach, friends, and family.[298]

BONE HEALTH AND YOUR CYCLE

Most of us think we need to start worrying about bone mass when we get older, but if you are a young, menstruating athlete or have a low BMI, there are a few things you should consider.

Stress fractures are common among menstruating athletes, especially those with low energy availability.

A prospective study in 2019 found that low energy availability, menstrual dysfunction (including not having a period for more than three months), and low bone mineral density were associated with an increased risk of developing a stress fracture, especially for athletes under the age of twenty.[299] Another study from 2017 found that twenty-nine percent of the college athletes studied were at moderate or high risk for having relative energy deficiency in sport (RED-S) and developing stress fractures.

Low BMI may also impact your likelihood of developing a stress fracture. A 2016 study found individuals below the fifth percentile for their age-specific BMI were *nine times* more likely to have low bone mass density compared to those in the fiftieth to eighty-fifth percentiles.[300]

Check out our next section, Injury Prevention and Your Cycle, to learn ways to decrease your risk of stress fractures!

INJURY PREVENTION AND YOUR CYCLE

Besides fractures, did you know menstruating people may be at a higher risk of other sport-related injuries?

FASCINATING FACT

Not only does being a menstruating athlete increase your risk of injury, period *irregularities* may be another factor contributing to the higher injury risk! In a 2012 cross-sectional study looking at 249 menstruating high school athletes, athletes with irregularities in their cycles had an increased risk of severe injuries when compared to their counterparts with normal menstrual cycles. About one in five of the high school athletes studied had menstrual irregularities, and more than six in ten experienced some sort of musculoskeletal injury, making both menstrual disturbances and musculoskeletal injuries topics that need to be considered in athletes who cycle.[301]

The most commonly studied injury showing disproportionate injury rates between menstruating and non-menstruating people is a knee injury to a ligament called the anterior cruciate ligament, or ACL. A

2005 analysis of college basketball and soccer statistics from 1990–2002 found that ACL injury rates were higher for menstruating athletes in both sports.[302]

PRO TIP

Don't let these stats stop you from playing! The rate of injury is still low for individuals with a menstrual cycle, and the risk of injury should not stop you from playing the sports you enjoy![303] We'll talk about ways to train smart and add some preventive strengthening into your routine later in this chapter.

This increase in injury risk may be partially due to hormones. A 2019 review found estrogen may decrease stiffness in tendons and ligaments, influencing the higher injury rates in individuals with a menstrual cycle.[304] Along with contributing to the rates of ACL injuries, the shifts in hormones throughout your cycle may also influence posture and the risk of ankle injuries.[305]

While we can't change the normal hormonal fluctuations throughout our menstrual cycles, some factors influencing injury risk are within our control. The risk of ACL injury may be related to lower extremity biomechanics, or *how* we move.

According to a 2017 review, two specific postural factors seen to influence injury risk include:

- Knee valgus: when our knees drop inward with our feet wider than our knees.
- Increased external rotation of our tibia: when our shin bone rotates outward.

FASCINATING FACT

Knee valgus has also been related to an increased risk of stress fractures, according to a 2020 review.[306]

To change how we move, it's important to strengthen stabilizing muscles, like your glutes and core!

Things to include in your routine throughout your cycle:

- any exercises standing on one leg
- balance work on a Bosu or balance board
- bridges
- plank and side plank
- anything else core-related or balance-related

PRO TIP

According to a 2012 review, warmups may be beneficial in reducing injury when they incorporate a combination of strengthening, stretching, balance work, and exercises focused on landing mechanics and sports-specific drills.[307] Starting your warmup program in the off-season and consistently performing it before games and practices will help maximize results and decrease injury risk.

DECREASING FRACTURE RISK

A 2017 review found that in order to promote optimal bone health, it is important to maintain adequate nutrition and exercise regularly, including weight-bearing exercises and strength training.[308]

PRO TIP

Although weight-bearing activity is thought to be beneficial for bone mass density, individuals with menstrual dysfunction may be at a higher risk for developing fractures, especially if they're experiencing more than thirty-five days between menstrual cycles.[309]

If you're concerned about bone health, we suggest keeping track of your cycle as it may be a good indicator of overall health and injury risk! We recommend gradually increasing high-impact activities, rather than jumping right into intense high-impact workouts, especially if you have low body fat or menstrual dysfunction.

Regarding nutrition, there are certain vitamins and minerals crucial for bone health. These include calcium, phosphorus, magnesium, fluoride, vitamin D, vitamin K, vitamin C, B vitamins, iron, zinc, copper, manganese, and boron.[310] Remember, the best way to ensure you're getting adequate nutrition is to get lots of whole foods, high in micronutrients and dietary fiber. If you're worried about your bone health, talk with a professional about getting lab work done!

PRO TIP

Soda, whether regular, diet, or decaf, may be detrimental to bone health. A 2006 study found soda intake was associated with low hip bone density,[311] so decreasing both sugary and diet drinks may be something to consider if you're worried about your bone health.

HORMONAL CONTRACEPTIVES AND INJURY RISK

What if you're on the pill or using another form of hormonal contraception? While in this book we're typically discussing menstrual cycles unaltered by synthetic hormones, we find it important to note that a 2018 study found about fifty percent of the 430 elite athletes they surveyed were on hormonal contraceptives, and almost seventy percent had been on hormonal contraceptives at some point.[312]

More studies need to be done on how hormonal contraceptives influence injury risk. Preliminary evidence suggests oral contraceptives may actually improve the gap in injury rate, which may be partially due to the lack of hormonal fluctuations when you're on hormonal contraceptives.[313]

We believe that once you understand your body and how to prevent injury through strengthening, you'll be more confident in whatever activities you do, whether you choose to use hormonal contraceptives or not.

INJURY PREVENTION TAKEAWAYS

So, what can you do if you want to improve your performance and overall health?

Fuel your body!

If you aren't getting your period regularly or are having menstrual problems, it may be time to consider adding more healthy carbohydrates, proteins, and fats into your diet!

FASCINATING FACT

A 2014 study analyzing a small group of individuals with exercise-related menstrual dysfunction found six months of increasing calories by 360 calories per day improved chances of regular menstruation and ovulation.[314]

We want to remind you that "looking" healthy and "being" healthy can be two different things. External appearances, BMI, and size aren't always good indicators of true mental and physical health, and being an athlete doesn't necessarily mean you are healthy. What healthy looks like and feels like for you may not be the same as the person next to you, and that's ok! If your goal is overall well-being, it's key to find a routine that works for you and feels good in *your* body.

While the injury risk for athletes is small and we aren't discouraging you from staying active, menstruating individuals have a higher risk of injuries such as ACL tears, ankle injuries, and stress fractures.[315]

The good news is, there are ways you can be proactive and decrease your risk of injury!

When it comes to reducing injury risk, strengthening the whole body is vital!

While hormones may influence injury risk, you can be proactive about adding whole-body strength training into your routine to decrease this risk. Proper warmups are key for athletes, and strengthening your core and glute muscles can help improve the quality of movement in your sport. Many athletes tend to strengthen by playing their sport and doing sport-related drills, but it's also important to include core strengthening, hip strengthening, and balance work into your routine. For those of you who "cross-train" with running or cardio, make sure to complement it with some strengthening and balance work!

FAD DIETS, SUGAR, AND YOUR CYCLE

If you've ever heard a company or influencer promoting a "magic" diet plan, claiming drastic and fast results, chances are, it's a fad diet.

Fad diets are popular eating plans, often offering quick but unsustainable results. Some fad diets emphasize removing entire food groups or macronutrients like carbs or fats from your diet, while others sell you their meal plans to keep your calorie intake impossibly low, resulting in a calorie deficit.

Fad diets don't take into consideration your individual needs, especially the ever-changing nutritional needs of those who menstruate. It is important to remember that each macronutrient has specific roles in your body, making consumption of each a necessary part of a well-rounded diet, and our gut needs a variety of foods to promote optimal gut and overall health.

So, what makes fad diets appealing?

Fad diets are popular because, let's face it, they're selling us the "quick-and-easy" approach to weight loss or health instead of emphasizing sustainable habits. The promise of near-immediate results is much more enticing than the long-term commitment to planning menus, grocery shopping, and cooking most of our food at home.

FASCINATING FACT

Social influence, interpersonal relationships, and media can be motivating factors when choosing to be on a fad diet.[1] It's definitely important to understand how food influences our bodies and health, but it's also vital to surround yourself with supportive community as you make positive lifestyle changes. Remember, what's right for your partner, friends, or family may not be right for you!

MARKETING AND FAD DIETS

Marketing also influences our food choices. Companies often use trendy words in their marketing, but just because a product says "organic," "all-natural," or "Paleo" doesn't mean it's healthy.

When a company takes something out of their products, such as sugar or fat, they often replace it with an ingredient that isn't necessarily a "healthy" choice. "Low sugar" can mean products have been sweetened with artificial sweeteners or flavors, and "low fat" can mean sugar was added to the product to make it taste better. This is why reading labels is key!

PRO TIP

If you're drawn to fad diets because you're concerned about weight management, it's important to find a food and exercise routine that you can be consistent with instead of following the fads and hoping for drastic results. A 2019 review proposes both "low carb" and "low fat" diets might not be the best options for weight management.[2]

We believe that a high-quality, well-rounded, non-restrictive diet that you can stick with is the best way to promote overall health.

Now, let's talk about some of the most popular fad diets and how they relate to the health and well-being of menstruating people.

THE PALEO DIET

The Paleolithic diet, called "Paleo" for short, has become a popular trend in recent years. The basic concept behind the Paleo diet is to eat like our ancestors did...without processed food and even certain whole foods that were not available to our ancestors.

The Paleo diet frames food intake from an anthropological perspective.[3] Our ancestors had much fewer preventable health problems than we do now, so what were they doing differently?

FASCINATING FACT

The American Paleo diet may not reflect what our ancestors were eating. While some people use the Paleo diet as an excuse to eat a diet high in meat, some projections suggest meat was only a small portion of the total food intake of our ancestors.[4] Based on several anthropological studies, a true Paleo diet would have consisted mainly of plants, insects, seafood, and animals, with animal intake being estimated at only around three percent of all food consumed.[5] In addition, the meat our ancestors ate was very lean compared to the factory-farmed meat common today. If you're following the Paleo diet, try to eat a variety of whole foods, including plenty of fruits and vegetables, and moderate amounts of animal proteins.

When compared to the Standard American Diet (SAD) it is true that many Americans would likely benefit from the general guidelines found in the Paleo diet, and the Paleo diet has been associated with decreased risk of mortality from all causes.[6]

While this may be true, we want to be careful not to claim any one way of eating as the best option for *all* people. Many diets emphasizing whole foods would show benefits compared to the Standard American Diet, which is full of processed and packaged foods. If the Paleo diet is followed strictly over a long period of time, it may lead to restrictive eating, nutrient depletion, changes in the gut microbiome, and cardiovascular changes.[7]

One list of "Foods to Avoid on the Paleo Diet" includes dairy, grains, starchy vegetables, legumes, foods with added salt, and fatty, cured, and processed meats.[8] Cutting these foods out completely may not be beneficial for every individual, especially if you have a history of disordered eating or an obsession with being healthy, known as orthorexia. If you're a menstruating athlete rigidly following these guidelines, you may not be getting enough nutrients to fuel your active body. Plus, athletes *need* carbs!

Overall, we like to encourage incorporating all tolerated foods into your diet and enjoying the food you consume. If you're generally active and don't have other health concerns, it may be best to keep sweet potatoes, regular potatoes, grains, and legumes in your diet.

SALT, THE PALEO DIET, AND YOUR CYCLE

One of the proposed benefits of the Paleo diet is the reduced intake of salt.

FASCINATING FACT

Table salt is made of sodium and chloride (NaCl). An estimated ninety percent of the sodium we consume comes from salt.[9]

The excess salt common in the Standard American Diet (SAD), may contribute to preventable health problems common in Western culture, such as cardiovascular disease, hypertension, changes in immune function, and chronic inflammation.[10]

To put things in perspective, the CDC recommends 2300 mg of sodium per day as part of a healthy diet.

- Most Americans consume far more than the recommended amount of sodium, averaging around 3400 mg per day.
- The CDC estimates over seventy percent of sodium intake in the American diet comes from processed foods and restaurant meals.[11]

While sodium can be harmful when consumed in excess, it is necessary for many biological processes and may even play a role in menstrual health! A 2018 study found sodium intake of less than 1500 mg per day may be related to decreased progesterone levels and increased risk of anovulation.[12]

Tips for maintaining healthy sodium levels include:

- Eat more whole foods, including fruits, veggies, and legumes
- Try to cook most of your meals at home
- Be mindful of packaged foods, including salad dressings, pasta sauces, and frozen entrees and side dishes; check the serving sizes to see how much sodium you're consuming
- When eating out, check if there are nutrition facts online for the restaurant to help you make more informed decisions about your food choices, including sodium content.[13]

THE KETOGENIC AND ATKINS DIETS

The ketogenic and Atkins diets have become very popular in recent years. These diets both emphasize low carbohydrate and high fat and protein intake.

THE KETOGENIC DIET

The ketogenic diet typically consists of high fat intake, with anywhere from fifty-five to seventy percent of daily calories coming from fat[14] and limited carbohydrate intake, with less than twenty to fifty grams of carbs consumed per day, which is equivalent to one-half to one cup of rice.

How does keto work?

Extreme restriction of carbohydrates causes our body to rely on our fat stores as a fuel source.[15] Fatty acids are brought to the liver where they are broken down to create ketone bodies, which can replace glucose as the primary energy source in times of low carbohydrate availability.[16]

While it sounds like a good thing to have your body using your fat stores as fuel, research is lacking in terms of how the ketogenic diet affects healthy menstruating people. Just because the keto diet might work for your non-menstruating partner or friend doesn't mean it will be beneficial for you, especially if you have menstrual problems.

Decreasing carbohydrates too much may negatively impact your cycle. A small 2003 study found that forty-five percent of the young menstruating people on a ketogenic diet suffered from menstrual disruption during the six-month study. Some individuals even stopped menstruating! Six of the twenty participants experienced missing periods, most likely as a result of the low-carbohydrate diet.[17] In a 2012 study, metabolic and hormone changes were examined in participants who followed three types of diets: low-fat, low glycemic index (low in processed sugars and refined carbohydrates), and very low-carbohydrate, which is similar to keto in that even carbohydrates from whole foods and natural sources were decreased. The very low-carbohydrate diet resulted in changes including increased markers of inflammation, increased levels of cortisol (our primary stress hormone), and issues regulating thyroid hormones, all of which are detrimental to a healthy cycle.[18] Another small 2021 study analyzing healthy young menstruating people found that following a four-week ketogenic diet plan had a negative impact on cholesterol levels, which the authors found to be a concerning change in health status.[19]

FASCINATING FACT

The keto diet may be beneficial for some individuals, especially those with pre-existing metabolic conditions including obesity, diabetes, and PCOS.[20] Switching from glucose metabolism to fat metabolism may help with cellular repair, and the byproducts of this process, known as ketones, have also been shown to decrease appetite, making fasting and weight management easier.[21] Potential downfalls include the breakdown of muscle and protein along with fat.[22]

Instead of going to extremes when it comes to limiting carbs, it may be beneficial to start by lowering sugar intake to the amount recommended by the World Health Organization (WHO). The WHO suggests getting less than five percent of your daily energy intake from added sugars.[23] When you realize how much sugar you are consuming during an average day, it's easy to understand how metabolic conditions like diabetes and insulin resistance are so common. We will talk all about this in the next few sections!

THE ATKINS DIET

The Atkins diet is similar to the keto diet, but it focuses less on high fat intake and has four phases, each with varying carbohydrate restrictions.

The first phase of the Atkins diet requires extreme restriction of carbohydrates to less than twenty grams per day for the first two weeks. The following three phases consist of gradually adding in whole food carbohydrate sources, slowly increasing caloric intake from carbohydrates.[24]

We want to remind you that carbs are not the enemy, and extreme carbohydrate restriction may not be the best option to promote health in menstruating people.

BENEFITS AND RISKS OF LOW CARB DIETS

Is decreasing carbohydrates from healthy, whole food sources really going to positively influence your health over the long term?

While many studies on low-carb diets demonstrate significant short-term weight loss, a 2006 review analyzing the Atkins diet found no *long-term* benefits in terms of weight loss, and because of the emphasis on decreasing carbohydrates, people on these diets may be lacking in fiber and crucial micronutrients found in fruits and veggies.[25] Other potential health risks include negative changes to cholesterol levels, kidney function, and cardiovascular health.[26]

Our stance doesn't change throughout the book: there is no quick fix for improving your health—change takes time and commitment. We encourage you to focus on whole foods and fuel your body in a way that feels good for *you*. When in doubt, work with a nutritionist to examine what foods are best for you. And always remember that your menstrual cycle is a great indicator of your overall health status—it's been coined as the fifth vital sign, after all![27]

THE MEDITERRANEAN DIET

The Mediterranean diet has become very popular in recent years and is one dietary plan that we can back! While it does contain the word "diet," it is more of a lifestyle than a true diet, emphasizing the consumption of quality whole foods and plenty of healthy fats in a non-restrictive way.

FASCINATING FACT

Though the modern version of the Mediterranean diet includes higher percentages of animal proteins, the traditional Mediterranean diet primarily focuses on plant-based foods, such as dark leafy greens, healthy fats like olive oil and nuts, and whole grains, with fish and poultry being the main sources of animal protein.[28]

Here is an example of what the Mediterranean diet looks like:

- Grains, 1-2 servings/meal
- Legumes, >2 servings/week
- Potatoes, <3 servings/week
- Vegetables, >2 servings/meal
- Fruits, 1-2 servings/meal
- Nuts, 1-2 servings/day
- Red meat, <2 servings/week
- White meat, 2 servings/week
- Dairy, 2 servings/day
- Eggs, 2-4 servings/week
- Olive oil, included in every meal
- Fish, >2 servings/week.[29]

The Mediterranean diet may decrease risk of mortality from all causes due to its emphasis on healthy whole foods.[30]

Regarding reproductive health, a 2018 study found that the Mediterranean diet may support fertility, and another study from 2019 found improved success with assisted reproductive technologies, such as in vitro fertilization (also known as IVF) when individuals were following the Mediterranean diet.[31] The high fiber intake and anti-inflammatory properties of foods within the Mediterranean diet are likely the reasons for the beneficial effects of this dietary plan.[32]

VEGETARIANISM AND VEGANISM

We know what some of you may be thinking. *Vegetarian and veganism aren't fad diets...I've been plant-based since fifth grade!*

We fully understand this is a lifestyle chosen by many, and it's not a fad diet if you're doing it for ethical reasons. We also realize that a well-planned, well-executed vegetarian or vegan diet can be successful. However, if weight loss or better general health are the sole reasons you're choosing to be vegetarian or vegan, keep reading.

Our goal in this chapter is to explain the science behind why vegetarianism and veganism might not be beneficial for everyone and to encourage readers to understand how the dietary choices they make can influence their overall health and menstrual cycle. Research has shown that cutting out animal products may not always be the most health-promoting choice, especially for individuals who have a menstrual cycle.

A 2007 comparative study found that while certain markers of health, such as being active and maintaining a healthy weight, were better in vegetarians, the vegetarians in the study reported more menstrual problems and worse mental health statuses than their non-vegetarian counterparts, with a higher rate of depression in both the vegetarian and semi-vegetarian groups.[33] This is why we don't equate numbers on a scale or high activity levels with well-being; these factors don't always correlate with optimal physical and mental health.

PLANT-BASED DIETS AND MICRONUTRIENT DEFICIENCIES

Cutting out entire food groups can put you at risk for nutrient deficiencies, and vegetarian and vegan diets may contain inadequate levels of zinc, copper, selenium, iron, and vitamin B12.[34]

Zinc and **copper** are both beneficial for menstrual health but may not be easily absorbed and utilized in vegetarian and vegan diets.[35] Low zinc may influence oxidative stress and inflammation[36] and copper plays multiple roles in the body, but some of the most important for menstruating people include assisting in the absorption of iron and influencing the regulation of blood clotting.[37]

Dietary sources of zinc include oysters, beef, crab, lobster, pork, chicken, pumpkin seeds, cashews, chickpeas, and other legumes such as lentils and beans.

Dietary sources of copper include beef liver, shellfish, chocolate, potatoes, mushrooms, cashews, sunflower seeds, turkey giblets, and tofu.[38]

Selenium plays a crucial role in hormone balance due to its positive effects on oxidative stress, helping balance inflammation and improve fertility,[39] and vegetarians and vegans may be at risk of having deficient selenium levels.[40]

Dietary sources of selenium include sunflower seeds, Brazil nuts, chicken liver, beef liver, oysters, clams, fish roe, sardines, salmon, eggs, and beef.

Iron is a critical micronutrient for menstrual health. A 2007 comparative study found iron levels were lower in both vegetarians and semi-vegetarians compared to non-vegetarians[41], and a 2020 review on veganism found vegan diets lack the iron most easily absorbed by the body, known as heme iron, due to the fact that it is found in animal-based products,[42] making this a critical micronutrient to watch if you're vegetarian or vegan!

Dietary sources of heme iron include beef, poultry, pork, and fish.

Dietary sources of non-heme iron include dark leafy greens such as spinach, kale, and collard greens. Remember to add some vitamin C, like fresh lemon or lime juice, to help with the absorption of non-heme iron.

Vitamin B12 plays a role in DNA synthesis, red blood cell formation, and neurological health, and it helps maintain healthy energy levels.[43]

A 2014 study found that an estimated eighty percent of vegans were vitamin B12 deficient, even in populations consuming a fair amount of processed foods with added B12.[44]

This is notable because the American population has come to rely heavily on fortified foods, or processed foods with nutrients added into them, as a primary source of nutrition. If you're consuming many of your nutrients from fortified foods, such as breakfast cereals, you may want to focus more on whole food sources of these vitamins and minerals instead of refined versions.

If you are vegan, you may want to get lab work done and supplement with B12 as indicated due to the lack of natural vegan sources of B12. As always, check with a healthcare provider before supplementing.

Dietary sources of vitamin B12 include animal products such as beef, pork, poultry, fish, shellfish, eggs, and small amounts in dairy products.[45]

PLANT-BASED DIETS AND PROTEIN

If you are a vegetarian or vegan, your diet is missing complete proteins which contain all nine essential amino acids, the building blocks of protein that can only be found in our diet. (Check out page 47 for a full review of essential amino acids and complete versus incomplete proteins.)

Because of this, it's important to combine incomplete protein sources to fill in the amino acid gaps. For example, combining legumes (black beans, lentils, peas, etc.) with whole grains (rice, quinoa, buckwheat, amaranth, etc.) results in two incomplete proteins coming together to make a complete protein.

Other examples of complete protein combinations include tofu and rice, hummus and bread, nuts/seeds and beans, and tempeh and noodles.

Planning your meals and food combinations is important if you're following a vegan or vegetarian diet in order to ensure you're getting enough nutrients to support your health.

PRO TIP

It's worth noting that most plant-based meat alternatives are highly processed in order to provide all nine essential amino acids. Because of the additives and the way these foods are processed, they aren't always the most health-supportive choices. So, when you're choosing plant-based alternatives, make sure to check the ingredient lists.

HEALTH BENEFITS OF VEGETARIAN AND VEGAN DIETS

There are some dietary benefits to plant-based and vegan diets. If you're eating the typical Standard American Diet, you will probably notice some improvements in overall health if you switch to a vegetarian or vegan diet, which tend to be high in fiber, antioxidants, and healthy fats.[46] In a 2018 controlled clinical analysis, eating a plant-based diet was correlated with improved insulin resistance and decreased visceral fat, which are both markers of metabolic health.[47]

Just remember, you can still get health benefits compared to the Standard American Diet by adding more whole foods into your diet.

If you go vegetarian or vegan, make sure to monitor both physical and mental health. If you have any health concerns, it's important to work with a nutritionist or healthcare provider to make sure you're getting sufficient protein and micronutrient intake, especially the micronutrients listed earlier in this chapter.

INTERMITTENT FASTING: THE TRUTH ABOUT FASTING AND YOUR CYCLE

You've probably heard of intermittent fasting, but what is it?

Intermittent fasting involves consuming all of your calories in a certain time frame, alternating between periods of eating and limiting food and drink intake.

Intermittent fasting can be confusing because there are several different protocols people follow. Some of the most common include the 16:8 method, Eat-Stop-Eat, the 5:2 method, and alternate-day-fasting (ADF).

- **The 16:8 Method:** one of the most common methods in which you eat all of your food for the day during an eight-hour window, drinking only water for the remaining sixteen hours.

- **The Eat-Stop-Eat Method:** a type of intermittent fasting in which you fast for twenty-four hours twice a week.

- **The 5:2 Method:** a type of intermittent fasting where you only eat 500-600 calories for two non-consecutive days of the week, eating normally on the other days.

- **The Alternate-Day-Fasting Method:** a type of intermittent fasting where you eat no food or less than twenty-five percent of your typical daily energy needs for a full day and return to normal energy consumption the day after, alternating days.

Intermittent fasting has been proposed to be a "cure-all." Many studies analyzing intermittent fasting claim it may help reduce the risk of diseases like cardiovascular disease, neurological disorders, cancer, and obesity.[48]

What isn't clear in these positive reports on intermittent fasting is the effect fasting has on the endocrine system, specifically on sex hormone regulation in individuals who menstruate.

The tricky, and quite unfortunate, thing about a lot of human science is that studies and clinical trials often do not include menstruating people. As for intermittent fasting, this reality remains true.

While there is some research supporting intermittent fasting if you have difficulty with weight management, high levels of androgens, or chronic health problems related to inflammation (which are all common symptoms of PCOS), we highly recommend talking to a healthcare provider before making any drastic changes to your lifestyle, especially if you are on medications.

Unfortunately, there is not enough research on intermittent fasting and the menstruating body to be able to give solid advice on whether or not it is something worth adopting. What we do know is that when you are hungry, you should eat. Ignoring hunger cues, dieting, and restricting calories signal to the brain that there are not enough resources available and that the body is not in a safe environment. When the menstruating body isn't safe, some of the first systems to shut down are the reproductive organs, which can lead to potential hormone disruption.[49]

PRO TIP

What may be beneficial is getting adequate sleep (seven to nine hours) and starting your morning with water prior to coffee to prime your system for your day! If you're getting adequate sleep, you're automatically fitting a seven to nine hour fasting window into your day, in which your body can get the benefits of fasting.

Our advice to you: if you're hungry, *eat.* Honor your body's wisdom as it communicates its needs to you.

SUGAR: REAL TALK

While moderate sugar consumption from whole food sources isn't bad for our health, most of us are consuming way more sugar than we realize!

Often, products marketed as healthy contain added sugar to enhance the taste; the added sugar in common products can really add up over the course of a day.

FASCINATING FACT

The World Health Organization (WHO) recently decreased their recommendations for daily sugar intake from ten percent of your daily caloric intake to less than five percent. They recommend less than twenty-five grams of added sugar per day, which is only six teaspoons.[50]

As an example, did you know that a Chobani® Fruit on the Bottom Greek Yogurt has nine grams of added sugar? If you're following the newer guidelines from the WHO, that's thirty-six percent of your daily recommended intake, and that doesn't include granola or sweetened creamer in your coffee, either! Most yogurts have more than this, making it important to read labels.

And if you find yourself reaching for soda or other sugary drinks, it's important to know that one twelve-ounce can of Pepsi has forty-one grams of sugar! This means just one soda alone almost doubles the daily recommendation from the WHO.

The good news is, this recommendation doesn't include "whole food" sources of sugar, such as fruits, veggies, and grains.

For your hormones and overall health, processed foods and sugary drinks, including soda and sweetened coffee drinks, are worth avoiding. And no, please don't substitute real sugar with fake sugar. This has its own health hazards that we will talk about in the next few sections. Keep reading to learn more!

WHY YOU SHOULD NOT EAT ANYTHING WITH HIGH-FRUCTOSE CORN SYRUP

Fructose, a sugar naturally found in fruits, is often added to processed foods to enhance the flavor. When fructose and other sugars are added into foods, they are often in highly concentrated forms such as high-fructose corn syrup.

High-fructose corn syrup is one of the most common sweeteners used in the United States, and it may be contributing to your health (and period) issues. A 2004 review found that consumption of high-fructose corn syrup in the U.S. increased by more than a thousand percent from 1970 to 1990.[51]

Why are added sugars, especially high-fructose corn syrup, such a big deal?

A 2013 article from *Global Public Health* found the rate of diabetes was *twenty percent higher* in countries like the U.S. where high-fructose corn syrup is readily available.[52]

Not only does high sugar intake influence blood sugar and insulin levels, but it can also influence liver health. When we consume excess sugar, it gets sent to the liver for later use and is turned into fat stores. Over time, these fat stores can negatively impact liver health, and high levels of added sugar may influence your likelihood of developing non-alcoholic fatty liver disease. A 2008 study found that in those with non-alcoholic fatty liver disease, consumption of fructose was two to three times higher than in controls.[53]

FASCINATING FACT

Did you know an estimated one in ten children in the U.S. have pediatric non-alcoholic fatty liver disease?[54] Current evidence suggests that the recent rise in this condition may be directly linked to high sugar consumption, specifically fructose. This makes sense when you realize soft drinks and snacks marketed to kids are usually full of added fructose.[55] Whether you're a kid or an adult, it may be best to check the sugar content in your snacks and beverages!

And if you think you might have symptoms of leaky gut but you're not sure why, check your sugar intake!

In the small intestine, high concentrations of fructose may lead to dysfunction of the epithelial barrier, which helps keep food particles and bacteria in the GI tract.[56] Poor epithelial barrier function may influence allergies, autoimmune disorders, and even some neurological conditions like Parkinson's, Alzheimer's, depression, and autism spectrum disorders.[57] If you've been diagnosed with any of these conditions, it's definitely worth examining your sugar intake.

On a brighter note, a special review from the Mayo Clinic suggests whole foods containing fructose, including fruits and veggies, are not related to health problems, but instead may be beneficial for overall health.[58] In a 2020 study, there were positive changes in the gut microbiome in menstruating individuals consuming a high-fructose diet in which the fructose came from fruits, whereas those who consumed high concentrations from high-fructose corn syrup demonstrated detrimental changes in their gut microbiome.[59] Another reason to increase your intake of whole foods!

SUGAR AND FOOD LABELS

One of the most frustrating parts of nutrition is label reading, especially since sugar and other additives are often disguised under a variety of names. While this is one of the reasons we promote eating whole foods, it's also important to be able to identify common sources of sugar on food labels, especially those high in fructose.

Some common ingredients and foods that are high in fructose include:

- Fructose
- High-fructose corn syrup
- Agave
- Honey
- Table sugar (which is half fructose and half glucose)
- Molasses
- Palm sugar
- Coconut sugar
- Invert sugar
- Pancake syrup[60]

Better options include:

- Raw sugar
- Turbinado sugar
- Maple syrup[61]

Other helpful tips are to read the label for "added sugar" *and* check portion sizes. Companies will often put more than one serving in a small container, which tricks individuals into thinking there is less sugar based on a quick glance at the nutrition facts on the packaging.

THE TRUTH ABOUT FAKE SUGARS

If something looks like sugar, tastes like sugar, and acts like sugar but isn't actually sugar, our motto is *"stay away."*

Although artificial sweeteners were created to promote weight management, a 2017 review found that artificial sweeteners may contribute to metabolic syndrome and obesity. They also disrupt the gut microbiome and may leave you feeling less full, leading to higher caloric consumption and weight gain.[62]

ARTIFICIAL SUGARS AND THE FDA

To our frustration, artificial sweeteners are still often recommended by healthcare professionals as a "safe" alternative to sugar,[63] but when you understand what's actually happening in your body when you consume fake sugars, you're able to make better, more health-promoting decisions.

Unfortunately, the FDA has approved artificial sweeteners as food additives, so it's up to you to protect yourself and check ingredients when you're grocery shopping.

> **PRO TIP**
>
> One of the big problems with fake sugar is that it can be added to foods without our awareness, which is why reading nutrition labels is so important.

Be on the lookout for these artificial sweeteners commonly found in processed foods:

- Acesulfame K (brand names: Sunett and Sweet One)
- Advantame
- Aspartame (two brand names: Equal and Nutrasweet)
- Neotame (brand name: Newtame)

- Saccharin (two brand names: Sweet 'N Low and Sweet Twin)

- Sucralose (brand name: Splenda)

- Sugar alcohols: Erythritol, Isomalt, Lactitol, Maltitol, Mannitol, Sorbitol, and Xylitol[64]

FAD DIETS, SUGAR, AND YOUR CYCLE TAKEAWAYS

Whether you're thinking about trying Paleo, keto, Atkins, the Mediterranean diet, intermittent fasting, vegetarianism, or veganism, we encourage you to ditch the "diet" ideologies of restrictive eating and strict guidelines. Instead, focus on consuming a wide variety of whole foods that make you feel good.

Health is not built by counting calories or keeping track of macros. Health is built from the steady commitment of making choices that are best for your mind, body, and spirit on a daily basis.

Read labels and be aware of extra added sugar—it adds up more quickly than you may realize! Sugar from real foods, such as fruit, is preferred, and don't assume that fake sugars are going to "solve" your sugar addiction—chances are, they'll probably make it worse.

Remember, it's all about balance.

We encourage you to let go of food rules and choose whole foods as often as possible; but remember, there's no such thing as a "perfect" diet, and it's good to enjoy your food!

THE BASICS OF HORMONAL BIRTH CONTROL

This section explains how hormonal contraceptives work with the goal of helping you make informed choices when it comes to your medical care.

A study from 2019 analyzing data from 2015-2017 found that sixty-five percent of menstruating people between the ages of fifteen and forty-nine were using some sort of birth control, including condoms, female sterilization, the pill, intrauterine devices (IUDs), and arm implants. Each form of birth control has different efficacy and side effects, which we'll talk about in this chapter.

While hormonal contraceptive use has been normalized, it's important to note that hormonal contraceptives inhibit your natural cycling and may have some less-than-desirable side effects.

For many individuals, hormonal contraceptives are presented as an answer to health problems such as acne, PMS, cramps, polycystic ovary syndrome, fibroids, and endometriosis. While they may be helpful for some symptoms, they may not get to the root cause of your issues, and many patients are not informed about potential side effects.

FASCINATING FACT

Although use of hormonal contraceptives is common among endometriosis patients, it may not always help with pain related to endometriosis if the pain is due to muscular problems. If pain is the primary reason you're choosing to be on hormonal contraceptives, we highly recommend following up with a pelvic health physical therapist. Pelvic health physical therapists can help identify any biomechanical or nerve-related issues contributing to your symptoms, regardless of your medical diagnosis.[1]

While some individuals use hormonal contraception to help manage health conditions or symptoms related to hormone imbalance, a large number of menstruating people are strictly using hormonal contraception for pregnancy prevention. This can seem like a "quick fix" for avoiding pregnancy, however, there may be undesirable side effects.

Hormonal contraceptives work by inhibiting ovulation. The consistent exposure to progestin (a synthetic version of progesterone), with or without estrogen, suppresses the release of gonadotropin-releasing hormone, luteinizing hormone, and follicle-stimulating hormone from the brain, stopping the natural hormonal cycling that occurs during the menstrual cycle. Progestin also thickens cervical mucus, influences fallopian tube motility, and may even induce thinning of the inner wall of the uterus.[2]

FASCINATING FACT

Your bone health may be negatively impacted if you start a hormonal contraceptive containing estrogen during adolescence.[3] For more information on injury prevention and bone health, check out page 196.

The most common types of hormonal contraception are:

- **The Pill**
    - Combined oral contraceptives (COCs)
    - Continuous or extended use oral contraceptives
    - Progestin-only oral contraceptives (POCs)
- **Long-Acting Reversible Contraceptives (LARCs)**
    - Intrauterine devices (IUDs)
    - Hormonal implants
    - Hormonal injections

Let's go into some details about each type!

ORAL CONTRACEPTIVES ("THE PILL"):

According to data from 2015-2017, 12.6% of women between fifteen and forty-nine in the United States were on the pill.[4]

There are three types of oral contraceptives: the combination pill, extended or continuous use pills, and the mini pill.[5]

The combination pill has both synthetic progesterone and synthetic estrogen and has "active" pills, containing the synthetic hormones, and "non-active" pills, which are just sugar pills. The "non-active" pills are taken to give you a withdrawal bleed, which mimics a period. While this can be reassuring for individuals trying to avoid pregnancy, the withdrawal bleed isn't actually your period and is not biologically necessary.[6]

Combined oral contraceptives work through a combination of progestin and synthetic estrogen. The progestin inhibits follicular development and ovulation (preventing pregnancy), and the estrogen influences the withdrawal bleed.[7] Combination oral contraceptives are ninety-one percent effective with normal use, meaning that nine out of one hundred people using this form of birth control become pregnant after a year of use.[8]

Common side effects from the combination pill include decreased libido, headaches, emotional changes, abdominal cramping, vaginal discharge, shorter periods, potential breakthrough bleeding or spotting, breast tenderness, and nausea. Remember to talk with your doctor if you have preexisting cardiovascular problems, including high blood pressure, as these can be exacerbated by the combination pill.[9]

Continuous or extended use contraceptives are combined oral contraceptives taken without monthly "non-active pills," leading to decreased frequency or lack of the monthly withdrawal bleeds. Extended use involves having a withdrawal bleed every three months, while continuous use involves only taking active pills, and therefore not getting a withdrawal bleed at all.[10] Since the withdrawal bleed isn't biologically necessary, these can be great options!

The **"mini pill"** contains only synthetic progesterone and has all "active" pills, meaning you don't get a withdrawal bleed. This oral contraceptive works by influencing the hormonal cascade associated with ovulation, changing the cervical mucus to inhibit sperm motility, and by altering the endometrium, decreasing the likelihood of implantation.[11] Progestin-only hormonal contraceptives stop ovulation only sixty to eighty percent of the time.[12]

The "mini pill" is a great option when estrogen is contraindicated but can lead to unscheduled bleeding or spotting. Other side effects include acne, undesired hair growth, and ovarian cysts.[13]

FASCINATING FACT

The morning after pill is a progestin-based pill that works to delay ovulation and thicken the cervical mucus, interfering with sperm transit. It should be taken within seventy-two hours of unprotected sex or a sexual encounter with failed protection to prevent pregnancy, but it does not provide protection against STIs. It's worth noting that the efficacy of the morning after pill declines forty-eight hours after unprotected sex, as well as in those with a BMI over thirty. Some of the most common side effects are irregular periods, headaches, acne, and sometimes nausea and vomiting.[14]

LONG-ACTING REVERSIBLE CONTRACEPTIVES

Long-acting reversible contraceptives (LARCs) have gained popularity in recent years. Once introduced into the body, they do not require action from the user, making them very user friendly and less prone to user-error.

The most common types of LARCs are IUDs, vaginal rings like the NuvaRing, implants, and injections.

PRO TIP

A 2018 study found the most common negative effects were reported with progestin-only contraceptives, including the mini pill, hormone shots, and hormone implants, and side effects were most frequently reported with the implant.[15] Nexplanon is the brand name of the most common hormonal implant approved for use in the U.S., so if you're using the Nexplanon, it's important to keep track of your symptoms.

If you're curious about the side effects of your birth control, just do a quick Google search for the brand and side effects. You might be surprised at what you find!

According to the CDC, one in ten women between the ages of fifteen and forty-nine in the United States were using intrauterine devices or contraceptive implants between 2015-2017.[16]

There are two types of IUDs: copper and hormonal.

- **Copper IUDs** work by inducing a local inflammatory response that inhibits implantation. We will talk more about the copper IUD in our non-hormonal birth control section on page 237.

- **Hormonal IUDs** rely on progestin to suppress endometrial growth and to help thicken the cervical mucus, inhibiting the motility of sperm.[17]

Benefits of IUDs include being user-friendly (once it's placed, you don't have to do anything until you get it replaced, which is usually three to five years later for hormonal IUDs and up to ten years later for copper IUDs), being ninety-nine percent effective in preventing pregnancy, and the fact that they are reversible.

While IUDs are often promoted in clinical practice due to the high efficacy and ease of use,[18] a 2018 cohort study found higher levels of anxiety and sleep problems in individuals using hormonal based IUDs versus non-hormonal based IUDs,[19] making it important to track any symptoms you experience related to mental health if you're on a hormonal IUD. Other potential side effects include pain with insertion, nausea and vomiting, decreased libido, weight gain, acne, depression, and ovarian cysts. They also don't reduce risk of sexually transmitted diseases,[20] so barrier method protection, such as condoms, may also be beneficial.

Vaginal rings are not as common as IUDs or implants, and there are only a few on the market. One of the benefits of the vaginal ring is that they can be used long term, but unlike IUDs, which require placement by a medical provider, the use of vaginal rings can be started and discontinued by the user without the involvement of a healthcare professional.[21] Because they are also hormonally based there is a chance of side effects, so it's important to do research on any type of hormonal contraceptives you're choosing.

Contraceptive implants are hormonal contraceptives that are placed under the skin, most commonly in the arm. The Nexplanon is the most common contraceptive implant available in the United States and is a small, rod-like implant that gets placed into the upper-inner arm and can remain there for up to three years.[22] Just like hormonal IUDs, the Nexplanon implant releases progestin,[23] which inhibits egg release, egg fertilization, and sperm motility by way of thickened cervical mucus. There is a list of serious side effects on Nexplanon's website, Nexplanon.com, but some complications associated with contraceptive implants include headaches, weight gain, acne, mood problems, decreased sex drive, dizziness, nausea and stomach pain, hair loss, nerve problems, pain at the implant site, and ovarian cysts.[24]

Depo-Provera is the most common injectable contraceptive in the United States, and just like IUDs, vaginal rings, and implants, also has a very high pregnancy prevention rate. With perfect use pregnancy prevention rate is 99.8%, however, injections are considered second tier because patients need to come back every twelve weeks for their injections, which can be a barrier to care. With typical use, Depo-Provera is ninety-four percent effective at preventing pregnancy.

While it has many benefits, this might not be the best option for individuals who want to get pregnant soon. Even though it's a reversible form of contraception, it may take twelve to eighteen months for fertility to return. Other side effects may include weight gain, decreased bone mass, and frequent or irregular bleeding at the start of use.[25]

EFFECTS OF BIRTH CONTROL ON MENTAL AND PHYSICAL HEALTH

If you have symptoms related to mental health, have an autoimmune condition, or struggle with weight management, you've probably been searching for answers as to why these issues may be occuring. But did you know hormonal contraceptives may be influencing your symptoms?

In order to promote body autonomy, it's important to understand that medications, *including hormonal contraceptives,* may affect your mental and physical health.

Let's talk about some of the potential side effects of hormonal contraceptives in the context of your overall health.

HORMONAL CONTRACEPTION AND DEPRESSION

According to the Center for Disease Control (CDC), one in ten women experience symptoms of depression,[26] but this risk may be higher if you've been on hormonal contraceptives. A study conducted in 2019 found that individuals who used hormonal contraception in their adolescent years were at higher risk for developing depression later in life.[27]

After examining 1,236 menstruating people in the United States, it was discovered that sixteen percent of the individuals who had taken hormonal oral contraceptives in their teens experienced symptoms of depression, whereas only six percent of the individuals who had never taken hormonal oral contraceptives experienced symptoms of depression.[28] That's a ten percent difference we're talking about!

In another study conducted in Denmark in 2016, it was found that there was an association between hormonal contraception and the use of antidepressant drugs.[29] Regarding severe depressive symptoms, a 2018 study found individuals who were on, or recently had been on, hormonal contraceptives had an increased risk of attempting or dying by suicide.[30]

We want to remind you that the studies above do not show causation and that there are other factors that may be contributing to this association, but the link between hormonal contraceptive use and depression is important to consider if you find yourself struggling with your mental health. We hope that by sharing this information, you can seek the care you need. If you're using hormonal contraceptives and are concerned about your mental well-being, it may be helpful to track and date your symptoms and share your findings with a mental health provider. It's often easier to determine the root cause of your symptoms if you can view how you've been feeling on a timeline.

FASCINATING FACT

Alterations in mood is one of the most common reasons why people stop the use of oral contraceptives.[31] Some of the changes in mood and mental health may be influenced by the way hormonal contraceptives affect neurotransmitter production and absorption of micronutrients related to depressive symptoms.[32] We talked in our PMDD chapter about the importance of tryptophan in the formation of serotonin; a 1979 article found individuals on oral contraceptives had abnormal processing of tryptophan, therefore altered serotonin production, as well as lower levels of folate and vitamin B12, which are associated with depression.[33] This is important to keep in mind as you work through any physical and mental symptoms you're experiencing.

HORMONAL CONTRACEPTIVES AND YOUR NERVOUS SYSTEM

Hormonal contraceptives may also influence your nervous system!

Although the hormones in hormonal contraceptives are synthetic, they are still able to bind to hormone receptors in the nervous system and body.[34]

Estrogen and progesterone may both influence nervous system activity. Estrogen receptors can be found in the parts of the brain associated with learning and memory,[35] and a 2015 study analyzing ninety individuals found changes in specific areas of the brain in individuals who were on hormonal contraceptives.[36] It has been proposed that hormonal contraceptives may play a role in cognitive and perceptual changes, mood, and changes in brain activation and structure in individuals using hormonal contraceptives compared to controls.[37]

While it has been suggested that hormonal contraceptives may influence our brains and nervous systems, better quality research needs to be done.[38] However, it's still important to keep track of your symptoms. If you're on hormonal contraceptives and are noticing any physical or mental symptoms that began after you started using hormonal contraceptives, it's important to put a timeline together and share it with your healthcare team!

HORMONAL CONTRACEPTIVES, WEIGHT, AND THE GUT

While you may have heard that hormonal contraceptives cause weight gain, the research isn't conclusive,[39] and it may depend on the type of contraceptives you're using.

FASCINATING FACT

A 2016 study suggests that some of the weight gain associated with hormonal contraceptives may actually be related to micronutrient deficiencies, which is something to keep in mind if you're on hormonal contraceptives and are struggling with your weight.[40]

Hormonal contraceptives are one of the most commonly prescribed classes of medications, however, most people aren't aware that hormonal contraceptives have been linked with changes in the gut microbiome and certain micronutrient deficiencies.[41] A very small 2021 study found minor changes in gut microbiome diversity and composition in individuals taking combined hormonal contraceptives,[42] and another small study from 2022 found changes in gut composition and function in individuals taking oral contraceptives.[43] Hormonal contraceptive use has also been correlated with deficiencies in folate, B2, B6, B12, vitamin C, vitamin E, zinc, selenium, and magnesium.[44] B vitamins play a crucial role in maintaining healthy energy levels, and vitamin C, vitamin E, zinc, selenium, and magnesium all have antioxidant properties.

If you're on the pill or have a hormonal IUD or arm implant and are struggling with your health, it may be worth talking to your provider about getting lab work done.

HORMONAL CONTRACEPTIVES AND AUTOIMMUNE DISEASE

Did you know an estimated eighty percent of individuals who are diagnosed with autoimmune disorders are menstruating people?[45]

Hormones may play a role in this![46]

A 2017 review found that use of hormonal contraceptives may influence risk of developing certain autoimmune diseases, such as lupus, Crohn's, interstitial cystitis, multiple sclerosis and ulcerative colitis, and that it's important to understand this risk prior to use.[47]

Autoimmune conditions often have vague symptoms and tend to be underdiagnosed, so keep track of your symptoms and keep your care team updated with any changes. If you've been diagnosed with an autoimmune disorder after starting hormonal contraceptives, it may be worth discussing other options with your provider. *Beyond the Pill* by Dr. Jolene Brighten is a great resource if you choose to discontinue use of hormonal contraceptives!

NON-HORMONAL BIRTH CONTROL

Now that we've talked about hormonal contraceptives, let's talk about some non-hormonal options!

In this section, we will provide information about alternative, non-hormonal birth control approaches. We think it's important to understand the benefits and risks of all options when making decisions about your health.

While our goal is to help you make informed decisions, we also want to remind you that we are not providing medical advice. Find the method that makes the most sense for you, and remember, abstinence is the only pregnancy prevention method that is 100% effective, and not all methods (including hormonal contraceptives) provide protection from sexually transmitted infections.

AM I REALLY FERTILE EVERY DAY?

You likely learned at a young age that if you have sex, no matter what day it is in your cycle, you will get pregnant. We're here to tell you this simply isn't true!

> In reality, there are only five to seven days in your cycle where you are fertile and have a chance of conceiving.

You may be surprised to learn this wonderful news just like we were!

Knowing this empowering information and understanding your cycle and fertility can help you make informed choices about what forms of contraception make the most sense for you.

PRO TIP

Ovulation may not always occur on day fourteen, so your fertile window may vary cycle to cycle. While you may think you can't get pregnant during your period, the last few days of your period may fall into your fertile window if you ovulate early.

We will never criticize anyone who chooses to use hormonal contraceptives. However, we do believe that individuals should be educated on decisions they are making about their bodies and how these decisions influence their health.

The following are some of the non-hormonal options we will discuss in greater detail in this chapter.

- **The Fertility Awareness Method (FAM)** is a method of birth control that focuses on education and bringing greater awareness to the signs of a menstruating person's "fertile window." This method utilizes the following factors to determine fertility status:
  - Cervical mucus
  - Basal Body Temperature (BBT)
  - Cervical positioning
- **Copper IUDs** are non-hormonal. Instead of relying on hormones to prevent pregnancy, the copper IUD causes local inflammation, which interferes with the ability of sperm to travel to the egg. An example of a copper IUD is Paraguard.[1]
- **Condoms** are put over the shaft of the penis before penetration and act as a physical barrier, preventing pregnancy and STIs.
- **Diaphragms** are worn in the vagina, near the cervix, and are a physical barrier preventing sperm from entering the uterus. Typically, spermicide is used simultaneously for maximum protection.

- **The Withdrawal, or Pull-Out Method,** is when the penis is removed from the vagina before ejaculation.

FAM: FERTILITY AWARENESS METHOD

FAM is a method of birth control that brings greater awareness to a menstruating person's fertile window.

This method utilizes three bodily signals of fertility:

1. Basal Body Temperature (BBT)
2. Cervical mucus (CM)
3. Cervical positioning

Paying attention to these signals helps you know when you are most fertile and, if you are trying to avoid pregnancy, when to use a barrier method or abstain from intercourse. We love this method because it helps you become more comfortable and acquainted with your body and menstrual cycle.

PRO TIP

Not all providers are trained in FAM. If you choose to use FAM, it's important to find a healthcare provider who is versed in this specific birth control modality. If you're having difficulty finding a provider in your area, it may be worth looking into utilizing a FAM educator to supplement the care of your provider.

BASAL BODY TEMPERATURE (BBT):

Your BBT is your body's lowest resting temperature. To utilize FAM, you take your BBT every day with a thermometer that goes out to the second decimal point. For the most accurate results, your BBT should be taken at the same time every day, preferably when you wake up in the morning.[2]

BBT shifts throughout your cycle, depending on what phase you are in and if you have ovulated:

- Menstruation: Your BBT usually drops significantly at the onset of your period, ranging from 97.00-97.70.

- Follicular Phase: Your BBT remains in the 97.00-97.70 range during the follicular phase.

- Ovulation: Your BBT increases just after ovulation. Remember, the increase in temperature can differ between individuals and from cycle to cycle.[3]

- Luteal Phase: Your BBT will be elevated, usually greater than 97.80 during the luteal phase.[4]

PRO TIP

While BBT is a good indicator of whether or not you've ovulated, if you're trying to avoid pregnancy, barrier protection may be a wise addition since your BBT doesn't indicate when your fertile window starts, making it challenging to prevent pregnancy if only relying on BBT.[5]

CERVICAL MUCUS (CM)

CM is the discharge you may notice in your underwear.

The white-ish stuff in your panties is *totally 100% normal* and is actually a sign of fertility!

FASCINATING FACT

Did you know you can only get pregnant when your cervix is releasing watery or egg-white-like CM? This is referred to as "fertile" mucus by those who follow FAM. The pH of your vagina is not a welcoming environment for sperm most of your cycle. Your vagina has a more acidic pH when fertile CM is absent, and this lower pH makes it harder for sperm to survive.[6]

Right after your period, you may notice less cervical mucus and experience some vaginal dryness, slowly transitioning to white and sticky, almost like residue from a sticker. When it becomes whiter and creamier, you are getting closer to ovulation, and usually, you are at the peak of ovulation when your CM resembles raw egg whites.

PRO TIP

Another helpful factor to consider if you're close to ovulation is if you have raw egg-white-like CM when you wipe after using the restroom. If this is the case, it's definitely best to avoid unprotected penetrative sex unless you are trying to get pregnant.

After ovulation, you may experience fertile cervical mucus for one or two more days, and then you will notice less for the remainder of your cycle until you start your period again. Your fertile window is only prior to and during ovulation, so once ovulation has passed, your fertile window is over for that menstrual cycle.

CERVICAL POSITION

The positioning of your cervix correlates with ovulation and therefore fertility. Tracking cervical position is one of the most challenging aspects of FAM.

The cervix sits at the top of your vagina at the opening of your uterus. To begin observing your cervical position, insert your pointer finger in your vagina and feel for your cervix. For some, it may be easier to reach while squatting low in the shower. Your cervical tissue feels much different than the tissue of your vaginal canal as it will be smooth and less "spongy" than your vaginal tissue. When you are fertile, your cervix will sit high in your vagina and be soft and slightly open, resembling a donut. You may have a hard time reaching it when you are fertile if you have a naturally deep vagina.

When you are not fertile, your cervix will sit lower in your vagina and feel harder and closed.

PRO TIP

Because examining your own cervical position is difficult, some FAM instructors consider it optional and rely on basal body temperature and cervical mucus to determine the days you're most fertile.

This section is just a *brief* overview of FAM, and if you are considering trying FAM, we highly recommend working with your healthcare team and a FAM educator for the best results. There are many great resources available to learn more about utilizing FAM as birth control. If you are interested in learning more so you can use this contraceptive method, check out the following resources:

- *Taking Charge of Your Fertility* by Toni Weschler, MPH

- *The Fifth Vital Sign* by Lisa Hendrickson-Jack

- FertilityFriday.com, Lisa Hendrickson-Jack's website

    - Check out the *Fertility Friday* podcast for educational tips if you're on the go!

NON-HORMONAL IUDS (INTRAUTERINE DEVICES)

The Paraguard is a non-hormonal IUD covered in copper. This device gets placed in the uterus and the copper covering deters sperm from getting to an egg due to a local inflammatory response.[7] The copper IUD can be ninety-nine percent effective in preventing pregnancy and can be worn for up to ten years but does not protect against STIs.[8]

The Paragard, though non-hormonal, has some negative side effects that are less than thrilling. According to Planned Parenthood, copper IUDs can lead to heavy periods and increase the intensity of cramps for the first three to six cycles after insertion. Remember, the copper IUD is a foreign object inserted into your uterus that remains there for years and elicits a local inflammatory response. Not everyone adjusts well to this form of birth control.

FASCINATING FACT

Copper IUDs may also influence the bacteria in the vagina, increasing the risk of bacterial vaginosis, according to a 2018 study.[9]

Bacterial vaginosis is a condition caused by disproportionate amounts of the "good" and "bad" bacteria in your vagina.[10] Symptoms of bacterial vaginosis include discharge, fishy odor, and irritation, and it is associated with a higher risk of developing HIV and other sexually transmitted infections. Treatments involve improving the vaginal flora and increasing lactobacilli populations back to their normal levels.[11]

It's important to monitor for any unusual health symptoms if you choose to use the Paraguard; some people do not tolerate copper well due to underlying conditions, such as Wilson's disease and sensitivity to copper.[12]

CONDOMS

Condoms can be a good barrier to use on fertile days if you are using FAM. They also help prevent STIs. Condoms are eighty-two percent effective at preventing pregnancy when used properly.

"Properly" is the key phrase here!

Proper use looks like rolling the condom completely down the shaft of the penis and remembering to "pinch an inch" at the top of the condom, leaving room for semen after ejaculation. It's key to put on the condom before there is any ejaculation of semen.

> **PRO TIP**
>
> If using lubricant, make sure it is made from the right base. Condoms are typically made of latex or polyurethane. When using condoms, you want to use water or silicone-based lubricants rather than oil-based lubricants. Using oils like coconut oil with a condom may lead to an increased likelihood of the condom breaking, creating an ineffective barrier.[13]

DIAPHRAGMS

Diaphragms are a shallow, flexible "cup" inserted in the vagina to cover the cervix. Diaphragms are eighty-eight percent effective at preventing pregnancy but do not prevent STIs.

For diaphragms to be most effective in preventing pregnancy, a spermicide should be used simultaneously. One of the great things about diaphragms is that they can be inserted up to eighteen hours prior to sexual contact. So, if you know you're going to be sexually active later that day, you can insert a diaphragm in the morning, toss some spermicide in your purse, and know you're protected from possible pregnancy. Also, if your partner isn't too excited about period sex, diaphragms can be a great barrier when you're bleeding!

FASCINATING FACT

While you should use spermicide with a diaphragm, it's important to choose a spermicide that both prevents pregnancy and is safe for your intimate parts and overall health.

Most spermicides contain a chemical called nonoxynol-9, which is often found in harsh cleaning products. Planned Parenthood states that nonoxynol-9 may irritate vaginal tissue, as well as the tissue of the penis, and that this irritation may make the users more susceptible to HIV and STIs. One study found a dose-dependent negative effect of nonoxynol-9 on bacterial balance in the vagina, leading to a higher likelihood of developing bacterial vaginosis.[14] So the more frequent use of spermicide containing nonoxynol-9, the higher risk you may have of developing unwanted side effects.

The good news is that there are some safer, more gentle spermicides on the market. If using a diaphragm with spermicide is your preferred method of birth control, we suggest looking into ContraGel, which is vegan and non-toxic.[15]

SPONGES

Contraceptive sponges are a less popular method of birth control. Sponges are round and made from a soft, squishy plastic that contains spermicide. The sponge acts as a barrier by covering the cervix while the spermicide kills or slows down the movement of sperm toward the opening of the uterus. Unfortunately, the only sponge available in the United States was the Today Sponge, which contained nonoxynol-9. As of the publication date of this book, the Today Sponge is no longer being manufactured.

THE WITHDRAWAL OR PULL-OUT METHOD

The Withdrawal, or the Pull-Out Method, is when the penis is removed from the vagina before ejaculation to prevent pregnancy from occurring. The Pull-Out Method does not prevent STIs.

This method is ninety-six percent effective when used correctly *every single time.* However, this method is not reliable and is likely only effective about seventy-eight percent of the time.

In other words, if this is your choice of birth control, you risk pregnancy one out of five times you have sex. In the heat of the moment, this method may not be as reliable due to the amount of willpower it requires from both parties involved.

A NOTE ON FEMININE HYGIENE PRODUCTS

Though feminine hygiene products are widely used, many of us use them without realizing there is a lack of regulation within the period product industry. Unfortunately, there is very little government oversight on what is in your period or personal hygiene products, making it difficult to make informed decisions.[16]

PRO TIP

Volatile organic compounds (VOCs) are a class of chemicals that have negative impacts on human health, with known toxic, irritating, or carcinogenic properties.[17] According to the EPA, VOCs are often found in petroleum fuels, hydraulic fluids, paint thinners, and dry-cleaning agents—even scarier, they can be found in period products!

For a list of volatile organic compounds found in tampons, pads, vaginal washes, sprays, powders, and moisturizers, check out the article by Lin and colleagues in our sources.[18]

With this information in mind, we recommend doing research on the companies you choose; while most products contain some volatile organic compounds, there are companies that are working to minimize the risk of exposure to toxic chemicals. Some of the companies worth researching are LOLA, Cora, Rael, Veeda, NatraCare, The Honey Pot, and Honest Co.

TAMPONS

While an estimated eighty-six percent of menstruating people in the United States use tampons, many don't realize that they could be a source of heavy metals and pesticides.[19]

A 2019 study found a possible link between higher levels of mercury and oxidative stress biomarkers in those who use tampons. While the findings weren't statistically significant, any increase in toxin exposure is concerning and needs to be kept in mind, especially when these exposures come from something that is so commonly used and in a very absorptive area of the body.[20]

PADS

The pros of using pads are that they are non-invasive and involve less exposure to the absorptive tissue in the vagina.

The cons of using pads are that they can be messy and bulky. If this is your period product of choice, it is important to change your pad before it gets excessively wet in order to avoid vaginal or urinary infections.

MENSTRUAL CUPS

Menstrual cups have become a popular period product due to the fact that they are non-toxic and environmentally friendly.

Made from silicone, menstrual cups can be reused for up to ten years, depending on the chosen brand and maintenance of the cup. The great thing about menstrual cups is that they can be left in your vagina for up to twelve hours when you have a normal bleed.

PRO TIP

Remember, typical period blood loss over the duration of your bleed should be equal to about two to three tablespoons of blood. Menstrual cups are meant to be changed two to three times in a twenty-four-hour period. If your menstrual cup is overflowing within a few hours or you have leakage even with a good seal between your menstrual cup and vaginal wall, this may be a sign of heavy menstrual bleeding. Check out our section on heavy menstrual bleeding to learn more!

Brands we like are Diva Cup, FLEX Menstrual Cup, and Lunette Menstrual Cup. Some brands, such as Diva Cup, have two sizes: one for someone who hasn't given birth vaginally and one for someone who has.

Menstrual cups can work for most people who menstruate. If you're just starting to use menstrual cups, be patient with yourself, and give it a few cycles to get used to it. Positioning the cup just right can be tricky at first, but if you stick with it, you will be a pro in no time. Be sure to properly clean your menstrual cup between each use and store it in a sanitary, dry location.

PERIOD PANTIES

Last but certainly not least, let's talk about period panties!

Cute underwear you can wear while you're bleeding without any other period protection is a revolutionary idea that is starting to become more popular.

Period panties are a great way to reduce waste and are cost effective since you can just throw them in the wash after wearing them. And thankfully, they have no resemblance to granny-panties or adult diapers—they're actually trendy and pretty comfortable!

PRO TIP

It's crucial to conduct your own thorough research on the menstrual products you choose to use. There have been several lawsuits against feminine hygiene companies based on safety and toxin-free claims that aren't necessarily true.

Some companies have falsely claimed that their products are free from PFAS, or per- and polyfluoroalkyl substances. PFAS are toxic compounds that can have long-term effects on lipid metabolism, the immune system, and most relevant to this book, the endocrine system.[21] This is especially relevant since PFAS are known as "forever chemicals" because they are not broken down easily.[22]

Knix period underwear was found to contain a PFAS called fluorine.[23] Thinx period underwear also contains PFAS, which have been associated with customers developing irregular menstrual cycles, UTIs, yeast infections, and thyroid and fertility issues.[24] There are likely other companies with similar toxins in their products, so we encourage you to do your research before purchasing period and personal hygiene products.

RESTORING YOUR CYCLE

By now, you know there are various ways you can naturally restore your cycle and balance your hormones. Small daily decisions can drastically impact your well-being and hormone health!

This chapter is full of helpful tips and tricks to help you feel good *throughout* your cycle and naturally manage any period problems you might be facing.

In the beginning of the book, we talked about the health pyramid consisting of basic aspects of health including nutrition, hydration, movement, sleep, stress management, and community. These are all pieces of the puzzle when we consider what types of lifestyle changes we can make to improve our hormone and overall health.

We'll cover each of these facets of health in this chapter.

NUTRITION

SEED CYCLING

Seed cycling involves eating different seeds during the different phases of your menstrual cycle to encourage hormone equilibrium. This is a simple tool that may have positive outcomes for individuals with menstrual cycle problems.

Seed cycling schedule:

- First Half of Your Cycle (Follicular Phase): two tablespoons of flax and/or pumpkin seeds per day

- Second Half of Your Cycle (Luteal Phase): two tablespoons of sesame and/or sunflower seeds per day

You might be wondering, *Is there evidence to support seed cycling?*

Though we couldn't find any peer-reviewed studies specifically looking at seed cycling, there *is* research on each individual seed, and the research we've compiled demonstrates the potential benefit of seed cycling. We hope more research will be conducted on this healing modality in the future, but for now, let's review some research regarding the health benefits of the seeds themselves and how these benefits relate to the menstrual cycle.

There are certain components of plants that are structurally similar to estrogen and can mimic estrogen in the body. These compounds are known as phytoestrogens. Phytoestrogens can have both estrogenic and/or antiestrogenic effects in the body, depending on the amounts of estrogen already in the body.[1]

Lignans and isoflavones are major types of phytoestrogens, and each of the seeds in the seed cycling schedule is high in lignans![2]

Lignans are powerful, perceptive agents that act according to the environment and what is most needed at the present time—either suppressing naturally occurring estrogens or helping increase the presence of estrogen in the body.

FASCINATING FACT

Isoflavones, another type of phytoestrogen, are found primarily in soy. A 2003 review proposed that while both have health benefits, greater consumption of lignans may be a marker of a healthier diet because dietary sources of lignans tend to be higher in fiber and complex carbs and lower in fat.[3] This is good news for those of you who are doing seed cycling!

Each seed is slightly different in its micronutrient profile. We'll discuss the various benefits of each seed below!

Flaxseeds

Flaxseed is a great source of a specific lignan called secoisolariciresinol diglucoside (SDG).[4] SDG acts both as an antioxidant, preventing cellular damage due to oxidative stress, and as a phytoestrogen, either promoting estrogenic or anti-estrogenic properties in the body.[5] Flaxseed may help shift estrogen metabolism down the more health promoting pathway due to it's high content of lignans such as SDG.[6]

Pumpkin Seeds

SDG, the major lignan found in flaxseed, is also found in pumpkin seeds. Because of this, pumpkin seeds and flaxseed may have similar estrogenic effects.[7] Pumpkin seeds are also high in omega-3[8] and micronutrients such as potassium, magnesium, zinc, and selenium.[9]

Sesame Seeds

Sesame seeds have both high antioxidant capacity and lignan concentration.[10] Sesame seeds have a different lignan content than flaxseeds and pumpkin seeds, and they tend to be higher in the lignans lariciresinol and pinoresinol. Sesame seeds also contain another lignan known as sesamin.

Even though they have different lignans, a 2005 study found that consumption of sesame seeds produces lignans in the gut in a similar multitude and manner to flaxseeds! A small study in 2005 found sesamin was a precursor of a lignan produced in the gut that may have beneficial estrogenic effects.[11]

Sunflower Seeds

Although sunflower seeds tend to have lower lignan content than sesame and flaxseed, of the four seeds involved in seed cycling, a

2017 study found sunflower seeds to have the highest antioxidant capacity.[12]

Sunflower seeds have been shown to have benefits outside of reproductive health as well. A 2018 review analyzing the health benefits of sunflower seeds found the seeds may have anti-inflammatory effects, encourage improved gut health, have antimicrobial properties and promote pain relief.[13] Sunflower seeds are also high in minerals like calcium, iron, magnesium, selenium, zinc, and potassium, which are vital to hormone and overall health.[14]

BONUS: Chia Seeds

Although chia seeds are not technically part of seed cycling, they contain omega-3 fatty acids, dietary fiber, antioxidants, and polyphenols—all of which are beneficial to individuals with a cycle. You can incorporate them throughout your cycle, and we love adding them into smoothies, salads, oatmeal, or using them to make chia seed pudding.[15]

If you are ready to give seed cycling a try, we suggest using the following guidelines:

- In the first half of your cycle, supplement with flax and/or pumpkin seeds.

- In the second half of your cycle, supplement with sesame and/or sunflower seeds.

- If you're not cycling regularly or are trying to get your period back, one tip is to use the moon phases as a place to start. Begin flax and pumpkin seeds with the new moon and switch to sesame and sunflower seeds with the full moon. You can do a quick Google search with the current month and new moon or full moon to figure out the best day to get started.

PRO TIP

When possible, use whole seeds and grind them into a powder just before consuming them to get optimal nutrition.[16] If this isn't feasible, it's still beneficial to include them in pre-ground or whole form!

Now, let's review how to use food to manage things like PMS, estrogen dominance, PCOS, endometriosis, heavy periods, and missing periods!

GENERAL NUTRITION GUIDELINES

Let's start with how we care for our bodies with food! By now, you probably understand that the foods you eat can influence your hormone health. Here are some general tips for anyone and everyone to consider when choosing foods to fuel and nourish their body.

Whole vs. Processed Foods

Whole foods are the best way to nourish our bodies. Cooking at home and eating whole foods promotes increased consumption of fiber and decreased consumption of processed fats, sugars, and other less-than-ideal additives!

Even packaged foods marketed as "healthy" may have some sneaky or undesirable ingredients in them! This is why we promote eating whole foods as often as possible. If you buy your groceries in their whole form (i.e.. a potato versus a bag of frozen, pre-cut French fries), you can see what ingredients go into the final product and know that you're avoiding unnecessary additives.

Carbs: Glycemic Index

Glycemic index is just a fancy term for the rating system used to measure how quickly our blood sugar rises after eating. Foods high in sugar and refined carbohydrates tend to have a high glycemic index, and whole foods tend to have a lower glycemic index.

A 2009 study found diets consisting of foods with a higher glycemic index negatively influenced ovulation and fertility in women who had never had children,[17] hammering home the concept that the types of foods we eat can influence our hormone balance and cycles.

Label Reading

One of the most frustrating aspects of nutrition is label reading. So many things are added to foods without us even realizing it, even in foods that are marketed as "health foods"!

If you don't already, we encourage you to start looking at ingredient lists on food labels, because sometimes "low fat" translates to "high sugar," and as we've reviewed multiple times in this book, high sugar is not ideal for hormone balance. It's also worth noting that sometimes "low sugar" simply translates to high levels of artificial sweeteners, and those are not beneficial either. Learning how to read labels can be made simple with this one helpful hint: if you can't pronounce an ingredient or you're unsure what an ingredient is, look it up!

Labels are ordered from highest content to lowest, so if one of the top three ingredients in a product is sugar or processed fats, it might be best to put that product down. Sugar, specifically in the form of fructose, can be tricky to find on labels, but some common ingredients that are high in fructose are agave, fructose, high-fructose corn syrup, honey, molasses, pancake syrup, palm sugar, coconut sugar, invert sugar, sorghum, and table sugar, which is half fructose and half glucose.

Remember, not all fats are created equal. Many foods that are marketed as "natural," "vegetarian," or "vegan" have processed fats such as canola, cottonseed, and soybean oil, which are all highly inflammatory. When it's an option, choose foods made with olive oil, coconut oil, or avocado oil instead.

> **PRO TIP**
>
> We're pro-butter! If you look at the ingredients on most margarine spreads, they're loaded with different types of processed oils. Real butter is always better than the fake stuff.

Eat Out Less

Note that while eating out isn't "bad" for you, it's best to dine out in moderation. Your hormones and your budget will thank you later!

Restaurant food is typically less nutritious than home-cooked food, and because organic foods tend to be more expensive, chances are the food you're eating at a restaurant will have been conventionally grown. A lot of delicious restaurant products are loaded with inflammatory fats and sugar to keep you coming back.

All in all, just be mindful, not obsessive, about the foods you put in your body.

Inflammatory Foods

We've talked a lot about how inflammation affects our cycle. Some simple dietary tips for decreasing inflammation include reducing intake of processed and packaged foods, eating out less, decreasing saturated and trans fats, eating plenty of fiber to regulate blood sugar, and incorporating liver supporting foods such as broccoli, cabbage, kale, Brussels sprouts, garlic, onions, and carrots into your diet.

Probiotics and Prebiotics

Going back to the very beginning of this book when we stated that what you eat greatly affects the way you feel, you can understand that overall well-being and health begins in the gut. If your gut is in a state of dysbiosis, meaning that there is an imbalance of good and bad bacteria, you will not be able to optimally digest and absorb nutrients from the foods you are eating.

Probiotics and prebiotics play a major role in gut health.

Probiotics promote "good" bacteria in our gut and dietary sources include supplements and foods like yogurt, kimchi, kombucha, sauerkraut, kefir, and fermented vegetables.[18]

Prebiotics are the dietary fiber sources that feed the good bacteria in our gut. Dietary sources of prebiotics include bananas, cow's milk, beans, oats, apples, barley, garlic, onions, leeks, artichokes, and asparagus.[19]

It's important to include probiotics and prebiotics in your diet to help with your gut microbiome, especially since the health of your gut microbiome can influence the health of your cycle!

Organic vs. Conventional

Sadly, pesticides and herbicides that are harmful to human health and the environment are commonly used on conventionally grown food. If you're in the U.S., where regulation is lacking, eating organic, when possible, does make a difference.[20] Eating organic helps you avoid many of the pesticides, antibiotics, and hormones that are sprayed or pumped into conventionally grown and produced foods. Extra bonus—you're supporting farmers that care about the health and sustainability of the environment!

PRO TIP

If eating completely organic seems a little bit overwhelming or outside of your budget, start by getting to know the Dirty Dozen and Clean Fifteen lists on EWG.org. The Dirty Dozen is a list of the top twelve conventionally grown produce items with the most contaminants and chemicals. The Clean Fifteen is a list of the top fifteen conventionally grown produce items with the smallest amounts of harmful contaminants. These are two great references to equip you with knowledge of which foods tend to be higher or lower in endocrine disruptors. These lists are updated annually, so be sure to check back each new year for the most up-to-date lists. The EWG also has an app called EWG's Healthy Living App with ratings for more than 120,000 foods and personal care products! Go to EWG.org to find more information.

Avoid Constipation

While some individuals may think their constipation is "normal," it is less than ideal for hormone health. One way to help ensure daily bowel movements is to aim for five servings of fruits and veggies per day. Morning hydration can also help "get things moving," so make sure to include a glass of water with your morning coffee!

Eat More, Not Less

Whether you're an athlete with menstrual cycle problems or you are just someone who has light, missing, or irregular periods, it may be a sign that you need to eat more, not less! In a 2014 study analyzing a small group of individuals with exercise-related menstrual dysfunction, a six-month period of increasing caloric intake by 360 calories per day improved chances of regular menstruation and ovulation.[21] Your body needs adequate fueling throughout the day to maintain health in all aspects.

Quit Counting Calories

Focus more on the ingredients in your food rather than the calorie content. Counting calories takes away your intuition and your body's innate ability to know when it's hungry and when it's full. You might also be missing out on necessary nutrients that fuel your body if you're focusing solely on counting calories. Just like we promote tossing the scale out, we also promote tossing out the habit of calorie counting!

Honor Your Hunger

If you're hungry, eat! One way to prevent binge eating is to honor your hunger cues. You may need to pack a few extra snacks or eat larger meals during your luteal phase since this is when your body needs the most energy in your cycle. It's okay if your appetite is constantly changing! Remember, as an individual with a menstrual cycle, your body is constantly changing, too!

Breakfast of Champions

Science supports the concept of eating a "breakfast of champions," and so do we!

Not only is eating a large, nutrient-filled breakfast going to fuel your day well, but it may also help prevent dinner-time binging. Eating a smaller dinner has been shown to improve aspects of overall health, including sleep and inflammation management.[22]

Alcohol

A 2017 review found that alcohol influences almost every system in the body, including the endocrine system. Alcohol can influence the communication between the hypothalamus, pituitary, and organs crucial to hormone health, disrupting hormonal balance.[23] Excess alcohol can also lead to liver problems, which is less than ideal for hormone health.[24] Alcohol may influence the GI system, negatively impacting our gut microbiome and potentially contributing to symptoms related to leaky gut.[25]

If you choose to drink alcohol, try to stay away from sugary drinks and cocktails, and limit alcohol to one to two drinks per day or five drinks per week. If you are a social drinker, try incorporating some non-drinking activities into your social routine such as inviting a friend on a hike or walk, or having friends over for tea or a home-cooked meal!

PRO TIP

Stick to the 1:1 rule when drinking alcohol. For every alcoholic drink you consume, drink a glass of water before reaching for another beverage. Another tip: you can always ask for sparkling water or club soda with a splash of cranberry juice or squeeze of lemon or lime after you've reached your drink limit. This will help you feel included in social drinking without abandoning your health goals.

*Note: Even though club soda has the word "soda" in it, it's actually sugar-free. Tonic water, on the other hand, has about the same sugar content as a regular soda. Good to know, right?

Hydration

Water comprises about fifty-five to seventy-five percent of a person's body weight, making water consumption a vital aspect of health.[26] Hydration is a key factor in body temperature regulation, cognitive function, mood regulation, bowel movement regulation, kidney function, heart health, skin health, and avoidance of some chronic diseases.[27] A good rule of thumb is to drink half your body weight in ounces of water per day at minimum and eat hydrating foods such as fruits and vegetables.

PRO TIP

If you're feeling a mid-afternoon slump, try drinking a tall glass of ice-cold water to wake up your body. Bonus points if you add in a big cup of either warm or cold water before your morning coffee!

NUTRITION GUIDELINES FOR PERIOD PROBLEMS

This section will provide a recap of how to address your period problems using nutrition. For deeper dives into each topic, refer back to our Problems with Your Cycle chapter.

ESTROGEN DOMINANCE, PMS, AND PMDD

Those struggling with estrogen dominance, PMS, and PMDD may benefit from the following nutrition tips:

- **Seed cycling:** Refer to the section on seed cycling on page 251 where we go into the science and research behind seed cycling.

- **Fiber:** Eat more fiber and less processed foods and refined seed or vegetable oils. Remember, constipation is not normal. Eating plenty of dietary fiber and drinking water will help maintain normal bowel movements.

- **Cruciferous vegetables:** Increase cruciferous vegetable intake with veggies such as cabbage, broccoli, kale, arugula, cauliflower, and Brussel sprouts.

- **Microbiome:** Improve your microbiome by eating a diet rich in both probiotics (fermented foods) and prebiotics (dietary fiber). Check out our section on probiotics and prebiotics on page 39. It's also important to address food allergies or intolerances in order to promote gut health, so if you're struggling to figure out your gut issues, working with a functional nutritionist is a great place to start!

Dietary sources of the micronutrients that may be beneficial for Estrogen Dominance, PMS, and PMDD symptoms include:

- **Calcium:** milk, cheese, and other dairy products, leafy greens (collard greens, broccoli rabe, kale), foods fortified with calcium (foods that have added calcium in them), and seafood.

- **Magnesium:** nuts, seeds, dark leafy greens, seaweed, legumes, dairy products, and whole grains.

- **Dietary sources of vitamin D:** Although we get vitamin D primarily through sunlight, dietary sources of vitamin D include fortified dairy products, fish such as salmon, herring, sardines, and tuna, egg yolks, mushrooms, fortified orange juice, and cod liver oil, which has the added benefit of being a great source of omega-3.

- **Vitamin B6:** chickpeas, beef liver, tuna, salmon, chicken, potatoes, turkey, bananas, acorn squash, and butternut squash.

- **Omega-3:** fatty fish (salmon, tuna, herring), fish oil, flaxseeds, chia seeds, and walnuts.

- **DIM:** cruciferous vegetables such as kale, cabbage, Brussels sprouts, bok choy, cauliflower, arugula, radish, turnip, broccoli, kohlrabi, watercress, rutabaga, maca, horseradish, and daikon.

- **Calcium-D-glucarate:** cruciferous vegetables, apple, grapefruit, and orange.[28]

- **Curcumin:** Turmeric is a spice that has high amounts of curcumin; be sure to pair it with black pepper to increase its bioavailability.[29]

PCOS

Individuals struggling with PCOS should focus on protein, fiber, and healthy fat intake.

- **Protein:**
  - Note: Aim for at least 0.8 grams of protein multiplied by body weight in kilograms (kg) or 0.36 grams for body weight in pounds (lbs) (i.e., if you weigh 150 lbs or 68 kg, you would aim for at least 54 grams of protein per day).
  - While current recommendation is usually 0.8 g/kg/day (.036g/lb/day), this is based on sedentary adults and menstruating people may need closer to 1.6 g/kg/day. Something to consider as you're adding protein into your diet![30]

- **Carbohydrates:**
  - Aim for at least twenty-five grams of fiber per day. Remember, constipation is not normal and it's important to eat enough fiber and drink enough water to support daily bowel movements. A great place to start is to try to add five servings of fruits and vegetables into your diet each day.
  - Track your sugar intake and try to follow the World Health Organization's recommendation of less than five percent of calories and no more than twenty-five grams of added sugar per day.

- **Fat:**
  - Incorporate healthy fats such as avocado oil and olive oil into your diet to reduce blood sugar spikes and help stabilize insulin. Refer to the section on dietary fat on page 49 for more information.

- Remember, type of fat matters! It's important to decrease packaged foods high in processed oils and cook at home when possible. Restaurant meals typically contain more saturated and processed fats than cooking at home.

- Reading labels can be really helpful for avoiding less-than-ideal fats. Check out the list on page 56 for our fat "friends" and "foes" list.

Dietary sources of the micronutrients that may be beneficial for PCOS include:

- **Calcium:** milk, cheese, and other dairy foods, leafy greens (collard greens, broccoli rabe, kale), foods fortified with calcium (foods that have added calcium in them), and seafood.

- **Magnesium:** nuts, seeds, dark leafy greens, seaweed, legumes, dairy products, and whole grains.

- **Potassium:** avocados, bananas, sweet potatoes, potatoes, peas, prunes, apricots, and legumes.

- **Iodine:** seaweed, seafood, iodized salt, dairy, and eggs.

- **Zinc:** oysters, beef, crab, lobster, pork, chicken, pumpkin seeds, cashews, and chickpeas and other legumes (lentils, beans, etc.).

- **Folic acid:** dark green leafy vegetables, liver, bread, yeasts, and fruits.

- **Vitamin C:** citrus fruits, strawberries, tomatoes, hibiscus tea, broccoli, spinach, bell peppers, and kiwi fruit.

- **Vitamin D:** Although we get vitamin D primarily through sunlight, dietary sources of vitamin D include fortified dairy products, fish such as salmon, herring, sardines, and tuna, egg yolks, mushrooms, fortified orange juice, and cod liver oil, which has the added benefit of being a great source of omega-3.

- **Vitamin B12:** beef, pork, poultry, fish, shellfish, eggs, and some traceable amounts in dairy products.

ENDOMETRIOSIS

Individuals struggling with endometriosis may benefit from the following nutrition tips:

Foods that may be beneficial for endometriosis include:

- **Fruits and vegetables:** There is conflicting evidence that certain fruits and veggies can help manage endometriosis, but there is research on individualized diet plans being beneficial for individuals with endometriosis. Check out page 170 to learn more!

- **Healthy fats:** It may be beneficial to increase your intake of healthy fats rich in omega-3 fatty acids such as fatty fish like salmon, tuna, and herring, fish oil, flaxseeds, and chia seeds.[31]

Foods that may be beneficial to avoid if you have endometriosis:

- **Processed foods:** Packaged foods and processed meats including beef and ham have been linked to increased risk of developing endometriosis.[32] These foods contain high amounts of saturated and trans fat and low amounts of omega-3.[33]

- **Alcohol:** Alcohol may negatively impact endometriosis.[34] We suggest replacing your evening glass of wine with another antioxidant-rich beverage such as tart cherry juice.

Dietary sources of the micronutrients that may be beneficial for endometriosis include:

- **Thiamine:** whole grains, meat, and fish.[35]

- **Folate:** dark green leafy vegetables, liver, bread, yeasts, and fruits.

- **Vitamin C:** citrus fruits, strawberries, tomatoes, hibiscus tea, broccoli, spinach, bell peppers, and kiwi fruit.[36]

- **Vitamin E:** nuts, egg yolks, cheese, oatmeal, avocados, olives, green leafy vegetables, and plant-based oils such as olive oil.[37]

  - It may be beneficial to get your vitamin E from foods rather than supplements due to the high concentrations of vitamin E in some supplements.[38]

- **L-arginine:** walnuts, peanuts, soy protein, and fish.[39]

HEAVY MENSTRUAL BLEEDING

Individuals struggling with heavy menstrual cycles may benefit from the following nutrition tips:

- **Managing inflammation:** Easy tips for managing inflammation include decreasing processed and packaged foods and increasing fruit and veggie intake.

  - **Ginger:** Has been shown to be one food that can help with inflammation and heavy menstrual cycles.[40]

- **Supporting hormone balance:** Estrogen dominance can be a common reason for heavy bleeding. Focus on foods that support healthy estrogen levels and liver detoxification. Refer to the previously listed tips on managing estrogen dominance for more information.

- **Nutrient-rich diet:** Since your bleed is heavy and likely longer than average, you might be losing greater amounts of nutrients than what is typical. It's important to focus on eating a well-rounded diet that incorporates a wide variety of foods to make up for this loss.

Some micronutrients that may be beneficial for managing heavy bleeding:

- **Vitamin E:** nuts, egg yolks, cheese, oatmeal, avocados, olives, green leafy vegetables, and plant-based oils such as olive oil.[41]

    - It may be beneficial to get your vitamin E from foods rather than supplements due to the high concentrations of vitamin E in some supplements.[42]

- **Zinc:** oysters, beef, crab, lobster, pork, chicken, pumpkin seeds, cashews, and chickpeas and other legumes (lentils, beans, etc.).

- **Heme iron:** beef, poultry, pork, and fish.

- **Non-heme iron:** dark leafy greens like spinach, kale, and collard greens.

    - Remember to add a source of vitamin C, such as lemon or lime juice, to improve absorption of non-heme iron.

Refer to our chapters on heavy menstrual bleeding and iron deficiency for more information about the importance of iron.

AMENORRHEA (MISSING PERIODS)

For individuals with no known underlying medical condition causing their missing periods, the main way to support the return of your cycle using nutrition involves:

- **Increasing caloric intake of nutrient-dense foods:** If you aren't getting your period regularly or are having menstrual problems, it may be time to consider adding more healthy carbohydrates, proteins, and fats into your diet! A 2014 study analyzing a small group of individuals with exercise-related menstrual dysfunction found six months of increasing calories by 360 calories per day improved chances of regular menstruation and ovulation.[43]

- **Seed cycling:** Refer to the section on seed cycling on page 251, where we go into the science and research behind seed cycling.

Note: Missing periods can be caused by many different factors such as eating disorders, malnourishment, or over-exercising. If you've been missing your period for several months, it is always a good idea to take a pregnancy test if you've been sexually active since your last bleed. If you aren't pregnant, it's wise to consult with a healthcare professional to gain further insight as to what may be causing your missing periods.

MOVEMENT

There is a lot of scientific research regarding the benefits of exercise, and we encourage you to get moving to experience the benefits yourself!

Remember, you don't have to go to the gym to get the benefits of exercise. Exercise can be in the form of short bursts of activity throughout the day, and a good baseline to start with is aiming for three thirty-minute workouts per week!

Check out page 95 for a full list of useful tips to help you get moving!

STRESS MANAGEMENT

Stress is another key player in our hormone response; we'll review some science and tips for stress management in this section!

START WITH SELF-REFLECTION

In order to make positive changes, self-reflection is key. It's important to examine how we respond to daily situations, whether they are good, bad, or neutral. When we look at negative experiences as an opportunity to learn and grow (and a normal part of living), we can move through challenges with ease and grace.

Our goal is to help you understand that good communication is vital. Both the external dialogues we have with others and the internal dialogues we have within our minds influence our outlook and interactions. We also want to help you understand that knowing your cycle can help you handle emotional ebbs and flows with less judgement of your emotional responses; when you understand these fluctuations you can improve your communication around your differing needs throughout your cycle.

We believe that it's important to acknowledge and experience your feelings. Being human means experiencing not just joy, excitement, and happiness, but also grief, sorrow, and loneliness. It's important to work through *all* of your emotions, feelings, and experiences, and understand that it is okay to feel exactly how you're feeling in a given moment. When you acknowledge a feeling, sometimes that makes it easier to move through it rather than get stuck in it. We are *all* working through these aspects of being human, and no one is immune from feeling the full spectrum of human emotions.

PRO TIP

It's important to keep in mind that there are a lot of reasons why we feel certain ways; culture, education, upbringing and socioeconomic status can influence our mindset. As you work through your own story, we highly recommend the book *The Body is Not an Apology: The Power of Radical Self-Love* by Sonya Renee Taylor.

BIG FEELINGS ARE OKAY

While we're going over practices to help you re-center and refocus your energy, we also want to remind you that it's *okay* to be upset.

By acknowledging and addressing how you feel, you will be less likely to bottle up your emotions, and that may help prevent a messy emotional outburst. Once you recognize your patterns, you can start to work through them and make changes in your life, as necessary, to promote optimal emotional, mental, and physical health.

PRO TIP

If everything in your life feels terrible (which we all experience at some point, and is a valid way to feel), have strategies in place to help. One strategy we like when we're having a bad day is to let it be. Say, "Welp, this day isn't great, and I'm just going to take care of myself so that tomorrow can be better." Or create a mantra, such as "tomorrow is a new day, a fresh start" and repeat this to yourself as you fall asleep.

Another strategy that can be helpful is counting your breath. Count to five as you inhale through your nose, count to five as you exhale through your nose. Take at least ten breaths doing this, increasing the number of breaths as you get used to it. The nice thing about this strategy is that you can do it wherever you are to get a quick nervous system reset.

THE BRAIN-CHANGING EFFECTS OF SELF-REFLECTION

Remember our feel-good neurotransmitter, serotonin? What we choose to focus our mind on may actually influence serotonin levels in the brain!

A 2007 study showed that when individuals were prompted to remember sadness, happiness, and neutral emotions, recalling memories that induced happiness was associated with increased serotonin synthesis while recalling the feeling of sadness was negatively associated with serotonin production.[44] This is especially relevant for those with PMDD, which, as we reviewed earlier, may be related to issues with serotonin.

Practices like journaling and meditation can help tap into this brain-changing potential.

PRO TIP

Here are a few journal prompts to help bring your focus to the positive things in life!

- What is one thing that always makes you laugh?
- List three of your favorite people and write a reason why you're grateful for each of them (bonus points if you tell them why you appreciate them!).
- What is one thing you can do this week to make someone else's life a little bit better?
- Think of five things that you're grateful for this week and then write about one of them in detail.
- Positive affirmations—make a list of positive "I am" statements. Pick one to focus on each morning this week.
    - Some of our personal favorites include I am strong, I am worthy, I am loved, I am whole.
- Pick a mantra or uplifting statement to read or recite to yourself before bed and in the morning.
- Write a positive affirmation on your bathroom mirror or somewhere in your space that you will see every day.

Along with journaling, meditation is also a great practice for regulating our emotional and neurological response! Meditation may positively influence dopamine, which is another neurotransmitter associated with motivation, reward, cognitive function, and certain aspects of behavior.[45]

These studies demonstrate the positive brain-changing effects of mindfulness practices such as meditation and journaling, so it may be worth adding a mindfulness practice into your daily or weekly routine!

MINDSET, POSTURE, AND BREATHING

Our physical body and emotional body are intricately linked, and posture may be part of this connection!

Posture may influence (or be influenced by) confidence, self-esteem, arousal, mood, and our perception of fear.[46]

FASCINATING FACT

While it's difficult to know if posture influences emotional response or vice versa, a 2017 study found changing posture influenced emotional status in individuals with mild to moderate depression. In this study, individuals with mild to moderate depression tended to have slumped posture compared to controls. Improving posture to an upright position decreased reports of fatigue and increased positive emotions,[47] showing that changing your posture may have positive effects on mental health!

Standing up tall with the chest forward and arms wide with palms forward is often referred to as "power posing," and some studies have found it may influence how individuals are perceived in social situations.[48] While there is conflicting research on the topic of the effects of power posing and posture,[49] changing your posture is an easy thing to incorporate into your life with minimal, if any, risks— why not give it a try and see how you feel?

Now, let's talk about the biomechanics of posture and how posture might relate to your nervous system response!

POSTURE, BREATHING, AND YOUR NERVOUS SYSTEM

Did you know that posture, breathing, your deep core muscles, and your nervous system are all linked?

Posture influences your ability to take deep breaths, which affects your vagus nerve as well as your nervous system and endocrine responses!

The diaphragm, your primary breathing muscle, contracts and moves downward as you inhale. Think about the diaphragm moving downward as a way to create more

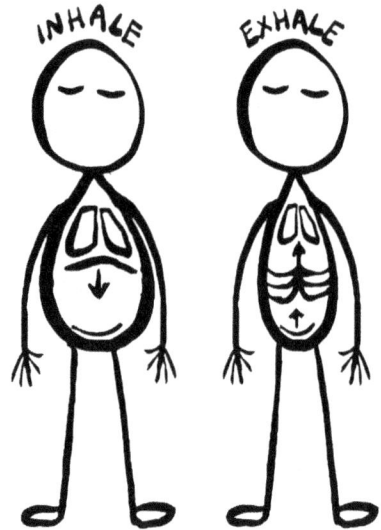

space for air in the lungs. As you inhale, the diaphragm moves down and your belly expands.

As you exhale, your deep core muscles and your pelvic floor contract, and your belly button gently draws towards your spine. The contraction of the deep core when you exhale is why you might hear the cues "exhale on the effort" during exercise.[50]

Your posture can either help or hinder your ability to get deep breaths and optimally use your diaphragm.

Let's do a little test at home to show you the difference:

- First, get into a slouched posture. Let your chin drop towards your chest and round your back. Now, try to take a deep breath. Notice how it's pretty challenging to get a deep breath in this position?

- Now, do the opposite motion, arching the low back as far forward as it will go and pushing your chest forward. Notice, this still may feel challenging to get a deep breath in.

- Now, sit up as tall as you can, with your head stacked over your shoulders and shoulders stacked over your hips. Take a deep breath. Does this feel easier?

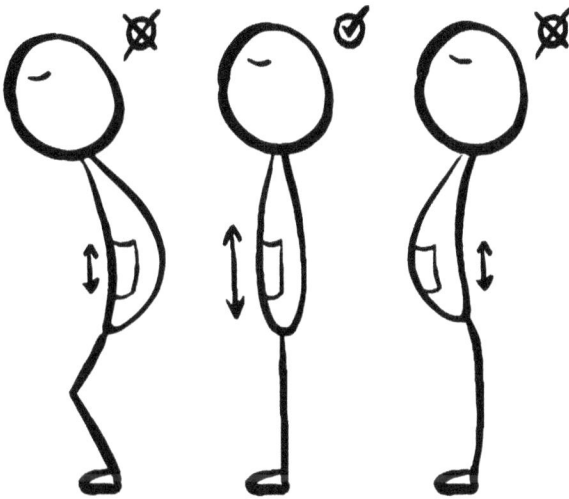

Breathing strategies may be even more important if you notice tension in your neck and shoulders. When we are stressed, we tend to slouch, making it harder to get full, deep breaths. When your diaphragm can't move downward efficiently, whether it's because of a muscular problem or your posture, the muscles around your neck and ribs have to lift the ribs up every time you breathe in, in order to create space for air in the lungs. This means your posture and breathing patterns may actually be the source of your neck tension, headaches, and migraines!

If you feel like you have a hard time getting a deep breath, have pelvic floor problems, or have constant tension in your neck and shoulders, we highly recommend finding a pelvic health physical therapist to help with these issues.

While breathing and posture may not be sexy or exciting, poor breathing strategies and management of intra-abdominal pressure is related to conditions like urinary incontinence and pelvic organ prolapse! This is why it's so important to work on the deep core, breathing, and posture in whatever activities you're doing. And to any cross fitters, runners, or gymnasts out there, leaking while you exercise is not normal. If you're having any leakage with exercise (or otherwise), call your local pelvic health PT!

RETRAINING YOUR POSTURE AND NERVOUS SYSTEM

Now that we've reviewed the science behind the benefits of mindfulness, meditation, and yoga, let's get into some ways you can incorporate them into your routine! The great news about these techniques is that you don't need any fancy equipment or a gym membership—all you need is your body and breath!

PRO TIP

Yoga doesn't have to be a super physical practice as it is often preached and practiced in Western society. One way to start integrating yoga techniques into your life is by adding deep belly breathing into your current movement routine. Plus, now you know there's actually scientific reasoning behind the old saying "take a deep breath."

Note: Remember, meditating and breathing deeply should not cause any dizziness, lightheadedness, headaches, or any other sort of body pains. If you have any questions about starting a breathing or meditation practice, yoga therapists specialize in creating yoga and meditation practices specific to your individual needs.

DAILY BREATHING PRACTICES

These easy daily practices are a great place to start your mindfulness routine!

> **PRO TIP**
>
> If you are anxious, you can use a little bit of weight (think a cork yoga block or medium-sized book) to help tap into a diaphragmatic breathing pattern. Start lying on your back (or with your legs up the wall) and place the weighted item on your abdomen. Now, focus on breathing in and out through the nose for a count of five. The weight will help to engage diaphragm with your breathing. (Remember, more is not necessarily better, and we recommend sticking with something the size of a cork yoga block or medium-sized book to start.)
>
> **Note:** To see the difference, first you can take a deep breath with one hand on your chest and one hand on your belly. See where the breath falls (if it's mainly chest or belly). After breathing with weight on your belly for ten to fifteen minutes, remove the weight and see if you notice any difference.

Seated Diaphragmatic Breathing

Sit as tall as you can. Tuck your chin back and bring it parallel to the ground. Now, find your lower ribs (underneath your bra line in the front) and let them sink towards the spine, drawing them down and back.

Place one hand on your belly and one on your chest. Inhale deeply through your nose and try to pull the air DOWN into your belly. Feel your belly rise under the hand on your abdomen while the hand on the chest remains mostly still.

Exhale through pursed lips, as if to blow out a candle across the room and feel the belly tense and draw in as you do so.

Seated Diaphragmatic Breathing with Lateral Rib Expansion

Sit as tall as you can. Tuck your chin back and bring it parallel to the ground. Now, find your lower ribs (underneath your bra line in the front) and let them sink towards the spine, drawing them down and back.

Bring your right hand to your right ribs and left hand to left ribs with fingers pointing forward and thumbs pointing back toward the spine. Squeeze the shoulder blades together and inhale through the nose for a count of five. Focus on letting the shoulders relax down away from the ears as you feel the ribs expand out into your hand with your inhale. Exhale for a count of five, feeling the ribs drop back down towards the body.

Seated Alternate Nostril Breathing

Coming to a comfortable seated position with good posture (see above), lift the right hand. Close the index and middle finger so that the thumb and ring finger can be used to block the nostrils. With the right thumb, gently press the right nostril closed, exhaling completely through the left nostril. After the exhale, inhale through the left nostril, closing the nostril with the right ring finger after the inhale, and exhaling through the right nostril. Complete several rounds, closing the nostril after the inhale and exhaling through the opposite nostril.

Standing Power Pose

Standing power pose is all about standing tall!

Stand with your feet hip-width apart and toes pointing forward. Bend your knees slightly. Now, find your lower ribs (underneath your bra line in the front) and let them sink towards the spine, drawing them down and back. You should feel your core engage here.

Squeeze the shoulders together and let your arms rest by your side, rolling your palms forward with the thumbs facing out. Stack your ears above the shoulders with your chin parallel to the ground.

Now that you're standing tall and in good posture, set a timer for three minutes and focus on taking deep breaths in and out through your nose. Inhale deeply through your nose and try to pull the air DOWN into your belly. Exhale through pursed lips, as if to blow out a candle across the room, and feel the belly tense and draw in as you do.

Legs up the Wall

Legs up the wall is as easy as it sounds—sit with your hips close to a wall and lie on your back, bringing your legs up the wall with your feet towards the ceiling.

Work on your belly breathing here.

PRO TIP

If you have glaucoma, fluid retention (as is common with heart, kidney, or liver failure), or high blood pressure that's not medically managed, stick with the other poses in this section! And make sure to check in with a provider before doing legs up the wall for longer durations—we recommend ten to fifteen minutes to start.

If you just tried any of the exercises above, congrats—you did it! You've successfully started a mindfulness practice. Try and incorporate both "exercise snacks" and "mindfulness snacks" into your routine.

SLEEP

SLEEP AND HORMONE HEALTH

Sleep hygiene isn't the first thing most people think of when they envision well-being, but quality sleep may be the missing piece of your health puzzle.

Sufficient sleep is essential for optimum health,[51] and virtually all bodily systems are negatively impacted by poor or inadequate sleep.[52]

Lack of sleep may be related to menstrual irregularity and psychiatric problems, especially when individuals are getting less than five hours per night,[53] and a 2018 study proposed sleep hygiene be added into the treatment plan when trying to address menstrual cycle dysfunction.[54]

FASCINATING FACT

Sleep deprivation increases cortisol, our primary stress hormone.[55] A reason lack of sleep may negatively impact hormone balance is that one of the major building blocks of progesterone is also one of the main building blocks of our stress hormone, cortisol. This building block can be "stolen" from progesterone in order to make more cortisol, causing decreased progesterone levels while we build cortisol during times of stress.[56] Melatonin, our primary sleep hormone, may also play a role in regulating estrogen and progesterone levels.[57]

We now know that lack of regular sleep can influence hormone production in more than one way, leading to a skewed ratio of estrogen to progesterone, potentially leading to estrogen dominance.

SLEEP AND TECHNOLOGY

With advances in technology, especially the amount of screen time that is common in our culture, our sleep cycles are much different than those of our ancestors.

Artificial lights, including blue light from light-emitting diodes (better known as LEDs), heavily influence our biological clocks. The changes in our sleep patterns and circadian rhythms are most influenced by artificial light at night.[58] This disruption of the biological clock can lead to fatigue, sleepiness, changes in behavior, and poorer academic achievement (arguably interchangeable with work achievement in adults).[59]

While the use of sleep aids is common, they can be addictive and may have negative side effects. There are some natural options such as melatonin and valerian root,[60] however, we encourage you to try the following tips before reaching for any over the counter or prescription medications.

TIPS FOR IMPROVING SLEEP

- **Get into a routine! This sounds cliche, but it *works.***
  - Try to start your bedtime routine around the same time each night.
  - Avoid screens in bed. Your bed should be reserved for sleep and intimacy.
  - One to two hours before bed, put your phone away for the evening and don't look at it.
  - If you use your phone for an alarm clock, put it across the room or out of reach. Bonus if you keep it in another room and get an old school alarm clock.

- **Reduce blue light exposure.**
    - Blue light blocking glasses are a great tool for reducing blue light exposure before bed.
    - F.lux is an app, among several others, designed to minimize blue light exposure as the sun goes down. While apps like these are a good option, they don't completely eliminate blue light emitted from electronic devices, so blue light blocking glasses may be the best option if you're trying to eliminate exposure.

- **Don't eat your biggest meal late at night.**
    - A 2018 study concluded that high-energy dinners, or consuming most of your calories at night, might disturb sleep. It may be best to consume most of your calories and nutrients earlier in the day and to keep your dinners light to improve sleep quality.[61]
    - Remember to eat a hearty breakfast and lunch, fueling throughout the day in order to avoid binging at dinner. And don't forget to pack extra healthy snacks in the second half of your cycle when you naturally need more energy.

- **Get your exercise in!**
    - As we reviewed earlier, it has been suggested that consistent exercise may be an effective way to improve sleep without the use of drugs, whether you choose aerobic exercise or resistance training.[62]
    - Bonus points for exercising if you have sleep apnea. A 2012 study found that twelve weeks of moderate-intensity aerobic and resistance exercise decreased obstructive sleep apnea symptoms in sedentary, overweight/obese adults, even in cases where there was minimal weight loss.[63]

COMMUNITY

The last vital aspect of health that we want to touch on is the importance of friendship and community.

In this day and age, it is easy to feel isolated, stressed, and inadequate, comparing ourselves to unrealistic ideals. Viewing the lives of others through the lens of social media or the internet can often make us feel less than worthy.

We want you to remember—you are so much more than how you look in a photo or the number of likes you get.

Think about the things you love about your friends...even if they're drop-dead gorgeous, it probably wasn't the first characteristic you listed. Believe it or not, your people think similarly about you!

What we see on social media is typically the highlight reel of someone's life and doesn't demonstrate the struggles they may be experiencing.

Here's the hard truth: social media can be incredibly toxic for our physical, mental, and emotional health. The constant and subtle competitive notes, the blatant bullying, the polarizing statements— it can quickly become all too much. That's why we need each other. We need community not just when we're doing well, but also during our times of struggle.

The people you surround yourself with can greatly affect your overall quality of life. Connection, belonging, and emotional and physical support are all aspects of community that influence your mental health and general well-being.

If you find yourself lacking in meaningful relationships, it may be time to get plugged into a community in close proximity to where you live, work, or play. Activities such as recreational sports, art or dance classes, clubs, or meet-up groups in your area may provide great opportunities for you to find your people organically.

If you're struggling to find your community or are feeling especially lonely, we want to remind you that it's a sign of strength to ask for help and add a mental health provider to your care team.

Ask yourself these questions to help direct you towards a supportive community:

- What do I want in the relationships in my life?
- What am I tolerating?
- What does it look like to live in alignment with my values?

Once you start living from a place rooted and secure in your values, you will naturally be drawn to people who share similar morals and interests.

Our final message is this: be YOU. There is no one else in the world quite like you with your unique skills and outlook on life. You will never have the exact same qualities as anyone else, and that's actually your superpower!

When you begin to accept yourself, flaws and all, you can begin to shed the layers of needing external approval and focus on your mental and physical health, becoming the person you were created to be.

Think of it this way: when you are healthy physically, mentally, spiritually, and emotionally:

- You can better serve your community and those around you.
- You can elevate other people in your life who need to be lifted up.
- And best of all, you can use your story to encourage others to commit to their own journey of health.

So find people who uplift you in this journey, and keep moving forward in health!

BE EMPOWERED

So many people want to make the step towards better health but don't know how or where to start. You've made it to the end of a book *full* of information. How are you feeling? Overwhelmed? Exhausted?

Take your time. Old habits die hard, and new habits aren't formed overnight.

Give yourself the grace of a year.

We suggest you mark the date one year from now on a calendar. You officially have one year to change your health and change your life. Can you do it? It's up to you!

For the next year, we want you to focus every day on the small decisions that really add up. Remember, so much of health comes from those tiny choices we make on a daily basis such as walking, taking the stairs, or adding an extra serving of fruits and veggies in. These small, conscious choices become easier each day and will eventually become sustainable, healthy habits.

Remember, life is anything but linear.

Nobody is perfect, and not every day is going to be your greatest. When you have setbacks or feel discouraged, don't let shame, guilt, or self-judgment overcome you. Instead, reach out to your community for support and encouragement, and know that you are doing an amazing job. Pick up from where you left off and keep going after the health you are so worthy of!

As you use this year to get to know yourself and live to your fullest potential, we think you'll be amazed at what you find out about yourself throughout the process! So get to it!

All of our love,

Heather and Kailee

RECIPES

THREE MEALS FOR MENSTRUATION

Note: The following recipes use fats for cooking such as butter, extra virgin olive oil (EVOO), and coconut oil. We listed our favorites for each recipe, but feel free to use the oil of your preference!

VEGETARIAN/VEGAN

Breakfast:	Lunch: meal-sized spinach	Dinner:
chickpea scramble with turmeric, ginger, onions, bell pepper, and avocado	salad with blueberries, raspberries, dried apricots, walnuts, and a homemade dressing with extra virgin olive oil (EVOO), apple cider vinegar, and ginger with a whole grain baguette/toast and EVOO to dip	lentil and mushroom stew with wild rice

CHICKPEA SCRAMBLE

INGREDIENTS:

- 2 Tbsp EVOO
- ½ yellow onion, chopped
- 1 orange, yellow, or red bell pepper, chopped
- 1 can chickpeas, drained, rinsed, and slightly mashed
- 1 inch fresh ginger root, grated
- 2 tsp turmeric
- 1 avocado, diced or sliced
- Salt and pepper to taste

INSTRUCTIONS:

Heat two tablespoons of EVOO in a large skillet over medium heat and add chopped onion and bell pepper. Cook for about five minutes until onions and peppers become soft. Add chickpeas, ginger, turmeric, black pepper and salt to the skillet and stir occasionally for five minutes on medium/high heat. Once everything is coated in turmeric and the chickpeas begin to brown, turn off heat, and transfer the scramble to a plate. Top with avocado, more salt and pepper, and, if you're feeling adventurous, a little hot sauce! Enjoy!

SPINACH BERRY SALAD FOR MENSTRUATION

INGREDIENTS:

- 1 cup spinach
- Blueberries
- Raspberries
- 1 Tbsp dried apricot, chopped
- ¼ cup walnuts
- Homemade Vinaigrette (see recipe below), with dash of ginger powder

INSTRUCTIONS:

Assemble all ingredients on top of the bed of spinach and drizzle with a generous amount of dressing. Enjoy with a slice of hearty, whole grain bread dipped in EVOO.

HOMEMADE VINAIGRETTE

INGREDIENTS:

- ½ cup EVOO
- ¼ cup apple cider vinegar (ACV)
- 2 cloves of garlic, minced
- 1 Tbsp honey or maple syrup
- 2 Tbsp of stone ground or Dijon mustard
- Salt and pepper to taste

INSTRUCTIONS:

Place all ingredients in a food processor and process for thirty seconds, or place all ingredients in a Mason jar and shake vigorously for about a minute. Store in the fridge for one to two months.

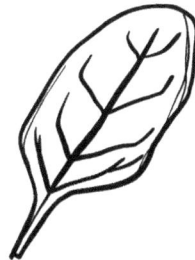

LENTIL AND MUSHROOM STEW

INGREDIENTS:

- 2 Tbsp EVOO
- 1 cup red onions, diced
- ½ cup carrots, sliced into coins
- ½ cup celery, diced
- 8 oz mushrooms, sliced
- 2 Tbsp tamari or soy sauce
- 2 Tbsp garlic, minced
- 2 Tbsp tomato paste
- ½ cup red wine (optional)
- ½ cup wild rice
- 1 cup dried uncooked lentils
- 2 cups vegetable broth
- 3 cups water (or more broth)
- 1 tsp garlic powder
- 1 tsp onion powder
- 2 tsp dried thyme
- 1 tsp dried rosemary
- 2 bay leaves
- 1 tsp cumin
- 3 cups baby spinach, chopped
- Salt and pepper to taste

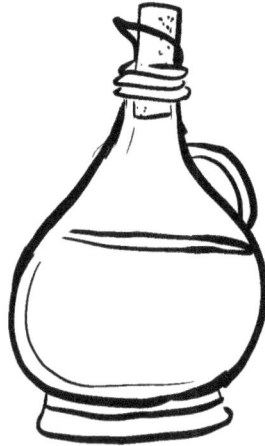

INSTRUCTIONS:

Begin by sautéing onion, carrots, celery, and mushrooms in EVOO in a large stock pot on medium heat until the onion and carrots are slightly softened. Add in tamari, garlic, and tomato paste. Stir until combined and garlic becomes fragrant. Add remaining ingredients except for the spinach and bring to a boil. Once boiling, turn to low heat, stir, and let simmer for twenty to twenty-five minutes until the lentils and rice are tender. Toss in spinach, and serve with whole grain bread for dipping.

NON-VEGETARIAN/VEGAN

Breakfast:	Lunch:	Dinner:
whole grain sprouted toast with mashed avocado, drizzle of EVOO, and smoked salmon with berries on the side	mushroom, broccoli, chicken and ginger stir-fry over brown rice topped with crushed walnuts	chickpea or lentil pasta with "jazzed-up" marinara (grass-fed ground beef, loads of garlic, and chopped collard greens)

AVOCADO AND SMOKED SALMON TOAST

INGREDIENTS:

- 1 avocado
- ½ lemon
- 2 pieces whole grain toast
- Smoked salmon, 1-2 pieces per slice of bread
- EVOO
- Salt and pepper
- Berries of choice, on the side

INSTRUCTIONS:

Mash avocado in a bowl and add juice of one-half lemon. Toast two whole grain pieces of bread and first top with a drizzle of EVOO and salt, then mashed avocado, salmon, and pepper. Enjoy with a side of fresh berries.

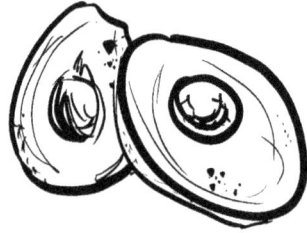

CHICKEN, BROCCOLI, AND MUSHROOM STIR-FRY

INGREDIENTS:

- 1 cup brown rice, uncooked
- 3 Tbsp EVOO
- 2 cups broccoli, chopped roughly
- 2 cloves garlic, minced
- 1 cup mushrooms, sliced
- 2 tsp ginger, freshly grated
- 1 lb chicken, cut into 1-inch pieces
- ¼ cup tamari sauce (or soy sauce)
- Black pepper
- Red pepper flakes
- ¼ cup crushed walnuts

INSTRUCTIONS:

Cook rice according to instructions on packaging and set aside. Heat one tablespoon of EVOO in a skillet over medium and add broccoli and garlic, cook for five minutes. Next, add mushrooms and ginger, cook for five more minutes until mushrooms become soft. Place the contents of the skillet in a bowl and set aside. Add two tablespoons of EVOO to the skillet on medium heat, add chicken. Cook all the way through, about eight minutes. Add to the contents of the bowl, tamari sauce, black pepper, and red pepper flakes, and stir well. Plate rice first and top with stir-fry mixture and crushed walnuts. Enjoy!

JAZZY CHICKPEA PASTA

INGREDIENTS:

- Chickpea or lentil pasta, 8 oz box
- 1 lb grass-fed beef, ground
- 1 Tbsp EVOO
- 2-3 cloves of garlic, minced
- 1 yellow onion, chopped
- 1 cup of collard greens, kale or turnip greens, chopped
- Marinara, 16 oz sugar-free

INSTRUCTIONS:

Cook pasta according to instructions on the box and set aside. Cook ground beef in a skillet on medium-high heat. Once cooked, drain liquid and set aside in a bowl. On medium heat, add one tablespoon of EVOO to the skillet. Once heated, add garlic and onion. Cook until the onions are translucent, then add greens and cook until wilted. Add cooked beef and marinara sauce into the skillet and stir until heated through and mixed well. Top pasta with the "jazzed-up" sauce and enjoy!

THREE MEALS FOR THE FOLLICULAR PHASE

VEGETARIAN/VEGAN

Breakfast: oatmeal with flaxseeds, pumpkin seeds, grated carrot or zucchini, and cashew butter drizzle and roasted grapefruit on the side	**Lunch:** meal-sized salad with romaine lettuce and spinach, roasted broccoli, black-eyed peas, hard boiled eggs, and EVOO and vinegar dressing with hummus and crackers	**Dinner:** collard wraps with lentils, kale sautéed in lemon juice and EVOO, grilled Portobello mushrooms, and vegan mayo-sriracha sauce

FUELED-UP OATMEAL

INGREDIENTS:

- ½ cup oatmeal, uncooked
- 1 Tbsp ground flaxseed
- ¼ cup carrot or zucchini, grated (½ cup if desired)
- 1 tsp maple syrup
- 1 Tbsp cashew butter
- 1 Tbsp pumpkin seeds

INSTRUCTIONS:

Cook oatmeal in one cup water in a small saucepan. Once cooked, add flaxseeds, carrot, or zucchini, and maple syrup. Top with cashew butter and pumpkin seeds. Enjoy with a side of one-half grapefruit, raw or broiled. See directions on the next page for broiled grapefruit.

BROILED GRAPEFRUIT

INGREDIENTS:

- Grapefruit, cut in half
- 1 tsp coconut sugar or raw sugar

INSTRUCTIONS:

Simply cut the grapefruit in half, sprinkle each half with one-half teaspoon coconut sugar or raw sugar, and broil in the oven on high for two to three minutes. Always be sure to watch the grapefruit closely so you do not burn it.

ROASTED BROCCOLI AND BLACK-EYED PEA SALAD

INGREDIENTS:

- ¾ cup broccoli, chopped
- Salt and pepper to taste
- Romaine lettuce, chopped
- Spinach
- ½ cup Black-Eyed Pea Salad, (see recipe on next page)
- 2 hard boiled eggs, sliced
- 1 Tbsp Homemade Vinaigrette, recipe on page 289

INSTRUCTIONS:

Preheat the oven to 375 degrees F/190 C. Coat the broccoli in EVOO, salt, and pepper, and roast for twenty-five minutes. Meanwhile, make a bed of chopped romaine lettuce and spinach and top with Black-Eyed Pea Salad, eggs, and dressing. Once broccoli is roasted, allow to cool for a minute or two and top the salad with it. Enjoy with a side of whole grain crackers and hummus or cheese.

BLACK-EYED PEA SALAD

INGREDIENTS:

- 1 can black-eyed peas, drained and rinsed
- 1 grapefruit, juiced and flesh shredded*
- ½ small red onion, diced finely
- 1 tsp molasses or 1 Tbsp maple syrup
- 1 Tbsp EVOO
- Salt and pepper to taste

INSTRUCTIONS:

Combine all ingredients in a bowl and mix well. Keep covered in the fridge for up to one week.

*A note on the grapefruit: to get "shredded flesh," cut in half and use a large fork to squeeze the juice out and scrape the flesh into the bowl. These bites of grapefruit will be little bites of heaven!

GRILLED PORTOBELLO COLLARD WRAPS

INGREDIENTS:

- 2 Portobello mushrooms, whole
- 1 Tbsp EVOO
- ½ tsp garlic powder
- 1 tsp cumin
- Salt and pepper to taste
- 1 cup kale, chopped
- 1 lemon, juiced
- Collard green leaves, fresh, whole, and rinsed
- 1 cup lentils, cooked according to instructions on package
- Vegan mayonnaise
- Sriracha

INSTRUCTIONS:

If grilling, heat up the grill to medium to medium-high heat. If oven roasting, preheat the oven to 400 degrees F/204 C. While the grill or oven is heating, cook the lentils according to the instructions on the package. Brush EVOO all over mushrooms. Mix garlic powder, cumin, salt, and pepper, and sprinkle over both sides of the mushrooms. If grilling, cook mushrooms for four to five minutes on both sides. If oven roasting, place right side up and roast for fifteen to twenty minutes. Once cooked, slice into half-inch slices. Next, sautéè kale in a skillet with lemon juice and EVOO until it wilts and becomes soft. Place a collard green leaf on a plate, spread vegan mayonnaise and sriracha, top with sliced mushrooms, lentils, and kale. Roll up like a burrito/wrap and enjoy!

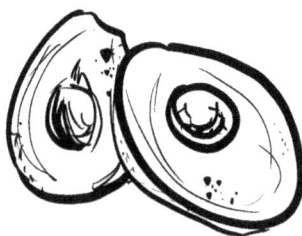

NON-VEGETARIAN/VEGAN

Breakfast: egg omelet with spinach/kale, mushrooms, whole-milk cheese, and toast with nut butter	**Lunch:** meal size salad with Romaine lettuce and spinach, roasted broccoli, grilled chicken, and EVOO and vinegar dressing with hummus and crackers	**Dinner:** baked salmon with roasted sweet potatoes, Brussels sprouts and quinoa

VEGGIE 'N CHEESE OMELET

INGREDIENTS:

- 2-3 eggs
- ½ cup kale or spinach, chopped
- 1/8 cup mushrooms, chopped
- ¼ cup whole-milk cheese, grated
- 1 piece whole grain toast
- 1 Tbsp nut butter

INSTRUCTIONS:

Heat oil of choice in a small pan on medium to medium-high heat. Scramble eggs in a bowl and pour into the pan, allowing the eggs to cook for two to three minutes before adding in the vegetables. Add the kale, mushrooms, and cheese, and flip one side of the omelet onto the other side so it resembles a taco. Continue cooking on medium heat while toasting the bread and spread nut butter onto the bread after toasted. Plate the omelet and nut butter toast. Enjoy!

MEAL SIZE CHICKEN SPINACH SALAD

INGREDIENTS:

- ½ crown of broccoli, separated or chopped
- 1 chicken breast
- Salt and pepper to taste
- Romaine lettuce, chopped
- Spinach
- 2 hard-boiled eggs, sliced
- 1 Tbsp Homemade Vinaigrette, recipe on page 289

INSTRUCTIONS:

Preheat the oven to 375 degrees F/190 C. Coat the broccoli and chicken breast in EVOO, salt, and pepper and roast for twenty-five minutes. While broccoli and chicken are roasting, hard boil eggs. Make a bed of chopped Romaine lettuce and spinach and top with eggs and dressing. Once broccoli and chicken are roasted, allow to cool for a minute or two, slice the chicken, and top the salad with the broccoli and chicken. Enjoy with a side of whole grain crackers and hummus, or cheese.

SIMPLE BAKED SALMON DINNER

INGREDIENTS:

- Quinoa
- Chicken broth, or bone broth
- 1 sweet potato, chopped
- 1 cup Brussels sprouts, chopped in half
- EVOO
- 1 tsp cumin
- 1/8 tsp red pepper flakes
- Salt and pepper to taste
- 4 oz salmon filet
- Lemon pepper seasoning

INSTRUCTIONS:

Cook quinoa according to package directions, swapping water with chicken/bone broth. Preheat the oven to 400 degrees F/204 C. Toss sweet potatoes and Brussels sprouts in EVOO to coat. Add cumin, red pepper flakes, salt, and pepper and bake for thirty minutes. In the meantime, prep salmon by brushing EVOO on the top of the fish and coating with lemon pepper seasoning. Once vegetables have cooked for thirty minutes, remove from the oven, stir around, add salmon to the baking sheet and return to the oven for twelve more minutes. Plate by making a bed of quinoa and placing the salmon on top and the vegetables on the side.

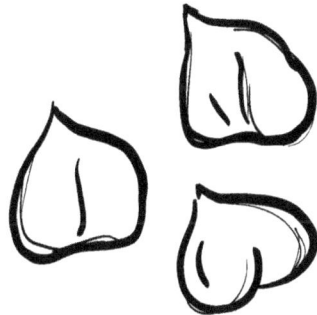

THREE MEALS FOR OVULATION

VEGETARIAN/VEGAN

Breakfast: baked pear with walnut, oat crumble and coconut cream	**Lunch:** salad with shredded cabbage, grapefruit, sliced pear and grilled tofu with an apple cider vinegar (ACV) and EVOO minty-herb dressing	**Dinner:** grilled cauliflower, zucchini, and leeks over a bed of lentils and whole grain rice

BAKED PEAR BREAKFAST

INGREDIENTS:

- 2 tsp butter or coconut oil
- 1 pear, Bartlett or Anjou, sliced in half with core scooped out
- ¼ cup oats
- 1 tsp coconut sugar, maple syrup, or honey
- Cinnamon
- Ginger
- Nutmeg
- 1 can full-fat coconut milk
- 2 Tbsp walnuts, crushed

INSTRUCTIONS:

Preheat the oven to 350 degrees F/176 C. Prepare a baking dish by smearing one teaspoon of butter or coconut oil on and place pears face down. Bake for fifteen minutes. While baking, mix oats, remaining teaspoon of butter or coconut oil, coconut sugar, and a dash of each spice. Remove the pear from oven and flip over so it is facing up. Top with oat crumble and bake for ten more minutes. While baking, make coconut cream by scooping coconut milk fat from top of can and whipping by hand or an electric mixer. Top baked pear with coconut cream and walnuts and enjoy!

MINTY CABBAGE AND GRAPEFRUIT SALAD

INGREDIENTS:

- 1 block of firm tofu, sliced ½-inch thick
- ½ cup EVOO
- 3 Tbsp tamari or soy sauce
- 1 Tbsp maple syrup
- 1 tsp garlic, minced
- 3 cups red cabbage, shredded
- 1 grapefruit, sectioned and diced
- 1 pear, sliced
- Minty Herb Dressing (recipe on next page)
- Fresh basil to taste

INSTRUCTIONS:

Marinate tofu in EVOO, tamari, maple syrup, and garlic for at least one hour. Heat grill to medium heat and grill tofu slices until charred. In a large mixing bowl, combine cabbage, grapefruit, and pear and massage with Minty Herb Dressing using hands. Serve salad topped with tofu and fresh basil.

MINTY HERB DRESSING

INGREDIENTS:

- ½ cup EVOO
- ¼ cup apple cider vinegar (ACV)
- 1 Tbsp mint, minced
- 1 Tbsp basil, chopped
- 1 Tbsp honey or maple syrup
- 1 tsp lemon juice
- Salt and pepper to taste

INSTRUCTIONS:

Place all ingredients in a Mason jar and shake vigorously for about a minute. Store in the fridge for one to two weeks.

GRILLED VEG AND LENTIL DINNER

INGREDIENTS:

- 1 cup lentils, uncooked
- 1 cup whole grain rice, uncooked
- Head of cauliflower, sliced into ½-inch thick slices
- 1 zucchini, sliced into ¼-inch thick slices lengthwise
- 2 leeks, washed, sliced in half, into 3-inch chunks
- EVOO
- 1 Tbsp garlic powder
- 1 Tbsp cumin
- ½ tsp smoked paprika
- Salt and pepper to taste
- Tahini
- Lemon juice

INSTRUCTIONS:

While the grill is heating to a medium-high heat, begin cooking lentils and rice according to package instructions. Prepare veggies by tossing them in EVOO, garlic powder, cumin, smoked paprika, salt, and pepper. Grill cauliflower heads and leeks for five minutes on each side, and zucchini for two to three minutes on each side. Serve grilled veggies over rice and lentils. Drizzle tahini and lemon juice on top and enjoy!

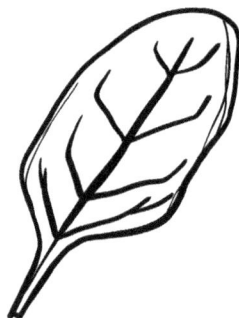

NON-VEGETARIAN/VEGAN

Breakfast: mushroom and cabbage sauté with breakfast chicken sausage	**Lunch:** whole grain sandwich with hummus, turkey/chicken, sautéed kale, and avocado with sliced pear and cherries on the side	**Dinner:** "pad thai" made with noodled carrots and zucchini, peanut sauce, fresh garlic, grilled chicken/tofu, and scrambled eggs

VEGGIE AND CHICKEN SAUSAGE SAUTÉ

INGREDIENTS:

- ½ cup mushrooms, sliced
- ½ cup purple cabbage, sliced thin
- ¼ cup yellow onion, chopped
- 1 Tbsp butter
- 4-5 oz chicken sausage, hormone and antibiotic free
- 1 cup spinach, chopped
- Salt and pepper to taste

INSTRUCTIONS:

Sauté mushrooms, cabbage, and onion in butter on medium heat until onions are translucent and soft. Add chicken sausage to the pan and cook until sausage is cooked through, or heated if pre-cooked. Toss in spinach and cook for another one to two minutes until spinach wilts. Salt and pepper to taste.

REVVED UP TURKEY SANDWICH

INGREDIENTS:

- 2 slices of whole grain bread
- ½ cup kale, chopped
- 1 tsp butter
- Salt and pepper to taste
- 2 Tbsp hummus
- 3 oz turkey or chicken breast, thinly sliced
- ½ avocado, mashed

INSTRUCTIONS:

While two slices of bread are toasting, heat a pan to medium heat and sauté kale in butter until the kale becomes slightly crispy, and add salt and pepper to taste. Once bread is toasted, spread hummus on one side and mashed avocado on the other. Add the crispy kale and turkey to the sandwich. Serve with sliced pear and cherries on the side.

VEGGIE NOODLE PAD THAI

INGREDIENTS:

- 2 cups carrots, spiralized or sliced with vegetable peeler
- 2 cups zucchini, spiralized or sliced with vegetable peeler
- ½ cup peanut butter
- 2 Tbsp tamari or soy sauce
- 1 Tbsp maple syrup or honey
- 1 tsp garlic, minced
- ½ lime, juiced
- 2 Tbsp water
- Grilled or pan-fried chicken or tofu
- 4 eggs, scrambled
- 2 Tbsp sesame seeds
- Green onion, chopped (optional)

INSTRUCTIONS:

Place veggie noodles (carrots and zucchini) in a large mixing bowl. In a smaller bowl, mix peanut sauce by combining peanut butter, tamari, maple syrup or honey, garlic, lime juice, and water. Coat noodles with peanut sauce and let sit to marinate. While the noodles are soaking in the flavors of the sauce, heat butter/EVOO in a sauté pan on medium heat and scramble the eggs. Once the eggs are cooked, combine noodles, eggs, chicken or tofu, and sesame seeds. Top with sliced green onions and extra sesame seeds and enjoy! This recipe makes two to three servings.

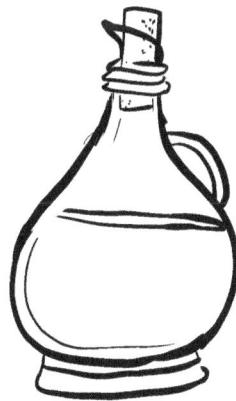

THREE MEALS FOR THE LUTEAL PHASE

VEGETARIAN/VEGAN

Breakfast: chickpea and sweet potato hash with garlicky kale	**Lunch:** cold quinoa and lentil salad with cabbage slaw	**Dinner:** stir-fried Brussels sprouts, cabbage, leeks, dandelion greens over brown rice or millet with crushed walnuts and tamari drizzle

CHICKPEA AND SWEET POTATO HASH

INGREDIENTS:

- 1 Tbsp butter or coconut oil
- 1 can chickpeas, drained, rinsed, and slightly mashed
- ½ onion chopped, red or yellow
- 1 tsp garlic, minced
- 1 sweet potato, grated
- 1 cup kale, chopped
- ½ tsp cumin
- ¼ tsp paprika
- Salt and pepper to taste

INSTRUCTIONS:

In a skillet, heat butter over medium heat. Add in chickpeas, onion, and garlic, and cook for two to three minutes. Add sweet potatoes and kale and cook until sweet potatoes are softened. Stir in cumin, paprika, and salt and pepper. Enjoy!

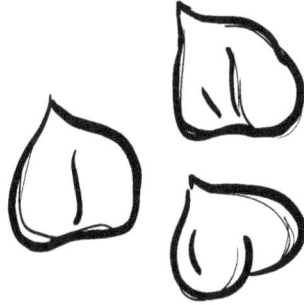

COLD QUINOA SALAD

INGREDIENTS FOR QUINOA SALAD:

- 2 cups quinoa, cooked and cooled
- 1 cup lentils, cooked and cooled
- 8 oz cherry tomatoes, halved
- 1 cup cucumbers, sliced
- ½ cup feta cheese (optional)
- 1 Tbsp italian seasoning
- ½ cup EVOO
- ¼ cup balsamic vinegar
- Salt and pepper to taste

INSTRUCTIONS:

In a large mixing bowl, combine all ingredients for quinoa salad. In another mixing bowl, combine all cabbage slaw ingredients. Set both in the fridge for at least one hour to cool and allow flavors to mix. Enjoy together or separate!

INGREDIENTS FOR CABBAGE SLAW:

- 1 cup purple cabbage, shredded
- 1 cup green cabbage, shredded
- ½ cup red onion, sliced paper thin
- 1 tsp fresh thyme
- 1 tsp garlic powder
- 2 Tbsp apple cider vinegar
- 3 Tbsp EVOO
- Salt and pepper to taste

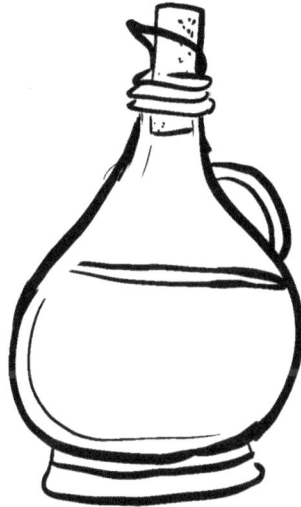

VEGGIE STIR FRY

INGREDIENTS:

- 2 Tbsp EVOO
- 1 ½ cup Brussels sprouts, quartered
- 1 ½ cup cabbage, chopped
- 1 cup leeks, sliced thin
- 2 tsp garlic, minced
- 2 tsp ginger, freshly grated
- ¼ cup tamari or soy sauce
- Red pepper flakes
- 1 cup dandelion greens, chopped
- 1 cup brown rice, cooked
- ¼ cup crushed walnuts
- Tahini, to drizzle on top (optional)

INSTRUCTIONS:

Heat EVOO in a skillet over medium heat and add Brussels sprouts, cabbage, and leeks. Cook for five minutes. While the vegetables are cooking, begin cooking the rice according to the instructions on the package. Next, add garlic, ginger, tamari, and red pepper flakes, and sauté until garlic is fragrant. Next, toss dandelion greens in the skillet and cook until wilted. Serve vegetables over brown rice and top with walnuts and tahini drizzle. Enjoy!

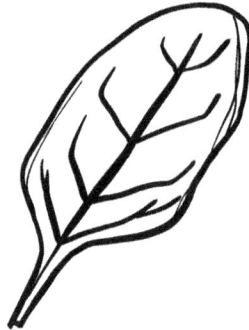

NON-VEGETARIAN/VEGAN

Breakfast: sweet potato and Brussels sprout hash with eggs	**Lunch:** : Quinoa bowl with grilled chicken, roasted squash and leeks, avocado, and crushed walnuts	**Dinner:** shrimp cooked in olive oil, garlic, turmeric, ginger powder, salt, black pepper, sautéed shredded red and green cabbage, and carrots

SWEET POTATO AND BRUSSELS HASH

INGREDIENTS:

- 1 cup Brussels sprouts, shaved or sliced thin
- ¼ cup yellow onion, chopped
- 1 tsp garlic, minced
- 1 sweet potato, grated
- 1 cup kale, chopped
- 1 Tbsp butter or coconut oil
- ½ tsp cumin
- ¼ tsp paprika
- Salt and pepper to taste
- 2-3 eggs, cooked to preference

INSTRUCTIONS:

In a skillet, heat butter over medium heat. Add in Brussels sprouts, onion, and garlic and cook for two to three minutes. Add sweet potatoes and kale and cook until sweet potatoes are softened. Stir in cumin, paprika, and salt and pepper. Set aside and cook eggs to preference. Serve eggs on top of hash and enjoy!

CHICKEN QUINOA BOWL

INGREDIENTS:

- 2 cups cooked quinoa
- 2 grilled chicken breasts, cubed or shredded
- 1 ½ cups butternut or kabocha squash, cut into 1-inch cubes
- 1 cup leeks, sliced thin
- ¼ cup + 2 Tbsp EVOO
- Salt and pepper to taste
- ¼ cup apple cider vinegar
- 8 oz feta cheese, crumbled
- 1 avocado, sliced or cubed
- ½ walnuts, crushed

INSTRUCTIONS:

Preheat oven to 375 degrees F/190 C. In a large mixing bowl, combine quinoa and chicken. Once the oven is preheated, place squash and leeks on a baking sheet and massage with two tablespoons of EVOO, salt, and pepper. Roast in the oven for twenty to twenty-five minutes or until the squash is soft and slightly browned. Once roasted, toss squash and leeks in with the quinoa and chicken. Add remaining one-quarter cup EVOO, apple cider vinegar, feta cheese, and salt and pepper to taste. Mix well. Top with sliced avocado and walnuts. Enjoy!

SHRIMP ZINGER

INGREDIENTS:

- 1 Tbsp EVOO
- 1 Tbsp butter
- 2 tsp garlic, minced
- ½ lb shrimp, frozen or fresh, shelled and deveined
- 1 tsp turmeric powder
- ½ tsp ginger powder, or 1 inch of fresh ginger, grated
- Salt and pepper to taste
- ¼ head of purple cabbage, shredded
- ¼ head of green cabbage, shredded
- 1 cup carrots, shredded

INSTRUCTIONS:

In a large skillet, heat EVOO and butter on medium heat. sauté garlic until fragrant, and stir in turmeric, ginger, and black pepper until the EVOO and butter are a bright yellow. Toss in shrimp and cook until pink but tender (about one to three minutes on each side). Once shrimp are cooked, remove them from the skillet and toss in the cabbage and carrots. Sauté until they begin to soften and are coated with remaining fats and spices in the pan. Toss the shrimp in the skillet with the vegetables and enjoy it warm and fresh!

INTERVAL TRAINING WORKOUTS FOR YOUR CYCLE

We want to remind you that you don't need fancy equipment or access to a gym to take care of your body!

That's why all of the workouts in this book require no equipment and have different options for modifications. If a certain exercise doesn't feel great, just replace it with another exercise that does! The most important thing is to get moving in a way that feels good for your body. You can mix and match to find a routine that works best for you.

THE BASICS:

This is the verbiage that will be used in almost every workout.

Stay Stacked: Find your basic posture, keeping your head stacked over your shoulders and your shoulders stacked over your hips. Think of good standing posture here.

Exhale on the Effort: This helps your deep core stabilizing muscles turn on during the most challenging part of the routine.

LEVEL I, LEVEL II, LEVEL III

We encourage you to start where you are and listen to your body—the most important thing is to get moving!

If you're new to exercise, start with level I! If that still feels like it might be too much, decrease the time to fifteen seconds for each exercise with a forty-five-second break.

If level I feels good, increase the intensity in level II.

For more of a challenge try level III, and if you want more intensity, feel free to up your time to forty-five seconds with a fifteen-second break.

INTERVAL TRAINING ROUTINE FOR MENSTRUATION

For this interval training workout, you'll perform the six exercises listed. Do each exercise for thirty seconds, taking a thirty-second break between exercises. Repeat the series five times. Be sure to stand up during the transition time between exercises to maximize benefits!

Bonus points if you give yourself five minutes after your workout to lie on your back for a mini-meditation! If you have a hard time meditating, you might find it a little bit easier after a good sweat session.

Check out eating-moving.com/workouts for a video version!

Exercises: Perform each exercise for 30 seconds, with a 30-second break

1. Standing Balance on the Right

2. Standing Balance on the Left

3. Shoulder Blade Squeezes Lying on Your Stomach

4. Modified Side Plank Glute Series Right

5. Modified Side Plank Glute Series Left

6. Chair Squats

*Repeat sequence 5x for a 30-minute workout

STANDING BALANCE ON THE RIGHT (30 SECONDS)

LEVEL I:

Stand with your hands on your hips and try to keep your upper body still as you lift your left foot off the ground. Slowly work on bringing your knee up to your hip at a 90-degree angle. Once your knee and hip are at 90 degrees, draw your toes up towards your nose. Remember to keep a slight bend in your right knee as you work on your balance. Hold for thirty seconds.

LEVEL II:

Start in the position from level I with your left leg lifted and your hands on your hips. As you inhale, shift your upper body forward and straighten your left leg behind you. The goal is to go from standing upright to having your upper body and left leg parallel to the ground. Your gaze should be down towards the ground and your chin tucked, keeping the neck nice and long. With your left leg straight, think about squeezing your booty as you press through your left heel, pointing your toes down toward the ground and rolling your inner thigh up towards the ceiling. As you exhale, come back to standing with the knee at 90 degrees. Remember to keep a slight bend in the right knee as you work on your balance. Repeat for thirty seconds.

LEVEL III:

Start in the position from level I with your left leg lifted and your arms overhead with your fingertips interlaced and first finger-pointing. As you inhale, shift the upper body forward and straighten the left leg behind you. The goal is to go from standing upright to having the upper body and left leg parallel to the ground. Exhale back to standing with the knee at 90 degrees and the fingertips still interlaced above your head. Repeat for thirty seconds for example: Remember to keep a slight bend in the right knee as you work on your balance. Repeat for thirty seconds.

30-SECOND BREAK

STANDING BALANCE ON THE LEFT (30 SECONDS)

Same as above, but to the left.

30-SECOND BREAK

SHOULDER BLADE SQUEEZES LYING ON YOUR STOMACH (30 SECONDS)

LEVEL I:

Lie on your stomach with your forehead supported by a rolled-up towel. Bring your arms by your sides with your palms facing down. With your arms on the ground, squeeze your shoulder blades together as you exhale. Inhale, relax. Repeat for thirty seconds.

LEVEL II:

Start in the position from level I, lying on your stomach with your arms by your sides and palms facing down. As you exhale, squeeze your shoulder blades together and lift your arms completely off the ground. Inhale, relax your arms back down to the ground. Repeat for thirty seconds.

LEVEL III:

Start in the position from level I, lying on your stomach with your arms by your sides and palms facing down. Squeeze your shoulder blades together and lift your arms completely off of the ground as you exhale. As you inhale, bring your arms away from the body at a 90-degree angle. As you exhale, bring your arms back to your sides. Keep your shoulder blades squeezed together and arms lifted the entire time. Repeat for thirty seconds.

30-SECOND BREAK

MODIFIED SIDE PLANK GLUTE SERIES RIGHT (30 SECONDS)

LEVEL I:

Start in a tall kneel with both knees on the ground and your upper body stacked. Bring your arms parallel to the ground. Now, tilt, bringing your left hand to the floor underneath your left shoulder and right hand up towards the ceiling with your right palm facing forward and your shoulder blades squeezing together. Extend your right leg out to the side with the foot on the ground, coming into your modified side plank. Stay here and work on belly breathing. Hold for thirty seconds.

LEVEL II:

Start in the position from level I, with your left hand on the ground and right leg extended. As you exhale, lift your right leg up, as you inhale, tap the foot down. Try to stay still, like you're between two panes of glass. Repeat for thirty seconds.

LEVEL III:

Start in the position from level I, with your left hand on the ground and right leg extended. Lift your right leg and hold there, pressing through the heels and drawing your toes up towards your nose. Now, draw the alphabet with the right heel in tiny letters—you should feel your glutes (booty muscles) working here! Repeat for thirty seconds.

30-SECOND BREAK

MODIFIED SIDE PLANK GLUTE SERIES LEFT (30 SECONDS)

Same as above, but to the left.

30-SECOND BREAK

CHAIR SQUATS (30 SECONDS)

LEVEL I:

Stand with your feet hip-width apart and toes pointing forward. Inhale while standing, and then sit back like you're sitting in a chair. Exhale as you press through the heels and big toe to stand back up. Try not to let your knees pass your toes when you're in your squat. Your legs should stay parallel throughout the exercise. Repeat for thirty seconds.

> **PRO TIP:**
>
> If you're new to exercise, try this with a chair. Instead of sitting back into your squat, sit down on the chair and stand back up. Make sure the chair is stable and in a place where it won't move. Remember, it's still important to keep your knees and toes pointing forward, so if your knees are dropping in, think about pressing them out. You should feel your glutes (booty muscles) working here.

LEVEL II:

Inhale in standing and sit back like you're sitting in a chair. As you exhale, stand up, adding a kick out to the side with the right leg. Repeat for thirty seconds, alternating sides.

LEVEL III:

Inhale in standing and sit back like you're sitting in a chair. As you exhale, take a small step out to the right. Stay in your squat and come back center, inhaling. As you exhale, take a small step out to the left. You want to stay in your squat for the whole exercise. Repeat for thirty seconds, alternating sides.

30-SECOND BREAK

*Repeat sequence 5x for a 30-minute workout

INTERVAL TRAINING ROUTINE FOR THE FOLLICULAR PHASE

For this interval training workout, you'll perform the six exercises listed. Do each exercise for thirty seconds, taking a thirty-second break between exercises. Repeat the series five times. Be sure to stand up during the transition time between exercises to maximize benefits!

Bonus points if you give yourself five minutes after your workout to lie on your back for a mini-meditation! If you have a hard time meditating, you might find it a little bit easier after a good sweat session.

Check out eating-moving.com/workouts for a video version!

Exercises: Perform each exercise for 30 seconds, with a 30-second break

1. Bridge

2. Leg Lifts Lying on Your Stomach

3. Chicken Wings

4. Side Plank (Right)

5. Side Plank (left)

6. Plie squat

*Repeat sequence 5x for a 30-minute workout

BRIDGE (30 SECONDS)

LEVEL I:

Lie on your back with your knees bent and your feet under your knees. Make sure your knees and feet are hip-width apart with your toes pointing forward. Lift the tops of your feet toward the ceiling so that your heel is the only part of your foot touching the ground. As you exhale, press through the heels and lift your hips into the air. Remember to stay in your stacked posture, creating a straight line from your shoulders to your knees. Hold for three seconds at the top. Repeat for thirty seconds.

PRO TIP:

We don't want this bridge to be a backbend. If you have any pain in your back, try tucking your tailbone under to take some of the stress off of your lower back. If you're still feeling discomfort, try performing the chair squat exercise from the menstruation routine in place of the bridge.

LEVEL II:

Lie on your back with your knees bent and your feet under your knees. Keep the bottoms of your feet on the ground. Use both of your arms to hug your left leg toward your chest. As you exhale, press through your right heel, engaging your glutes (booty muscles) as you lift your hips, coming into a variation of a single leg bridge (also known as Cook hip bridge). Try to keep your hips level and maintain one long line between your right knee and shoulders. Hold for three seconds at the top. Repeat for thirty seconds.

If you do level II, repeat on the opposite side as your next exercise.

LEVEL III:

Start lying on your back with both knees bent. Straighten your left leg out. Keep your left leg straight with the foot flexed (toes toward your nose) and lift the leg 45 degrees. As you exhale, press through the right heel and push up into your bridge. Try to keep your hips level and maintain one long line between your left leg and shoulders. Hold for three seconds at the top. As you inhale, gently lower your hips to the ground, keeping the left leg at a 45-degree angle. Repeat for thirty seconds.

If you do level III, repeat on the opposite side as your next exercise.

30-SECOND BREAK

LEG LIFTS LYING ON YOUR STOMACH (30 SECONDS)

LEVEL I:

Lie on your stomach with your arms by your sides. Make sure to keep your hip bones pressed into the ground and keep your legs straight. As you exhale, lift your left leg one centimeter off the ground. Inhale, relax. Repeat for thirty seconds, alternating sides.

> **PRO TIP:**
>
> You should feel this in your glutes (booty muscles), not your low back. If you're feeling it in the back, press the hip bones and ribs into the ground and don't lift the leg as high.

LEVEL II:

Same as level II from previous exercise, but hugging your right leg in towards the chest.

LEVEL III:

Same as level III from previous exercise, but lifting your right leg at a 45-degree angle.

30-SECOND BREAK

CHICKEN WINGS LYING ON YOUR STOMACH (30 SECONDS)

LEVEL I:

Lie on your stomach with your forehead supported by a rolled-up towel. Bring your hands behind your ears. As you exhale, squeeze your shoulder blades together and lift your elbows. As you inhale, relax. Repeat for thirty seconds.

LEVEL II:

Start in the position from level I, lying on your stomach with your hands behind your ears. As you exhale, squeeze your shoulder blades together and lift your elbows. Keep the elbows lifted, and as you inhale, bring your hands away from your ears so that your elbow is at a 90-degree angle. As you exhale, touch the back of your head. Repeat for thirty seconds.

LEVEL III:

Start in the position from level I, but with your elbows at 90 degrees and your forearms parallel to each other. As you exhale, lift your arms and draw the elbows to the ribs. As you inhale, come back to the starting position. Repeat for thirty seconds.

30-SECOND BREAK

SIDE PLANK RIGHT (30 SECONDS)

LEVEL I:

Lie on your right side. Bend your knees to 90 degrees. You should be one long line between your knees and the top of your head. Bring your right elbow under your right shoulder with your forearm on the floor pointing forward at a 90-degree angle to your shoulder. As you exhale, lift your hips off the ground, squeeze your shoulder blades together, and reach your left arm up toward the ceiling with your palm facing forward. Think about pressing the hips forward to engage your glutes (booty muscles). Hold for thirty seconds.

LEVEL II:

Start in the position from level I, but with your knees straight instead of bent. As you exhale, lift the hips off the ground, squeeze your shoulder blades together, and reach your left arm up toward the ceiling with your palm facing forward. Think about pressing the hips forward to engage your glutes (booty muscles). Hold for thirty seconds.

LEVEL III:

Start in the position from level II. Think about pressing the hips forward to engage your glutes (booty muscles). As you exhale, lift your left leg up. Hold for thirty seconds.

30-SECOND BREAK

SIDE PLANK LEFT (30 SECONDS)

Same as above, but to the left.

30-SECOND BREAK

PLIE SQUAT (30 SECONDS)

LEVEL I:

Bring your feet a little bit wider than hip-width apart. Turn your toes and knees out 45 degrees, with your arms straight down toward the ground and your palms together. Press through the outer edges of your feet (lifting the arches). Bend your knees and sit your butt back, touching your fingertips to the floor in between your feet. As you exhale, press through your heels and big toe to stand back up. Repeat for thirty seconds.

LEVEL II:

Start in the position from level I. Bend your knees and sit your butt back, touching your fingertips to the floor in between your feet. As you exhale, press through your heels and big toe to stand back up. As you stand up, reach your arms overhead. Repeat for thirty seconds.

LEVEL III:

Start in the position from level I. Bend your knees and sit your butt back, touching your fingertips to the floor in between your feet. As you exhale, stand back up, adding a jump with both feet coming off the ground and your hands reaching up toward the ceiling. Land softly with your hands at your chest and repeat. Repeat for thirty seconds.

30-SECOND BREAK

* Repeat sequence 5x for a 30-minute workout

INTERVAL TRAINING ROUTINE FOR OVULATION

For this interval training workout, you'll perform the six exercises listed. Do each exercise for thirty seconds, taking a thirty-second break between exercises. Repeat the series five times. Be sure to stand up during the transition time between exercises to maximize benefits!

Bonus points if you give yourself five minutes after your workout to lie on your back for a mini-meditation! If you have a hard time meditating, you might find it a little bit easier after a good sweat session.

Check out eating-moving.com/workouts for a video version!

Exercises: Perform each exercise for 30 seconds, with a 30-second break

1. Lunge Chops Right

2. Low Lunge Chops Left

3. Push-ups

4. Goddess Pose Hold

5. Knees to Elbow

6. Swimmies Lying on Stomach

*Repeat sequence 5x for a 30-minute workout

LOW LUNGE CHOPS RIGHT (30 SECONDS)

LEVEL I:

Start in a half kneel with your right foot forward and your left knee on the ground directly under your left hip. Your front knee should be at a 90-degree angle. Remember to keep your stacked posture. Now, bring your hands in front of you with your palms touching and arms parallel to the ground. Keeping your legs where they are, exhale and bring your hands just over the right thigh (only rotating your arms two to three inches). As you inhale, come back center. Repeat for thirty seconds.

LEVEL II:

Start in the same position as level I. Tuck your back toes under and lift your back knee off the ground. With your arms in front of you, exhale and bring your hands just over the right thigh (only rotating your arms two to three inches). As you inhale, come back center. Repeat for thirty seconds.

LEVEL III:

Start in the position from level II. Exhale and bring your hands just over the right thigh (only rotating your arms two to three inches). As you inhale, back to center. Now, as you exhale, bring your left leg forward (standing up) and bring your left knee up to tap the outstretched hands. As you inhale, come back into your high lunge. Repeat for thirty seconds.

30-SECOND BREAK

LOW LUNGE CHOPS LEFT (30 SECONDS)

Same as above, but to the left.

30-SECOND BREAK

PUSH-UPS (30 SECONDS)

LEVEL I:

The first level is an elevated push-up to help build strength with good form. Start at a stable, elevated surface (think countertop) in a plank position with your hands a little bit wider than your shoulders. Keep your stacked posture with your heels lifted and a slight bend in your knees. Bend your elbows to 90 degrees, keeping your plank position stable as you do so. Exhale, push back up to your elevated plank. Repeat for thirty seconds.

Note: make sure your elbows are at the level of your body before moving to level II or III.

LEVEL II:

Lie on your stomach with your hands just outside your chest. Your thumbs should be by your armpits and your fingertips under your shoulders. Keep your knees on the ground and press your body straight up. Remember to stay stacked throughout the whole motion. Repeat for thirty seconds.

PRO TIP:

Use a yoga block (at medium height) or two rolled-up towels under your chest to see how deep you're going into your push-up. Try to touch your chest to the towel, or block, with every repetition. Until you can do several reps with full range of motion, don't move on to the next variation. You're better served doing quality reps at a lower level than compromised ones at a higher level.

LEVEL III:

Start in the position from level II. Press straight up to the top of your push-up position. Perform push-ups from a high plank, keeping stacked and making sure your chest doesn't go lower than your arms. Repeat for thirty seconds.

30-SECOND BREAK

GODDESS POSE HOLD (30 SECONDS)

LEVEL I:

Bring your feet wider than hip-width apart with your toes and knees pointing out 45 degrees. Your hands will be pressed together in front of you at the sternum or breastbone (think prayer hands). Pushing your hips back, sit down into a squat. Make sure to keep your knees pressed outward. Hold for thirty seconds.

LEVEL II:

Start in the position from level I, but bring your arms out wide with your elbows bent at 90 degrees. Make sure to squeeze your shoulder blades together and keep your knees pressed outward. Hold for thirty seconds.

LEVEL III:

Start in the position from level I, but bring your arms overhead with the arms parallel. Hold for thirty seconds.

30-SECOND BREAK

KNEE TO ELBOW (30 SECONDS)

LEVEL I:

Level I is downward-facing dog. Start in a tabletop position (with your hands under your shoulders and your knees under your hips) and press through your hands to lift your hips and straighten your legs. Downward-facing dog is an upside-down V. You should be one line from your hips to your heels, allowing a slight bend in your knees, and one line from your hips to your hands. Your shoulders should be dropping away from your ears and your shoulder blades drawing together and toward the tailbone. Think about pressing your chest towards your legs. Hold for thirty seconds.

> **PRO TIP:**
>
> If the backs of your legs are tight, bend your knees! As you bend your knees, focus on pressing into the ground and pushing your hips up and back. Remember, it's okay if your heels don't touch the ground here. Notice if it feels any easier to keep your back in a straight line and upper body engaged if you bend your knees and let your heels lift off the ground.

LEVEL II:

Start in the position from level I (downward-facing dog). As you inhale, lift your right leg, keeping the leg straight. As you exhale, bring the leg back down, coming back into downward-facing dog. Repeat for thirty seconds, alternating legs.

LEVEL III:

Start in the position from level I (downward-facing dog). As you inhale, lift your right leg, keeping the leg straight. As you exhale, shift forward into plank and tap your right knee to your right elbow. As you inhale, lift the leg again. Exhale back to downward-facing dog. Repeat for thirty seconds, alternating legs.

30-SECOND BREAK

SWIMMIES LYING ON STOMACH (30 SECONDS)

LEVEL I:

Lie on your stomach with your arms extended forward and thumbs pointing towards the ceiling. Make sure to keep your hip bones pressed into the ground here. Tuck your chin and lift your left arm a centimeter off the ground as you exhale. As you inhale, put your left arm back down. As you exhale, lift the opposite arm. Repeat for thirty seconds.

LEVEL II:

Start in the position from level I. Tuck your chin, and as you exhale, lift your left arm and right leg a centimeter off the ground. As you inhale, put the arm and leg down. As you exhale, lift the opposite arm and leg. Repeat for thirty seconds.

> **PRO TIP:**
>
> Keep your ribs and hips glued to the ground. Remember, you should have no discomfort in your lower back here.

LEVEL III:

Start in the position from level I. Tuck your chin, and as you exhale, lift both arms and legs a centimeter off the ground. Keep both arms and legs lifted and quickly alternate the opposite arm and leg. Repeat for thirty seconds.

30-SECOND BREAK

*Repeat sequence 5x for a 30-minute workout

INTERVAL TRAINING ROUTINE FOR THE LUTEAL PHASE

For this interval training workout, you'll perform the six exercises listed. Do each exercise for thirty seconds, taking a thirty-second break between exercises. Repeat the series five times. Be sure to stand up during the transition time between exercises to maximize benefits!

Bonus points if you give yourself five minutes after your workout to lie on your back for a mini-meditation! If you have a hard time meditating, you might find it a little bit easier after a good sweat session.

Check out eating-moving.com/workouts for a video version!

Exercises: Perform exercise each for 30 seconds with a 30-second break

1. Low Lunge Rotation Right

2. Low Lunge Rotation Left

3. Forearm Plank

4. Wall Sit

5. Snow Angels

6. Bird Dog

*Repeat sequence 5x for a 30-minute workout

LOW LUNGE ROTATION RIGHT (30 SECONDS)

LEVEL I:

Start in a half kneel with your right foot forward and your left knee on the ground directly under your left hip. Your front knee should be at a 90-degree angle. Make sure you remain in your stacked position. Bring your palms together at your breastbone and rotate, hooking the back of your left arm over your right leg. Hold for thirty seconds.

LEVEL II:

Start in the position from level I. Bring your palms together at your breastbone and rotate, hooking the back of your left arm over your right leg. Now, tuck your left toes under and lift your back knee. Hold for thirty seconds.

LEVEL III:

Start in the position from level II. Staying in your twist, squeeze your shoulder blades together and open your arms. Hold for thirty seconds.

30-SECOND BREAK

LOW LUNGE ROTATION LEFT (30 SECONDS)

Same as above, but to the left.

30-SECOND BREAK

FOREARM PLANK (30 SECONDS)

LEVEL I:

Start in a tabletop position with your hands under your shoulders and your knees under your hips. Drop your elbows to the ground underneath your shoulders with your palms and forearms on the ground, facing forward. Keep your forearms parallel. Straighten your legs into a plank to find your leg position, and then drop your knees to the ground. Remember to stay stacked here and work on your belly breathing. Hold for thirty seconds.

> **PRO TIP:**
>
> Remember, your abdomen will move as you breathe here! There should be a gentle expansion of your abdomen as you inhale, and your low belly should draw in as you exhale.

LEVEL II:

Start in the position from level I without your knees dropped to the ground. Work on your belly breathing. Hold for thirty seconds.

LEVEL III:

Start in the position from level II. Holding this position, as you exhale, tap your right foot six inches out to the side. As you inhale, come back to center. Repeat for thirty seconds, alternating sides.

30-SECOND BREAK

WALL SIT (30 SECONDS)

*If you don't have a wall available, just do the chair squats from the menstruation workout!

LEVEL I:

Sit against a wall with your hips and knees at 90 degrees and your back and head against the wall. Bring your elbows into your ribs with the palms facing up and thumbs out, like you're holding a tray. Remember to squeeze your shoulder blades together and work on your belly breathing. Hold for thirty seconds.

LEVEL II:

Start in the position from level I, but as you exhale, reach your arms in front of you with the arms parallel to the ground and the palms facing toward the floor. Remember to squeeze your shoulder blades together and work on your belly breathing. Hold for thirty seconds.

LEVEL III:

Same as level I, but with your arms out wide against the wall with your elbows bent to 90 degrees. As you exhale, keep your shoulders back against the wall, touch your hands to your shoulders. As you inhale, come back to the starting position. Repeat for thirty seconds.

30-SECOND BREAK

SNOW ANGELS (30 SECONDS)

LEVEL I:

Lie on your stomach with your forehead supported by a rolled-up towel. Bring your hands wider than your ears with your elbows bent and pointing towards your legs. As you exhale, squeeze your shoulder blades, and lift your arms. As you inhale, relax. Repeat for thirty seconds.

LEVEL II:

Start from the position from level I. As you exhale, squeeze your shoulder blades and lift your arms, hugging your elbows down to your ribs. Keep your arms lifted throughout the entire exercise. As you inhale, come back to your original position. Repeat for thirty seconds.

LEVEL III:

Start in the position from level I. As you exhale, squeeze your shoulder blades and lift your arms, hugging your elbows down to your ribs. As you inhale, reach your arms as far above your head as you can. Keep the arms lifted the entire time. Repeat for thirty seconds.

30-SECOND BREAK

BIRD DOG (30 SECONDS)

LEVEL I:

Start in a tabletop position with your hands under your shoulders and your knees under your hips. As you inhale, straighten and lift your right leg. Think about pointing your toes down towards the ground and rolling your inner thigh up towards the ceiling. As you exhale, come back into tabletop position. As you inhale, straighten your left leg. Repeat for thirty seconds, alternating sides.

> **PRO TIP:**
>
> Keep your lower ribs pressing toward the spine (in other words, stay stacked) to prevent too much arch in the lower back.

LEVEL II:

Start in the position from level I. As you inhale, lift your left leg and right arm. As you exhale, come back into tabletop position. Repeat for thirty seconds, alternating sides.

LEVEL III:

Start in the position from level I. As you inhale, straighten and lift the right leg and left arm. As you exhale, bring your arm and leg out to the side six inches, keeping your core stable. As you inhale, back to center. As you exhale, come back into tabletop position. Repeat for thirty seconds, alternating sides.

30-SECOND BREAK

*Repeat sequence 5x for a 30-minute workout

YOGA WORKOUTS

If you're new to yoga, don't worry—we all start somewhere! Feel free to modify and move in ways that feel good for your body.

It's important to note you shouldn't have any joint pain, discomfort, numbness, or tingling in any of the postures. If you have glaucoma or hypertension (if you're taking high blood pressure medication, this means you, too!), talk to your doctor before practicing positions where your head is below your heart or your legs are above your heart. As always, if you have any questions about whether an exercise program is right for you, talk to your physician or physical therapist.

> Before you start with the postures, let's begin with some easy breath work. To work on your breathing, start in a sitting or standing position. Place one hand on your belly and one on your chest. Inhale deeply through your nose and try to pull the air down into your belly. Feel your belly rise under your hand while the hand on your chest remains mostly still. Exhale through pursed lips, as if to blow out a candle across the room, and feel your belly tense and draw in as you do. Try to find this same breathing pattern in all of the postures.

If you've never done yoga before, start with five deep belly breaths in each posture. If you've been practicing and feel comfortable with the postures, hold for ten breaths in each pose.

A NOTE FROM THE AUTHORS:

Remember, there are many different types and styles of yoga, and this section is just meant as an introduction to the physical postures.

If you're curious and want to learn more about the full practice, we highly recommend exploring different teachers and studios in your area! If you find a space that resonates with your physical, mental, and spiritual needs, you are more likely to stick with it.

Yoga with Adriene on YouTube is a great place to start, especially if it's challenging for you to make it to group or in-person classes. Bonus—she offers classes that are different time lengths. A twenty-minute practice is so much better than no practice!

And remember, yoga is not a religion but a practice that emphasizes self-awareness and exploration of the self through breath, movement, and stillness.

YOGA AND STRETCHING ROUTINE FOR MENSTRUATION

THE BASICS

This is the verbiage that will be used in almost every workout.

Stay Stacked: Find your basic posture, keeping your head stacked over your shoulders and your shoulders stacked over your hips. Think of good standing posture here.

OPTIONS FOR MODIFICATIONS:

Less Heat: options for a more restful practice.

More Heat: options to increase the intensity of your practice.

Flow for Menstruation (hold each posture for five to ten breaths):

1. Child's Pose

2. Child's Pose with Side Reach (Right)

3. Child's Pose with Side Reach (Left)

4. Cat/Cow

5. Low Lunge (Right)

6. Low Lunge Side Reach (Right)

7. Lizard Lunge (Right)

8. Low Lunge (Left)

9. Low Lunge Side Reach (Left)

10. Lizard Lunge (Left)

11. Double Knee to Chest

12. Modified Happy Baby Pose

13. Figure Four Stretch (Right)

14. Figure Four Stretch (Left)

15. Supine Butterfly

16. Resting Pose (Savasana)

1. CHILD'S POSE

Start on your yoga mat with your hands under your shoulders and your knees under your hips. This is known as tabletop position. From here, press your hips back towards your heels, letting them rest there. Your arms can be reaching forward or by your sides. Let your neck relax. Hold for five to ten deep belly breaths.

> **PRO TIP:**
>
> If you have knee pain or hip issues, you can bring your knees wider. If you have shoulder discomfort you can rest your arms by your sides or cross your forearms over each other and rest your forehead on your arms.

2. CHILD'S POSE WITH SIDE REACH (RIGHT)

From child's pose, stretch your hands forward. As you inhale, reach a little bit further forward, lengthening your spine. From there, gently walk your hands to the right side of the mat until you feel a stretch down the left side of your body. Hold for five to ten deep belly breaths and then come back to child's pose.

3. CHILD'S POSE WITH SIDE REACH (LEFT)

Same as above, but to the left.

4. CAT/COW

From child's pose, come back into tabletop position, bringing your hands under your shoulders and knees under your hips. Make sure that your lower back isn't dropping too far towards the ground.

As you inhale, let your lower spine and belly drop towards the ground, chest reaching forward, looking in front of your mat. Think about stretching the front of your body.

As you exhale, press your hands into the ground, tuck your chin to your chest, and round your back like an angry cat. Think about stretching the back of your body and pulling your shoulder blades apart here.

With each inhale, lower your belly, and with each exhale, round your back towards the ceiling. Perform each movement five to ten times, moving with your inhales and exhales.

PRO TIP:

Don't look all the way up towards the ceiling, as this may put too much stress on the neck. Think about bringing your gaze in front of your mat or to the wall in front of you as you inhale. As you exhale, tuck your chin to your chest and bring the gaze towards your belly button.

5. LOW LUNGE (RIGHT)

Come back into tabletop position with your hands under your shoulders and your knees under your hips. Step your right foot between your hands. From there, bring your hands to your right thigh and stack your shoulders above your hips. Your right knee should be above your ankle with your knee at a 90-degree angle; your knee should not go over your toes. Remember to stay stacked. Hold for five to ten deep belly breaths.

Note: perform whole low lunge series before switching to the opposite side.

More Heat

To work on balance and increase the intensity, reach your fingertips up towards the ceiling with your palms facing each other. Remember to stay stacked. You can also tuck your back toes under your heel and lift your knee to bring this into a high lunge for even more heat! Squeezing your booty here will help keep your lower back from arching.

6. LOW LUNGE SIDE REACH (RIGHT)

From your low lunge with the right leg forward, bring your right hand to your right thigh, and lift your left fingertips up towards the ceiling with the palm towards your ear. As you inhale, reach your arm up and over towards the right, feeling the stretch along the left side of your body. Hold for five to ten deep belly breaths. When you're done, come back to your low lunge with both hands reaching up towards the ceiling.

7. LIZARD LUNGE (RIGHT)

Start in low lunge with both palms reaching up towards the ceiling. As you exhale, bring your hands to the floor on the inside of your right foot. You can move your front foot out slightly and modify your leg position to your comfort. Your front knee should not go past the ankle, and there should be no pain or discomfort in your knee or hip. Take five to ten deep belly breaths. Once you have finished your five to ten deep breaths, bring your hands on either side of your front foot. Step your right leg back into tabletop position.

PRO TIP:

For more of an inner thigh stretch, roll onto the outside edge of your foot and push your knee out.

8. LOW LUNGE (LEFT)

Same sequence, starting with low lunge on the left.

9. LOW LUNGE SIDE REACH (LEFT)

Same as above, but to the left.

10. LIZARD LUNGE (LEFT)

Same as above, but to the left.

11. DOUBLE KNEE TO CHEST STRETCH

Transition from tabletop to lying on your back. Once on your back, hug both knees to your chest. You can spend a few breaths rocking side to side, gently massaging your low back. Hold for five to ten deep belly breaths.

12. MODIFIED HAPPY BABY POSE

Start with both knees hugged in towards your chest, and let your big toes touch and your knees fall to the sides. Your hands can be on the inside of your shins or around your knees. Hold for five to ten deep belly breaths, and then draw your knees back towards each other.

PRO TIP:

You can also grab the outer edges of your feet and bring the soles of your feet up to face the ceiling. You can keep your feet hip-width apart or a little bit wider. Feel free to rock side to side or bend and straighten your knees here. Do whichever variation feels best in your body!

13. SUPINE FIGURE FOUR STRETCH (RIGHT)

From knees to chest, place your feet on the ground with your knees bent. Cross your right ankle over your left knee. You can stay there or interlace your hands behind your left leg to gently pull your legs in towards your body. You should feel the stretch in the back of your right hip. Hold for five to ten deep belly breaths. Uncross your legs and place both feet on the ground.

14. SUPINE FIGURE FOUR STRETCH (LEFT)

Same as above, but to the left.

15. SUPINE BUTTERFLY STRETCH

With both feet back on the ground, bring the soles of your feet together and let your knees fall gently out to the sides, supporting your knees with pillows or blankets if needed for comfort. If you're experiencing discomfort in your low back, try placing a bolster under your back for more support. Place your hands on your belly or by your sides. Hold for five to ten deep belly breaths.

16. RESTING POSE (SAVASANA)

Lying on your back, straighten your legs and let them relax. Let your arms rest by your sides, palms facing up. Hold for ten to twenty deep belly breaths or set a timer for an amount of time that feels good for you!

PRO TIP:

As thoughts, feelings, emotions, or sensations come up (which they definitely do; after all, we're human!), come back to your breathing. You can count in for five and out for five as you breathe in and out through the nose. Maybe notice a gentle "saw" sound as you inhale through the nose, a gentle "haw" sound as you exhale, or notice the cooling sensation as air enters the nose on the inhale, the warming sensation as air leaves the nose on the exhale.

YOGA AND STRETCHING ROUTINE FOR THE FOLLICULAR PHASE

THE BASICS

This is the verbiage that will be used in almost every workout.

Stay Stacked: Find your basic posture, keeping your head stacked over your shoulders and your shoulders stacked over your hips. Think of good standing posture here.

OPTIONS FOR MODIFICATIONS:

Less Heat: options for a more restful practice.

More Heat: options to increase the intensity of your practice.

Flow for the Follicular Phase (hold each posture for 5-10 breaths):

1. Standing Power Pose (Mountain Pose)

2. Standing Side Stretch (RIGHT)

3. Standing Side Stretch (LEFT)

4. Forward Fold

5. Plank

6. Downward-Facing Dog

7. Baby Cobra

8. Downward-Facing Dog

9. Forward Fold

10. Triangle Pose (RIGHT)

11. Triangle Pose (LEFT)

12. Goddess Pose

13. Modified Half Lord of the Fishes (RIGHT)

14. Modified Half Lord of the Fishes (LEFT)

15. Seated Forward Fold (with legs crossed)

16. Resting Pose (Savasana)

1. STANDING POWER POSE (MOUNTAIN POSE)

Stand with your feet hip-width apart and toes pointing forward. Bend your knees slightly. Bring one hand to your front ribs right under your bra line and the other to your tailbone. Press your ribs towards your spine, and hips forward. You should feel your core engage here. Squeeze your shoulders together, and with your arms by your sides, roll your palms forward with the thumbs facing out. Lift through the back of your neck and draw your chin back, keeping your chin parallel to the ground and your ears over your shoulders. Remember to stay stacked here. Hold for five to ten deep belly breaths.

PRO TIP:

Remember, your belly should expand as you inhale and gently draw in towards your spine as you exhale.

2. STANDING SIDE STRETCH (RIGHT)

As you inhale, reach your arms up towards the ceiling with your palms facing each other or your fingers interlaced with your first finger pointing upward. Rock from side to side for a few breaths, feeling the stretch in the sides of your body. On an inhale, come back to center and stand as tall as you can with your fingertips reaching towards the ceiling. As you exhale, reach your hands to the right, pressing through your left foot and feeling the stretch in the left side of your body. You can keep your left arm lifted or let your left arm drop to your left side. Hold for five to ten deep belly breaths, and then come back to center.

PRO TIP:

Keep all of the other elements of your mountain pose while you're in this posture! Try to stand like you're in between two panes of glass, and remember, we're stretching both sides here, not just the left.

If interlacing your fingers is challenging, reach both hands as far upward as is comfortable and do your side stretch from there.

3. STANDING SIDE STRETCH (LEFT)

Same as above, but to the left.

4. FORWARD FOLD

Start in a standing position with your arms reaching towards the ceiling. Bend your upper body over your legs, coming into a forward fold. Keep your knees bent to take pressure off of your low back and improve the stretch in the back of your legs. As you inhale, think about lengthening your spine, and as you exhale, let your upper body relax over your legs. Hold for five to ten deep belly breaths.

5. PLANK

From forward fold, bend your knees and bring your hands to the floor, stepping back into plank. Stay stacked here, and remember, it's okay for your abdomen to move with your breathing, but we want to keep the back nice and still. Planks should be challenging! Hold for five to ten deep belly breaths.

PRO TIP:

Plank involves the same principles as mountain pose, so think about all the tips for finding good standing posture and you'll be in an amazing plank! Slightly bend your knees, press your hips down towards the ground, and draw your lower ribs back towards your spine. Another way to think about this is lifting your belly button away from the floor. Now, think about drawing your kneecaps up and squeezing those glutes (booty muscles).

Less Heat

From your high plank, drop your knees to the ground. Stay stacked here, keeping your body in one long line from your knees to the top of your head.

6. DOWNWARD-FACING DOG:

In plank, with your fingertips spread wide, press through your hands to push your hips up and back towards the wall behind you. Downward-facing dog is an upside-down V. You should be one line from your hips to your heels, allowing a slight bend in your knees, and one line from your hips to your hands. Your shoulders should be dropping away from your ears and your shoulder blades drawing together and towards the tailbone. Think about pressing your chest towards your legs. Hold for five to ten deep belly breaths.

PRO TIP:

If the backs of your legs are tight, bend your knees! As you bend your knees, focus on pressing into the ground and pushing your hips up and back. Remember, it's okay if your heels don't touch the ground here. Notice if it feels any easier to keep your back in a straight line and upper body engaged if you bend your knees and let your heels lift off the ground.

Less Heat

Child's pose is a great modification for downward-facing dog. Just drop your knees towards the ground, press your hips to your heels, and focus on your slow deep breathing.

You can also do downward-facing dog against a wall! Place your hands at shoulder height on a wall and walk your feet back, bending at your hip. Press your hips back until you are one line from your hips to your heels and one line from your hips to your hands.

6. PLANK

From downward-facing dog, shift back into high plank or low plank with your knees touching the ground. Hold for five to ten deep belly breaths.

Less heat

If you're already feeling the burn, feel free to skip the hold and go right to the next posture in the series, baby cobra!

7. BABY COBRA

From plank, drop your knees to the ground and slowly lower your body all the way down to the ground, keeping your elbows tight to your ribs and trying to keep your upper body and torso in a straight line from your knees to the top of your head. Once you are on the ground, bring your hands by your shoulders, keeping your elbows by the ribs. As you inhale, squeeze your shoulder blades together and lift the front of your shoulders and chest off of the mat. Your gaze should be two to three inches in front of the mat, and remember, you're not pressing up into a big backbend, you're using your back muscles to lift your shoulders and chest, keeping your shoulder blades down and back (away from the ears). Keep the connection between your hips and the ground, thinking about pressing down through your hips and belly button as you lift and squeeze your shoulders. Hold for five to ten deep belly breaths. From your baby cobra, press back up to your knees, tuck the toes, and lift your hips, finding your downward-facing dog.

PRO TIP:

You should have no discomfort with baby cobra or any other backbends. If you have any pain or discomfort, try coming out of the posture a little bit, finding a place where you don't have any pain.

8. DOWNWARD-FACING DOG

From plank, with your fingertips spread wide, press through your hands to push your hips up and back into your downward-facing dog. Hold for five to ten deep belly breaths.

9. FORWARD FOLD

From your downward-facing dog, walk your hands to your feet or step your feet to your hands, coming into your forward fold. Keep your knees bent to take pressure off your low back and improve the stretch in the back of your legs. As you inhale, think about lengthening your spine, and as you exhale, let your upper body relax over your legs. Hold for five to ten deep belly breaths.

10. TRIANGLE POSE (RIGHT)

Turn towards the left long edge of your mat. Bring your arms out wide and parallel to the ground, and step your feet wide, about three to five feet apart. Turn your right toes towards the right short edge of your mat with the left toes pointing slightly towards the right foot. Keeping the right arm parallel to the ground, reach the right arm as far as you can over the right leg. When you can't reach any further, drop your arm down towards your leg, coming into triangle pose. Hold for five to ten deep belly breaths. Now, turn so that your feet are facing towards the long edge of the mat with your arms parallel to the ground.

PRO TIP:

Your right leg will stay relatively straight, but remember to keep a tiny bend in your knee to protect your knee joint from overstretching. For this posture, you should be positioned like you're in between two panes of glass. Remember, you don't have to touch the ground! In fact, if you try, you might notice that your upper body has to bend to get there. This is why you reach the arm as far as it will go first and drop your arm after—it keeps your spine from dropping too far into the posture. Keep your upper body engaged by thinking about squeezing your shoulder blades together. You can even use your leg to create resistance as you press the back of your right hand or forearm into your leg.

11. TRIANGLE POSE (LEFT)

Same as above, but to the left.

12. GODDESS POSE

From your wide-legged stance, bring your hands together at your heart. Now, take a small step in, with your feet wider than hip-width apart. Bring your heels in, and keep your toes out at a 45-degree angle—your knees should be pointing with your toes here, not dropping in. Now, sit back into your goddess squat (similar to a plie squat). Think about pressing your knees out to engage your hip muscles. Your knees shouldn't go past the toes, so think about sitting back into your squat. Hold for five to ten deep belly breaths.

More heat

Bring your arms to goal post or cactus arms to build a little bit more heat here!

13. MODIFIED HALF LORD OF THE FISHES (RIGHT)

From standing, make your way into a seated position with your legs stretched out in front of you. Bend your right knee and place your right foot on the ground on the outside of the left thigh. Hug your right knee in towards your body to feel the stretch in your right hip. If that feels good, reach your right hand behind you and twist to the right. As you inhale, think about sitting as tall as you can. As you exhale, hug your leg toward your body and twist. Hold for five to ten deep belly breaths. When you're done, straighten your leg out in front of you.

> **PRO TIP:**
>
> You can also hook your left elbow over your right thigh to deepen the twist. Make sure you can still sit up tall when in this position!

14. MODIFIED HALF LORD OF THE FISHES (LEFT)

Same as above, but to the left.

15. SEATED FORWARD FOLD (WITH LEGS CROSSED)

Start with your legs straight out in front of you. Bend your knees and come into an easy seated position with your knees bent and legs crossed (think criss-cross applesauce). Before coming into your forward fold, grab onto your shins, and as you exhale, roll onto your tailbone, tuck your chin to your chest, and round your back towards the wall behind you. Option to stay here for a few breaths or inhale, sit as tall as you can, and exhale to fold over your legs, reaching the fingertips forward and letting your upper body relax over your legs. Hold for five to ten deep belly breaths.

16. RESTING POSE (SAVASANA)

Lying on your back, straighten your legs and let them relax. Let your arms rest by your sides, palms facing up. Hold for ten to twenty deep belly breaths or set a timer for an amount of time that feels good for you!

PRO TIP:

As thoughts, feelings, emotions, or sensations come up (which they definitely do; after all, we're human!), come back to your breathing. You can count in for five and out for five as you breathe in and out through the nose. Maybe notice a gentle "saw" sound as you inhale through the nose, a gentle "haw" sound as you exhale, or notice the cooling sensation as air enters the nose on the inhale, the warming sensation as air leaves the nose on the exhale.

YOGA AND STRETCHING ROUTINE FOR OVULATION

THE BASICS

This is the verbiage that will be used in almost every workout.

Stay Stacked: Find your basic posture, keeping your head stacked over your shoulders and your shoulders stacked over your hips. Think of good standing posture here.

OPTIONS FOR MODIFICATIONS:

Less Heat: options for a more restful practice

More Heat: options to increase the intensity of your practice

Flow for the Follicular Phase (hold each posture for 5-10 breaths):

1. Standing Power Pose (Mountain Pose)
2. Chair Pose
3. Chair Pose with Mini Twist (Right)
4. Chair Pose with Mini Twist (Left)
5. Forward Fold
6. Plank
7. Modified Locust Pose
8. Downward-Facing Dog
9. Forearm Plank
10. Forward fold
11. Warrior II (right)
12. Modified Side Angle (Right)
13. Warrior II (Left)
14. Modified Side Angle (Left)
15. Wide Legged Forward Fold
16. Resting Pose (Savasana)

1. STANDING POWER POSE (MOUNTAIN POSE)

Stand with your feet hip-width apart and toes pointing forward. Bend your knees slightly. Bring one hand to your front ribs right under your bra line and the other to your tailbone. Press your ribs towards your spine, and hips forward. You should feel your core engage here. Squeeze your shoulders together, and with your arms by your sides, roll your palms forward with the thumbs facing out. Lift through the back of your neck and draw your chin back, keeping your chin parallel to the ground and your ears over your shoulders. Remember to stay stacked here. Hold for five to ten deep belly breaths.

PRO TIP:

Remember, your belly should expand as you inhale and gently draw in towards your spine as you exhale.

2. CHAIR POSE

Start in your mountain pose with your feet hip-width apart and knees and toes pointing forward. Bring your arms in front of you, parallel to the ground with your palms facing down. Squeeze your shoulder blades together and tuck your chin, keeping it parallel to the ground. Now, sit back like you're sitting in a chair and the chair is really far behind you; make sure your knees don't go past your toes here. Hold for five to ten deep belly breaths and then return to mountain pose.

PRO TIP:

Think about pressing your knees out and lifting the arches of your feet here. Your legs should be parallel and your knees and toes should be facing forward in this pose.

Less Heat

Start in a standing position, remembering correct posture. Bring your palms together with your hands at your heart. Sit back into your chair pose from there. You can also go less deep into your squat to decrease the work in your legs.

More heat

Start in a standing position (with good posture, of course!) and reach your arms overhead with your palms facing each other. Sit back into your chair from there.

3. CHAIR POSE WITH A MINI TWIST (RIGHT)

Start in mountain pose with your hands at your heart and drop your hips back, coming into chair pose. From chair pose, bring your left hand to the inside of the left knee and right hand to your low back or tailbone. Now, turn to the right and gaze directly to the right or over the right shoulder. Hold for five to ten deep belly breaths and then return to mountain pose.

4. CHAIR POSE WITH A MINI TWIST (LEFT)

Same as above, but to the left.

5. FORWARD FOLD

Start in a standing position with your arms reaching towards the ceiling. Bend your upper body over your legs, coming into a forward fold. Keep your knees bent to take pressure off your low back and improve the stretch in the back of your legs. As you inhale, think about lengthening your spine, and as you exhale, let your upper body relax over your legs. Hold for five to ten deep belly breaths.

6. PLANK

From forward fold, bend your knees and bring your hands to the floor, stepping back into plank. Stay stacked here, and remember, it's okay for your abdomen to move with your breathing, but we want to keep the back nice and still. Planks should be challenging! Hold for five to ten deep belly breaths.

PRO TIP:

Plank involves the same principles as mountain pose, so think about all the tips for finding good standing posture and you'll be in an amazing plank! Slightly bend your knees, press your hips down towards the ground, and draw your lower ribs back towards your spine. Another way to think about this is lifting your belly button away from the floor. Now, think about drawing your kneecaps up and squeezing those glutes (booty muscles).

Less Heat

From your high plank, drop your knees to the ground. Stay stacked here, keeping your body in one long line from your knees to the top of your head.

7. MODIFIED LOCUST POSE

From plank, drop your knees to the ground and slowly lower your body all the way down to the ground, keeping your elbows tight to your ribs and trying to keep your upper body and torso in a straight line from your knees to the top of your head. Once you are on the ground, bring your arms by your sides with your palms down. Squeeze your shoulder blades and lift your arms. Your gaze will be down towards your mat and you can support your forehead with a towel roll if that feels best. Keep the connection between your hips and the ground, thinking about pressing down through your hips and belly button as you squeeze your shoulders together and lift your arms. Hold for five to ten deep belly breaths.

More Heat

Keep your hips pressed into the mat. With your legs straight, lift your legs up off the mat.

8. DOWNWARD-FACING DOG

From plank, with your fingertips spread wide, press through your hands to push your hips up and back towards the wall behind you. Downward-facing dog is an upside-down V. You should be one line from your hips to your heels, allowing a slight bend in your knees, and one line from your hips to your hands. Your shoulders should be dropping away from your ears and your shoulder blades drawing together and towards the tailbone. Think about pressing your chest towards your legs. Hold for five to ten deep belly breaths.

PRO TIP:

If the backs of your legs are tight, bend your knees! As you bend your knees, focus on pressing into the ground and pushing your hips up and back. Remember, it's okay if your heels don't touch the ground here. Notice if it feels any easier to keep your back in a straight line and upper body engaged if you bend your knees and let your heels lift off the ground.

Less Heat

Child's pose is a great modification for downward-facing dog. Just drop your knees towards the ground, press your hips to your heels, and focus on your slow deep breathing.

You can also do downward-facing dog against a wall! Place your hands at shoulder height on a wall and walk your feet back, bending at your hip. Press your hips back until you are one line from your hips to your heels and one line from your hips to your hands.

9. FOREARM PLANK

From downward-facing dog, shift into plank or modified plank. Drop your elbows to the ground underneath your shoulders with your palms and forearms on the ground, facing forward. Keep your forearms parallel. Remember to stay stacked and keep your chin tucked. Hold your plank for five to ten deep belly breaths. When you're done, walk your hands back under your shoulders and press up into your downward-facing dog.

10. FORWARD FOLD

From your downward-facing dog, walk your hands to your feet or step your feet to your hands, coming into forward fold. Keep your knees bent to take pressure off of your low back and improve the stretch in the back of your legs. As you inhale, think about lengthening your spine, and as you exhale, let your upper body relax over your legs. Hold for five to ten deep belly breaths. When you're done, come back to standing.

11. WARRIOR II POSE (RIGHT)

Turn towards the left long edge of your mat. Bring your arms out wide and parallel to the ground, and step your feet wide, about three to five feet apart. Turn your right toes towards the right short edge of your mat with your left toes pointing slightly towards your right foot. Now, bend your right knee so that it's at a 90-degree angle; your right knee should not go past the ankle here. Think about pressing your knee out so you can see your big toe. Keep your upper body stacked over your hips and try not to lean forward. Now, think about pressing through the outer edge of your back foot and notice the arch of the back foot gently lifting as you do so. Once you're settled, hold for five to ten deep breaths. Keep your legs where they are as we build into the next posture, side angle pose!

12. MODIFIED SIDE ANGLE POSE (RIGHT)

From your Warrior II pose with your right knee bent, bend your right elbow and place your right forearm on your right thigh. Reach your left arm up towards the ceiling with your palm facing forward. Squeeze your shoulder blades here and think about drawing your front ribs back and down. Hold for five to ten deep belly breaths.

PRO TIP:

See if you can lift your right arm just a millimeter above your leg. Balance here and notice how strong your core is!

More Heat

Reach the left fingertips over your head with the palm facing towards the ground. You should be one long line from the left fingertips to the outer edge of the left foot. With the left arm overhead, straighten and lift your right arm so that it's parallel to the left arm. Hold there and focus on your slow, deep belly breathing.

13. WARRIOR II POSE (LEFT)

Same as above, but to the left.

14. MODIFIED SIDE ANGLE POSE (LEFT)

Same as above, but to the left.

15. WIDE-LEGGED FORWARD FOLD

From your wide-legged stance, bend your knees and let your upper body fold over your legs. As you inhale, imagine your spine lengthening, and as you exhale, feel your upper body relaxing over your legs. Hold for five to ten deep belly breaths, and then make your way onto your back.

PRO TIP:

You can also add a side reach here. As you inhale, think about lengthening your upper body and spine, reach the fingertips as far forward as they'll go, and as you exhale, walk your hands to the left. Hold for five to ten breaths and switch sides.

16. RESTING POST (SAVASANA)

Lying on your back, straighten your legs and let them relax. Let your arms rest by your sides, palms facing up. Hold for ten to twenty deep belly breaths or set a timer for an amount of time that feels good for you!

PRO TIP:

As thoughts, feelings, emotions, or sensations come up (which they definitely do; after all, we're human!), come back to your breathing. You can count in for five and out for five as you breathe in and out through the nose. Maybe notice a gentle "saw" sound as you inhale through the nose, a gentle "haw" sound as you exhale, or notice the cooling sensation as air enters the nose on the inhale, the warming sensation as air leaves the nose on the exhale.

YOGA AND STRETCHING ROUTINE FOR THE LUTEAL PHASE

THE BASICS

This is the verbiage that will be used in almost every workout.

Stay Stacked: Find your basic posture, keeping your head stacked over your shoulders and

your shoulders stacked over your hips. Think of good standing posture here.

OPTIONS FOR MODIFICATIONS:

Less Heat: options for a more restful practice

More Heat: options to increase the intensity of your practice

Flow for the Luteal Phase (hold each posture for 5-10 breaths):

1. Standing Power Pose (Mountain Pose)

2. Forward Fold

3. Plank

4. Downward-Facing Dog

5. Cat/Cow

6. Low Lunge (Right)

7. Low Lunge Twist (Right)

8. Lizard Lunge (Right)

9. Low Lunge (Left)

10. Low Lunge Twist (Left)

11. Lizard Lunge (Left)

12. Double Knee to Chest

13. Supine Hip Internal Rotation Stretch (right)

14. Supine Hip Internal Rotation Stretch (left)

15. Supine Butterfly Stretch

16. Resting Pose (Savasana)

1. STANDING POWER POSE (MOUNTAIN POSE)

Stand with your feet hip-width apart and toes pointing forward. Bend your knees slightly. Bring one hand to your front ribs right under your bra line and the other to your tailbone. Press your ribs towards your spine, and hips forward. You should feel your core engage here. Squeeze your shoulders together, and with your arms by your sides, roll your palms forward with the thumbs facing out. Lift through the back of your neck and draw your chin back, keeping your chin parallel to the ground and your ears over your shoulders. Remember to stay stacked here. Hold for five to ten deep belly breaths.

PRO TIP:

Remember, your belly should expand as you inhale and gently draw in towards your spine as you exhale.

2. FORWARD FOLD

Start in a standing position with your arms reaching towards the ceiling. Bend your upper body over your legs, coming into a forward fold. Keep your knees bent to take pressure off your low back and improve the stretch in the back of your legs. As you inhale, think about lengthening your spine, and as you exhale, let your upper body relax over your legs. Hold for five to ten deep belly breaths.

3. PLANK

From forward fold, bend your knees and bring your hands to the floor, stepping back into plank. Stay stacked here, and remember, it's okay for your abdomen to move with your breathing, but we want to keep the back nice and still. Planks should be challenging! Hold for five to ten deep belly breaths.

PRO TIP:

Plank involves the same principles as mountain pose, so think about all the tips for finding good standing posture and you'll be in an amazing plank! Slightly bend your knees, press your hips down towards the ground, and draw your lower ribs back towards your spine. Another way to think about this is lifting your belly button away from the floor. Now, think about drawing your kneecaps up and squeezing those glutes (booty muscles).

Less Heat

From your high plank, drop your knees to the ground. Stay stacked here, keeping your body in one long line from your knees to the top of your head.

4. DOWNWARD-FACING DOG:

From plank, with your fingertips spread wide, press through your hands to push your hips up and back towards the wall behind you. Downward-facing dog is an upside-down V. You should be one line from your hips to your heels, allowing a slight bend in your knees, and one line from your hips to your hands. Your shoulders should be dropping away from your ears and your shoulder blades drawing together and towards the tailbone. Think about pressing your chest towards your legs. Hold for five to ten deep belly breaths.

PRO TIP:

If the backs of your legs are tight, bend your knees! As you bend your knees, focus on pressing into the ground and pushing your hips up and back. Remember, it's okay if your heels don't touch the ground here. Notice if it feels any easier to keep your back in a straight line and upper body engaged if you bend your knees and let your heels lift off the ground.

Less Heat

Child's pose is a great modification for downward-facing dog. Just drop your knees towards the ground, press your hips to your heels, and focus on your slow deep breathing.

You can also do downward-facing dog against a wall! Place your hands at shoulder-height on a wall and walk your feet back, bending at your hip. Press your hips back until you are one line from your hips to your heels and one line from your hips to your hands.

5. CAT/COW

From downward-facing dog, drop your knees and come back into tabletop position, bringing your hands under your shoulders and knees under your hips. Make sure that your lower back isn't dropping too far towards the ground.

As you inhale, let your lower spine and belly drop towards the ground, chest reaching forward, looking in front of your mat. Think about stretching the front of your body.

As you exhale, press your hands into the ground, tuck your chin to your chest, and round your back like an angry cat. Think about stretching the back of your body and pulling your shoulder blades apart here.

With each inhale, lower your belly, and with each exhale, round your back towards the ceiling. Perform each movement five to ten times, moving with your inhales and exhales.

PRO TIP:

Don't look all the way up towards the ceiling, as this may put too much stress on the neck. Think about bringing your gaze in front of your mat or to the wall in front of you as you inhale. As you exhale, tuck your chin to your chest and bring the gaze towards your belly button.

6. LOW LUNGE (RIGHT)

Come back into tabletop position with your hands under your shoulders and your knees under your hips. Step your right foot between your hands. From there, bring your hands to your right thigh and stack your shoulders above your hips. Your right knee should be above your ankle with your knee at a 90-degree angle; your knee should not go over your toes. Remember to stay stacked. Hold for five to ten deep belly breaths.

Note: perform whole low lunge series before switching to the opposite side.

More Heat

To work on balance and increase the intensity, reach your fingertips up towards the ceiling with your palms facing each other. Remember to stay stacked. You can also tuck your back toes under your heel and lift your knee to bring this into a high lunge for even more heat! Squeezing your booty here will help keep your lower back from arching.

7. LOW LUNGE TWIST (RIGHT)

From your low lunge with your right leg forward, bring your arms out wide and parallel to the ground. As you exhale, twist to the right, reaching your right arm back and left arm towards the front leg. Hold for five to ten deep belly breaths. When you're done, come back to center, reaching your arms up towards the ceiling.

8. LIZARD LUNGE (RIGHT)

Start in your low lunge with both palms reaching up towards the ceiling. As you exhale, bring your hands to the floor on the inside of your right foot. You can move your front foot out slightly and modify your leg position to your comfort. Your front knee should not go past the ankle, and there should be no pain or discomfort in your knee or hip. Take five to ten deep belly breaths. Once you have finished your five to ten deep breaths, bring your hands on either side of your front foot. Step your right leg back into tabletop position.

PRO TIP:

For more of an inner thigh stretch, roll onto the outside edge of your foot and push your knee out.

9. LOW LUNGE (LEFT)

Same sequence, starting with low lunge on the left.

10. LOW LUNGE TWIST (LEFT)

Same as above, but to the left.

11. LIZARD LUNGE (LEFT)

Same as above, but to the left.

12. DOUBLE KNEE TO CHEST STRETCH

Transition from tabletop to lying on your back. Once on your back, hug both knees to your chest. You can spend a few breaths rocking side to side, gently massaging your low back. Hold for five to ten deep belly breaths.

13. SUPINE HIP INTERNAL ROTATION STRETCH (RIGHT)

Lie on your back with your knees bent and your feet on the ground. Keeping your knees bent to 90 degrees, walk your right foot out to the right long edge of the mat, letting your knee drop in towards the midline. If this feels okay on your knee and hip, you can bring your left foot over your right knee to add a little extra stretch. Remember, you should have no knee or hip pain here. Hold for five to ten deep belly breaths and when you're done, walk your feet back to center with your feet on the ground.

14. SUPINE HIP INTERNAL ROTATION STRETCH (LEFT)

Same as above, but to the left.

15. SUPINE BUTTERFLY STRETCH

With both feet back on the ground, bring the soles of your feet together and let your knees fall gently out to the sides, supporting your knees with pillows or blankets if needed for comfort. If you're experiencing discomfort in your low back, try placing a bolster under your back for more support. Place your hands on your belly or by your sides. Hold for five to ten deep belly breaths.

16. RESTING POSE (SAVASANA)

Lying on your back, straighten your legs and let them relax. Let your arms rest by your sides, palms facing up. Hold for ten to twenty deep belly breaths or set a timer for an amount of time that feels good for you!

PRO TIP:

As thoughts, feelings, emotions, or sensations come up (which they definitely do; after all, we're human!), come back to your breathing. You can count in for five and out for five as you breathe in and out through the nose. Maybe notice a gentle "saw" sound as you inhale through the nose, a gentle "haw" sound as you exhale, or notice the cooling sensation as air enters the nose on the inhale, the warming sensation as air leaves the nose on the exhale.

ENDNOTES

THE SCIENCE BEHIND YOUR CYCLE

1. Louise Dickerson, "Hormones," Encyclopedia.com, June 18, 2018, https://www.encyclopedia.com/science-and-technology/biochemistry/biochemistry/hormone#2830101168.

2. "The Endocrine System," Encyclopedia.com, n.d., https://www.encyclopedia.com/medicine/news-wires-white-papers-and-books/endocrine-system.

3. Dale Purves et al., "The Limbic System," essay, in *Neuroscience*, 2nd ed. (Sunderland, MA: Sinauer Associates, 2001), https://www.ncbi.nlm.nih.gov/books/NBK11060/.

4. Cristy Phillips, "Lifestyle Modulators of Neuroplasticity: How Physical Activity, Mental Engagement, and Diet Promote Cognitive Health during Aging," *Neural Plasticity* 2017 (June 12, 2017): 1–22, https://doi.org/10.1155/2017/3589271.

5. Dale Purves et al., "The Limbic System," essay, in *Neuroscience*, 2nd ed. (Sunderland, MA: Sinauer Associates, 2001), https://www.ncbi.nlm.nih.gov/books/NBK11060/.

6. "Pituitary Gland: What It Is, Function & Anatomy," Cleveland Clinic, October 8, 2020, https://my.clevelandclinic.org/health/body/21459-pituitary-gland.

7. S Caleb Freeman, Ahmad Malik, and Hajira Basit, "Physiology, Exocrine Gland," essay, in *StatPearls [Internet]* (Treasure Island, FL: StatPearls Publishing, 2021), https://www.ncbi.nlm.nih.gov/books/NBK542322/.

8. Shaul Feldman, Nissim Conforti, and Joseph Weidenfeld, "Limbic Pathways and Hypothalamic Neurotransmitters Mediating Adrenocortical Responses to Neural Stimuli," *Neuroscience & Biobehavioral Reviews* 19, no. 2 (1995): 235–40, https://doi.org/10.1016/0149-7634(94)00062-6.

9. Sherry Gaba, "Understanding Fight, Flight, Freeze and the Fawn Response," Psychology Today, August 22, 2020, https://www.psychologytoday.com/us/blog/addiction-and-recovery/202008/understanding-fight-flight-freeze-and-the-fawn-response.

10. Johannes Hertel et al., "Evidence for Stress-like Alterations in the Hpa-Axis in Women Taking Oral Contraceptives," *Scientific Reports* 7, no. 14111 (October 26, 2017), https://doi.org/10.1038/s41598-017-13927-7.

11. Shannon Whirledge and John A Cidlowski, "Glucocorticoids, Stress, and Fertility," *Minerva Endocrinologica* 35, no. 2 (June 2010): 109–25, https://doi.org/https://www.ncbi.nlm.nih.gov/pmc/articles/PMC3547681/.

12. Anselm Doll et al., "Mindful Attention to Breath Regulates Emotions via Increased Amygdala–Prefrontal Cortex Connectivity," *NeuroImage* 134 (July 1, 2016): 305–13, https://doi.org/10.1016/j.neuroimage.2016.03.041.

13. Baldwin M. Way et al., "Dispositional Mindfulness and Depressive Symptomatology: Correlations with Limbic and Self-Referential Neural Activity during Rest.," *Emotion* 10, no. 1 (February 2010): 12–24, https://doi.org/10.1037/a0018312.

14. Dale Purves et al., "The Limbic System," essay, in *Neuroscience*, 2nd ed. (Sunderland, MA: Sinauer Associates, 2001), https://www.ncbi.nlm.nih.gov/books/NBK11060/.

15. E Agostoni et al., "Functional and Histological Studies of the Vagus Nerve and Its Branches to the Heart, Lungs and Abdominal Viscera in the Cat," *J. Physiol* 135, no. 1 (January 23, 1957): 182–205, https://doi.org/10.1113/jphysiol.1957.sp005703.

16. Richard Câmara and Christoph J. Griessenauer, "Anatomy of the Vagus Nerve," *Nerves and Nerve Injuries* 1 (December 2015): 385–97, https://doi.org/10.1016/b978-0-12-410390-0.00028-7.

17. Richard Câmara and Christoph J. Griessenauer, "Anatomy of the Vagus Nerve," *Nerves and Nerve Injuries* 1 (December 2015): 385–97, https://doi.org/10.1016/b978-0-12-410390-0.00028-7.

18. Javier A. Bravo et al., "Ingestion of Lactobacillus Strain Regulates Emotional Behavior and Central GABA Receptor Expression in a Mouse via the Vagus Nerve," *Proceedings of the National Academy of Sciences* 108, no. 38 (August 29, 2011): 16050–55, https://doi.org/10.1073/pnas.1102999108.

19. Sophie C. Payne et al., "Anti-Inflammatory Effects of Abdominal Vagus Nerve Stimulation on Experimental Intestinal Inflammation," *Frontiers in Neuroscience* 13 (May 8, 2019), https://doi.org/10.3389/fnins.2019.00418.

20. Joshua A. Waxenbaum, Vamsi Reddy, and Matthew Varacallo, "Anatomy, Autonomic Nervous System," essay, in *StatPearls [Internet]* (Treasure Island, FL: StatPearls Publishing, 2023), https://www.ncbi.nlm.nih.gov/books/NBK539845/.
Heather Gerrie, "Our Second Brain: More than a Gut Feeling," UBC Neuroscience, October 15, 2021, https://neuroscience.ubc.ca/our-second-brain-more-than-a-gut-feeling/#:~:text=Comprised%20of%20100%20million%20neurons,spinal%20cord%20or%20peripheral%20nervous.

21. Omar A Bamalan and Yasir Al Khalili, "Physiology, Serotonin," essay, in *StatPearls [Internet]* (Treasure Island, FL: StatPearls Publishing, 2021), https://www.ncbi.nlm.nih.gov/books/ NBK545168/.

22. Suhrid Banskota, Jean-Eric Ghia, and Waliul I. Khan, "Serotonin in the Gut: Blessing or a Curse," *Biochimie* 161 (June 2019): 56–64, https://doi.org/10.1016/j.biochi.2018.06.008.

23. Graeme Eisenhofer et al., "Substantial Production of Dopamine in the Human Gastrointestinal Tract," *The Journal of Clinical Endocrinology & Metabolism* 82, no. 11 (November 1, 1997): 3864–71, https://doi.org/10.1210/jcem.82.11.4339.

24. Marianne O. Klein et al., "Dopamine: Functions, Signaling, and Association with Neurological Diseases," *Cellular and Molecular Neurobiology* 39, no. 1 (November 16, 2018): 31–59, https://doi.org/10.1007/s10571-018-0632-3.

25. Pia M. Vidal and Rodrigo Pacheco, "Targeting the Dopaminergic System in Autoimmunity," *Journal of Neuroimmune Pharmacology* 15, no. 1 (January 19, 2019): 57–73, https://doi.org/10.1007/s11481-019-09834-5.

26. Young Sun Kim and Nayoung Kim, "Sex-Gender Differences in Irritable Bowel Syndrome," *Journal of Neurogastroenterology and Motility* 24, no. 4 (October 1, 2018): 544–58, https://doi.org/10.5056/jnm18082.

27. Nicolas Patel and Karen Shackelford, "Irritable Bowel Syndrome," essay, in *StatPearls [Internet]* (Treasure Island, FL: StatPearls Publishing, 2021), https://www.ncbi.nlm.nih.gov/books/NBK534810/.

28. Nicolas Patel and Karen Shackelford, "Irritable Bowel Syndrome," essay, in *StatPearls [Internet]* (Treasure Island, FL: StatPearls Publishing, 2021), https://www.ncbi.nlm.nih.gov/books/NBK534810/.

29. Young Sun Kim and Nayoung Kim, "Sex-Gender Differences in Irritable Bowel Syndrome," *Journal of Neurogastroenterology and Motility* 24, no. 4 (October 1, 2018): 544–58, https://doi.org/10.5056/jnm18082.

30. Yao-Tung Lee et al., "Risk of Psychiatric Disorders Following Irritable Bowel Syndrome: A Nationwide Population-Based Cohort Study," *PLOS ONE* 10, no. 7 (July 29, 2015), https://doi.org/10.1371/journal.pone.0133283.

31. Shi-Rui Zhao et al., "Effect of Cognitive Behavior Therapy Combined with Exercise Intervention on the Cognitive Bias and Coping Styles of Diarrhea-Predominant Irritable Bowel Syndrome Patients," *World Journal of Clinical Cases* 7, no. 21 (November 6, 2019): 3446–62, https://doi.org/10.12998/wjcc.v7.i21.3446.

32. John D. Betteridge et al., "Inflammatory Bowel Disease Prevalence by Age, Gender, Race, and Geographic Location in the U.S. Military Health Care Population," *Inflammatory Bowel Diseases* 19, no. 7 (June 2013): 1421–27, https://doi.org/10.1097/mib.0b013e318281334d.

33. Christopher McDowell, Umer Farooq, and Muhammad Haseeb, "Inflammatory Bowel Disease," essay, in *StatPearls [Internet]* (Treasure Island, FL: StatPearls Publishing, 2021), https://www.ncbi.nlm.nih.gov/books/NBK470312/.

34. Adi Lahat et al., "Change in Bowel Habits during Menstruation: Are IBD Patients Different?," *Therapeutic Advances in Gastroenterology* 13 (June 10, 2020): 175628482092980, https://doi.org/10.1177/1756284820929806.

35. Fang Xu et al., "Health-Risk Behaviors and Chronic Conditions among Adults with Inflammatory Bowel Disease — United States, 2015 and 2016," *MMWR. Morbidity and Mortality Weekly Report* 67, no. 6 (February 16, 2018): 190–95, https://doi.org/10.15585/mmwr.mm6706a4.

36. Vincenzo Monda et al., "Exercise Modifies the Gut Microbiota with Positive Health Effects," *Oxidative Medicine and Cellular Longevity* 2017 (March 5, 2017): 1–8, https://doi.org/10.1155/2017/3831972.

37. Mehrbod Estaki et al., "Cardiorespiratory Fitness as a Predictor of Intestinal Microbial Diversity and Distinct Metagenomic Functions," *Microbiome* 4, no. 1 (August 8, 2016), https://doi.org/10.1186/s40168-016-0189-7.

38. Corrie M. Whisner et al., "Diet, Physical Activity and Screen Time but Not Body Mass Index Are Associated with the Gut Microbiome of a Diverse Cohort of College Students Living in University Housing: A Cross-Sectional Study," *BMC Microbiology* 18, no. 1 (December 12, 2018), https://doi.org/10.1186/s12866-018-1362-x.

39. H P Peters et al., "Potential Benefits and Hazards of Physical Activity and Exercise on the Gastrointestinal Tract," *Gut* 48, no. 3 (March 1, 2001): 435–39, https://doi.org/10.1136/gut.48.3.435.

40. H P Peters et al., "Potential Benefits and Hazards of Physical Activity and Exercise on the Gastrointestinal Tract," *Gut* 48, no. 3 (March 1, 2001): 435–39, https://doi.org/10.1136/gut.48.3.435.

41. Carl V. Gisolfi, "Is the GI System Built for Exercise?," *Physiology* 15, no. 3 (June 1, 2000): 114–19, https://doi.org/10.1152/physiologyonline.2000.15.3.114.

42. Roma Pahwa, Amandeep Goyal, and Ishwarlal Jialal, "Chronic Inflammation," essay, in *StatPearls [Internet]* (Treasure Island, FL: StatPearls Publishing, 2021), https://www.ncbi.nlm.nih.gov/books/NBK493173/.

43. G.R. Johnston and N.R. Webster, "Cytokines and the Immunomodulatory Function of the Vagus Nerve," British *Journal of Anaesthesia* 102, no. 4 (April 2009): 453–62, https://doi.org/10.1093/bja/aep037.

44. Aaron N. Hata and Richard M. Breyer, "Pharmacology and Signaling of Prostaglandin Receptors: Multiple Roles in Inflammation and Immune Modulation," *Pharmacology & Therapeutics* 103, no. 2 (August 2004): 147–66, https://doi.org/10.1016/j.pharmthera.2004.06.003.

45. Zofia Barcikowska et al., "Inflammatory Markers in Dysmenorrhea and Therapeutic Options," *International Journal of Environmental Research and Public Health* 17, no. 4 (February 13, 2020): 1191, https://doi.org/10.3390/ijerph17041191.

46. Zofia Barcikowska et al., "Inflammatory Markers in Dysmenorrhea and Therapeutic Options," *International Journal of Environmental Research and Public Health* 17, no. 4 (February 13, 2020): 1191, https://doi.org/10.3390/ijerph17041191.

47. K. G. Nygren and G. Rybo, "Prostaglandins and Menorrhagia," *Acta Obstetricia et Gynecologica Scandinavica* 62, no. s113 (1983): 101–3, https://doi.org/10.3109/00016348309155208.

48. N. Torres, A.E. Vargas-Castillo, and A.R. Tovar, "Adipose Tissue: White Adipose Tissue Structure and Function," *Encyclopedia of Food and Health*, 2016, 35–42, https://doi.org/10.1016/b978-0-12-384947-2.00006-4.

49. N. Torres, A.E. Vargas-Castillo, and A.R. Tovar, "Adipose Tissue: White Adipose Tissue Structure and Function," *Encyclopedia of Food and Health*, 2016, 35–42, https://doi.org/10.1016/b978-0-12-384947-2.00006-4.

50. Tohru Funahashi, Iichiro Shimomura, and Yuji Matsuzawa, "Adipocytokines," *Encyclopedia of Endocrine Diseases*, 2004, 41–44, https://doi.org/10.1016/b0-12-475570-4/01460-8.

51. Susan K. Fried, Dove A. Bunkin, and Andrew S. Greenberg, "Omental and Subcutaneous Adipose Tissues of Obese Subjects Release Interleukin-6: Depot Difference and Regulation by Glucocorticoid1," *The Journal of Clinical Endocrinology & Metabolism* 83, no. 3 (March 1, 1998): 847–50, https://doi.org/10.1210/jcem.83.3.4660. Yang Luo and Song Guo Zheng, "Hall of Fame among Pro-Inflammatory Cytokines: Interleukin-6 Gene and Its Transcriptional Regulation Mechanisms," *Frontiers in Immunology* 7 (December 19, 2016): 604, https://doi.org/10.3389/fimmu.2016.00604.

52. N. Torres, A.E. Vargas-Castillo, and A.R. Tovar, "Adipose Tissue: White Adipose Tissue Structure and Function," *Encyclopedia of Food and Health*, 2016, 35–42, https://doi.org/10.1016/b978-0-12-384947-2.00006-4.

53. Masayuki Saito et al., "High Incidence of Metabolically Active Brown Adipose Tissue in Healthy Adult Humans," *Diabetes* 58, no. 7 (April 28, 2009): 1526–31, https://doi.org/10.2337/db09-0530.

54. Maria Chondronikola et al., "Brown Adipose Tissue Is Associated with Systemic Concentrations of Peptides Secreted from the Gastrointestinal System and Involved in Appetite Regulation," *European Journal of Endocrinology* 177, no. 1 (July 1, 2017): 33–40, https://doi.org/10.1530/eje-16-0958. Mariëtte R. Boon and Wouter D. van Marken Lichtenbelt, "Brown Adipose Tissue: A Human Perspective," *Metabolic Control*, 2015, 301–19, https://doi.org/10.1007/164_2015_11.

55. CJ Ley, B Lees, and JC Stevenson, "Sex- and Menopause-Associated Changes in Body-Fat Distribution," *The American Journal of Clinical Nutrition* 55, no. 5 (May 1, 1992): 950–54, https://doi.org/10.1093/ajcn/55.5.950.

56. Carla Horvath and Christian Wolfrum, "Feeding Brown Fat: Dietary Phytochemicals Targeting Non-Shivering Thermogenesis to Control Body Weight," *Proceedings of the Nutrition Society* 79, no. 3 (April 15, 2020): 338–56, https://doi.org/10.1017/s0029665120006928.

YOUR CYCLE EXPLAINED

1. Beverly G. Reed, Bruce R. Carr, and Alison Boyce, "The Normal Menstrual Cycle and the Control of Ovulation," essay, in *Endotext [Internet]*, ed. Kenneth R. Feingold and Bradley Anawalt (South Dartmouth, MA: MDText.com, Inc., 2000), https://www.ncbi.nlm.nih.gov/books/NBK279054/.

2. A. Thijssen et al., "'Fertility Awareness-Based Methods' and Subfertility: A Systematic Review," *Facts, Views & Vision in ObGyn* 6, no. 3 (2014): 113–23, https://www.ncbi.nlm.nih.gov/pmc/articles/PMC4216977/.

3. Beverly G. Reed, Bruce R. Carr, and Alison Boyce, "The Normal Menstrual Cycle and the Control of Ovulation," essay, in *Endotext [Internet]*, ed. Kenneth R. Feingold and Bradley Anawalt (South Dartmouth, MA: MDText.com, Inc., 2000), https://www.ncbi.nlm.nih.gov/books/NBK279054/.

4. Beverly G. Reed, Bruce R. Carr, and Alison Boyce, "The Normal Menstrual Cycle and the Control of Ovulation," essay, in *Endotext [Internet]*, ed. Kenneth R. Feingold and Bradley Anawalt (South Dartmouth, MA: MDText.com, Inc., 2000), https://www.ncbi.nlm.nih.gov/books/NBK279054/.

5. Su-Mi Kim and Jong-Soo Kim, "A Review of Mechanisms of Implantation," *Development & Reproduction* 21, no. 4 (December 31, 2017): 351–59, https://doi.org/10.12717/dr.2017.21.4.351.

6. Beverly G. Reed, Bruce R. Carr, and Alison Boyce, "The Normal Menstrual Cycle and the Control of Ovulation," essay, in *Endotext [Internet]*, ed. Kenneth R. Feingold and Bradley Anawalt (South Dartmouth, MA: MDText.com, Inc., 2000), https://www.ncbi.nlm.nih.gov/books/NBK279054/.

7. Julie E. Holesh, Autumn N. Bass, and Megan Lord, "Physiology, Ovulation," essay, in *StatPearls [Internet]* (Treasure Island, FL: StatPearls Publishing, 2022), https://www.ncbi.nlm.nih.gov/books/NBK441996/.

8. Su-Mi Kim and Jong-Soo Kim, "A Review of Mechanisms of Implantation," *Development & Reproduction* 21, no. 4 (December 31, 2017): 351–59, https://doi.org/10.12717/dr.2017.21.4.351.

9. Beverly G. Reed, Bruce R. Carr, and Alison Boyce, "The Normal Menstrual Cycle and the Control of Ovulation," essay, in *Endotext [Internet]*, ed. Kenneth R. Feingold and Bradley Anawalt (South Dartmouth, MA: MDText.com, Inc., 2000), https://www.ncbi.nlm.nih.gov/books/NBK279054/.

10. Beverly G. Reed, Bruce R. Carr, and Alison Boyce, "The Normal Menstrual Cycle and the Control of Ovulation," essay, in *Endotext [Internet]*, ed. Kenneth R. Feingold and Bradley Anawalt (South Dartmouth, MA: MDText.com, Inc., 2000), https://www.ncbi.nlm.nih.gov/books/NBK279054/.

11. Nicole Telfer and Maegan Boutot, "Estrogen 101: Getting to Know Our Hormones," *Hormones & Your Cycle*, May 20, 2019, https://helloclue.com/articles/cycle-a-z/estrogen-101.

12. Benjamin J. Delgado and Wilfredo Lopez-Ojeda, "Estrogen," essay, in *StatPearls [Internet]* (Treasure Island, FL: StatPearls Publishing, 2022), https://www.ncbi.nlm.nih.gov/books/NBK538260/.
    Angelica Lindén Hirschberg, "Sex Hormones, Appetite and Eating Behaviour in Women," *Maturitas* 71, no. 3 (January 16, 2012): 248–56, https://doi.org/10.1016/j.maturitas.2011.12.016.
    Jun Ho Kim, Hyung Taek Cho, and Young Jun Kim, "The Role of Estrogen in Adipose Tissue Metabolism: Insights into Glucose Homeostasis Regulation [Review]," *Endocrine Journal* 61, no. 11 (November 28, 2014): 1055–67, https://doi.org/10.1507/endocrj.ej14-0262.

13. Benjamin J. Delgado and Wilfredo Lopez-Ojeda, "Estrogen," essay, in *StatPearls [Internet]* (Treasure Island, FL: StatPearls Publishing, 2022), https://www.ncbi.nlm.nih.gov/books/NBK538260/.

14. Jie Cui, Yong Shen, and Rena Li, "Estrogen Synthesis and Signaling Pathways during Aging: From Periphery to Brain," *Trends in Molecular Medicine* 19, no. 3 (March 2013): 197–209, https://doi.org/10.1016/j.molmed.2012.12.007.

15. Beverly G. Reed, Bruce R. Carr, and Alison Boyce, "The Normal Menstrual Cycle and the Control of Ovulation," essay, in *Endotext [Internet]*, ed. Kenneth R. Feingold and Bradley Anawalt (South Dartmouth, MA: MDText.com, Inc., 2000), https://www.ncbi.nlm.nih.gov/books/NBK279054/.

16. Beverly G. Reed, Bruce R. Carr, and Alison Boyce, "The Normal Menstrual Cycle and the Control of Ovulation," essay, in *Endotext [Internet]*, ed. Kenneth R. Feingold and Bradley Anawalt (South Dartmouth, MA: MDText.com, Inc., 2000), https://www.ncbi.nlm.nih.gov/books/NBK279054/.

17. Richard B. McCosh, Kellie M. Breen, and Alexander S. Kauffman, "Neural and Endocrine Mechanisms Underlying Stress-Induced Suppression of Pulsatile LH Secretion," *Molecular and Cellular Endocrinology* 498 (December 1, 2019): 110579, https://doi.org/10.1016/j.mce.2019.110579.

NUTRITION OVERVIEW

1. Ralf Jäger et al., "International Society of Sports Nutrition Position Stand: Probiotics," *Journal of the International Society of Sports Nutrition* 16, no. 1 (January 15, 2019), https://doi.org/10.1186/s12970-019-0329-0.
    Huey Shi Lye et al., "Beneficial Properties of Probiotics," *Tropical Life Sciences Research* 27, no. 2 (August 2016): 73–90, https://doi.org/10.21315/tlsr2016.27.2.6.

2. Timothy G. Dinan, Catherine Stanton, and John F. Cryan, "Psychobiotics: A Novel Class of Psychotropic," *Biological Psychiatry* 74, no. 10 (November 15, 2013): 720–26, https://doi.org/10.1016/j.biopsych.2013.05.001.
    Amar Sarkar et al., "Psychobiotics and the Manipulation of Bacteria–Gut–Brain Signals," *Trends in Neurosciences* 39, no. 11 (November 2016): 763–81, https://doi.org/10.1016/j.tins.2016.09.002.

3. Gareth Gordon Syngai et al., "Probiotics - the Versatile Functional Food Ingredients," *Journal of Food Science and Technology* 53, no. 2 (November 9, 2015): 921–33, https://doi.org/10.1007/s13197-015-2011-0.
    Karolina Jakubczyk et al., "Chemical Profile and Antioxidant Activity of the Kombucha Beverage Derived from White, Green, Black and Red Tea," *Antioxidants* 9, no. 5 (May 22, 2020): 447, https://doi.org/10.3390/antiox9050447.

4. Samantha M. Ervin et al., "Gut Microbial β-Glucuronidases Reactivate Estrogens as Components of the Estrobolome That Reactivate Estrogens," *Journal of Biological Chemistry* 294, no. 49 (December 6, 2019): 18586–99, https://doi.org/10.1074/jbc.ra119.010950.

5. Malou P. Schreurs et al., "How the Gut Microbiome Links to Menopause and Obesity, with Possible Implications for Endometrial Cancer Development," *Journal of Clinical Medicine* 10, no. 13 (June 29, 2021): 2916, https://doi.org/10.3390/jcm10132916.

6. Sara Dizzell et al., "Protective Effect of Probiotic Bacteria and Estrogen in Preventing HIV-1-Mediated Impairment of Epithelial Barrier Integrity in Female Genital Tract," *Cells* 8, no. 10 (September 21, 2019): 1120, https://doi.org/10.3390/cells8101120.

7. Gerald W. Tannock, "Probiotics: Time for a Dose of Realism," *Current Issues in Intestinal Microbiology* 4, no. 2 (September 2003): 33–42, https://pubmed.ncbi.nlm.nih.gov/14503687/.

8. Joanne Slavin, "Fiber and Prebiotics: Mechanisms and Health Benefits," *Nutrients* 5, no. 4 (April 22, 2013): 1417–35, https://doi.org/10.3390/nu5041417.

9. Dorna Davani-Davari et al., "Prebiotics: Definition, Types, Sources, Mechanisms, and Clinical Applications," *Foods* 8, no. 3 (March 9, 2019): 92, https://doi.org/10.3390/foods8030092.

10. Rafael Ballan et al., "Chapter Nine - Interactions of Probiotics and Prebiotics with the Gut Microbiota," essay, in *Progress in Molecular*

Biology and Translational Science, ed. Jun Sun, 1st ed., vol. 171 (Cambridge, MA: Academic Press, 2020), 265–300.

Dorna Davani-Davari et al., "Prebiotics: Definition, Types, Sources, Mechanisms, and Clinical Applications," *Foods* 8, no. 3 (March 9, 2019): 92, https://doi.org/10.3390/foods8030092.

11. Dorna Davani-Davari et al., "Prebiotics: Definition, Types, Sources, Mechanisms, and Clinical Applications," *Foods* 8, no. 3 (March 9, 2019): 92, https://doi.org/10.3390/foods8030092.

12. Jeremy M. Berg, John L. Tymoczko, and Lubert Stryer, *Biochemistry*, 5th ed. (New York, NY: Freeman, 2002).

13. Claire Fromentin et al., "Dietary Proteins Contribute Little to Glucose Production, Even under Optimal Gluconeogenic Conditions in Healthy Humans," *Diabetes* 62, no. 5 (April 16, 2013): 1435–42, https://doi.org/10.2337/db12-1208.

14. Cara B. Ebbeling et al., "Effects of Dietary Composition on Energy Expenditure during Weight-Loss Maintenance," *JAMA* 307, no. 24 (June 27, 2012): 2627–34, https://doi.org/10.1001/jama.2012.6607.

15. Mackenzie A. Mady et al., "The Ketogenic Diet: Adolescents Can Do It, Too," *Epilepsia* 44, no. 6 (June 9, 2003): 847–51, https://doi.org/10.1046/j.1528-1157.2003.57002.x.

16. Devinder Dhingra et al., "Dietary Fibre in Foods: A Review," *Journal of Food Science and Technology* 49, no. 3 (April 12, 2011): 255–66, https://doi.org/10.1007/s13197-011-0365-5.

17. Dorna Davani-Davari et al., "Prebiotics: Definition, Types, Sources, Mechanisms, and Clinical Applications," *Foods* 8, no. 3 (March 9, 2019): 92, https://doi.org/10.3390/foods8030092.

18. *Dietary Guidelines for Americans, 2020-2025*, 9th ed. (Washington D.C: U.S. Department of Agriculture and U.S. Department of Health and Human Services, 2020), https://www.dietaryguidelines.gov/sites/default/files/2020-12/Dietary_Guidelines_for_Americans_2020-2025.pdf.

19. Marc P. McRae, "Effectiveness of Fiber Supplementation for Constipation, Weight Loss, and Supporting Gastrointestinal Function: A Narrative Review of Meta-Analyses," *Journal of Chiropractic Medicine* 19, no. 1 (March 2020): 58–64, https://doi.org/10.1016/j.jcm.2019.10.008. Samantha M. Ervin et al., "Gut Microbial β-Glucuronidases Reactivate Estrogens as Components of the Estrobolome That Reactivate Estrogens," *Journal of Biological Chemistry* 294, no. 49 (December 6, 2019): 18586–99, https://doi.org/10.1074/jbc.ra119.010950.

20. Sareen S. Gropper, Jack L. Smith, and Timothy P. Carr, *Advanced Nutrition and Human Metabolism*, 7th ed. (Boston, MA: Cengage Learning, 2018).

21. Fabrizio Ferretti and Michele Mariani, "Simple vs. Complex Carbohydrate Dietary Patterns and the Global Overweight and Obesity Pandemic," *International Journal of Environmental Research and*

Public Health 14, no. 10 (October 4, 2017): 1174, https://doi.org/10.3390/ijerph14101174.

22. Michelle Mouri and Madhu Badireddy, "Hyperglycemia," essay, in *StatPearls [Internet]* (Treasure Island, FL: StatPearls Publishing, 2022), https://www.ncbi.nlm.nih.gov/books/NBK430900/#_NBK430900_pubdet_.

23. J E Chavarro et al., "A Prospective Study of Dietary Carbohydrate Quantity and Quality in Relation to Risk of Ovulatory Infertility," *European Journal of Clinical Nutrition* 63, no. 1 (September 19, 2007): 78–86, https://doi.org/10.1038/sj.ejcn.1602904.
   Michael L Traub, "Assessing and Treating Insulin Resistance in Women with Polycystic Ovarian Syndrome," *World Journal of Diabetes* 2, no. 3 (March 15, 2011): 33–40, https://doi.org/10.4239/wjd.v2.i3.33.

24. J E Chavarro et al., "A Prospective Study of Dietary Carbohydrate Quantity and Quality in Relation to Risk of Ovulatory Infertility," *European Journal of Clinical Nutrition* 63, no. 1 (September 19, 2007): 78–86, https://doi.org/10.1038/sj.ejcn.1602904.

25. Cholsoon Jang et al., "The Small Intestine Converts Dietary Fructose into Glucose and Organic Acids," *Cell Metabolism* 27, no. 2 (February 6, 2018): 351–61, https://doi.org/10.1016/j.cmet.2017.12.016.

26. Xiaosen Ouyang et al., "Fructose Consumption as a Risk Factor for Non-Alcoholic Fatty Liver Disease," *Journal of Hepatology* 48, no. 6 (June 1, 2008): 993–99, https://doi.org/10.1016/j.jhep.2008.02.011.

27. Johanna K. DiStefano and Gabriel Q. Shaibi, "The Relationship between Excessive Dietary Fructose Consumption and Paediatric Fatty Liver Disease," *Pediatric Obesity* 16, no. 6 (December 11, 2020): e12759, https://doi.org/10.1111/ijpo.12759.

28. George A Bray, Samara Joy Nielsen, and Barry M Popkin, "Consumption of High-Fructose Corn Syrup in Beverages May Play a Role in the Epidemic of Obesity," *The American Journal of Clinical Nutrition* 79, no. 4 (April 1, 2004): 537–43, https://doi.org/10.1093/ajcn/79.4.537.

29. Heather J Leidy et al., "Beneficial Effects of a Higher-Protein Breakfast on the Appetitive, Hormonal, and Neural Signals Controlling Energy Intake Regulation in Overweight/Obese, 'Breakfast-Skipping,' Late-Adolescent Girls," *The American Journal of Clinical Nutrition* 97, no. 4 (February 27, 2013): 677–88, https://doi.org/10.3945/ajcn.112.053116.

30. Eva V. Osilla, Anthony O. Safadi, and Sandeep Sharma, "Calories," essay, in *StatPearls [Internet]* (Treasure Island, FL: StatPearls Publishing, 2022), https://www.ncbi.nlm.nih.gov/books/NBK499909/.

31. Eva V. Osilla, Anthony O. Safadi, and Sandeep Sharma, "Calories," essay, in *StatPearls [Internet]* (Treasure Island, FL: StatPearls Publishing, 2022), https://www.ncbi.nlm.nih.gov/books/NBK499909/.

32. Eva V. Osilla, Anthony O. Safadi, and Sandeep Sharma, "Calories," essay, in *StatPearls [Internet]* (Treasure Island, FL: StatPearls Publishing, 2022), https://www.ncbi.nlm.nih.gov/books/NBK499909/.

33. Sareen S. Gropper, Jack L. Smith, and Timothy P. Carr, *Advanced Nutrition and Human Metabolism*, 7th ed. (Boston, MA: Cengage Learning, 2018).

34. Priya Reddy and Ishwarlal Jialal, "Biochemistry, Fat Soluble Vitamins," essay, in *StatPearls [Internet]* (Treasure Island, FL: StatPearls Publishin, 2022), https://www.ncbi.nlm.nih.gov/books/NBK534869.

35. Amy E Griel et al., "An Increase in Dietary N-3 Fatty Acids Decreases a Marker of Bone Resorption in Humans," *Nutrition Journal* 6, no. 1 (January 16, 2007), https://doi.org/10.1186/1475-2891-6-2.

36. Antonio Camargo et al., "Dietary Fat Differentially Influences the Lipids Storage on the Adipose Tissue in Metabolic Syndrome Patients," *European Journal of Nutrition* 53, no. 2 (August 7, 2013): 617–26, https://doi.org/10.1007/s00394-013-0570-2.

37. So-Yun Yi et al., "Added Sugar Intake Is Associated with Pericardial Adipose Tissue Volume," *European Journal of Preventive Cardiology* 27, no. 18 (December 1, 2020): 2016–23, https://doi.org/10.1177/2047487320931303.
     Eva V. Osilla, Anthony O. Safadi, and Sandeep Sharma, "Calories," essay, in *StatPearls [Internet]* (Treasure Island, FL: StatPearls Publishing, 2022), https://www.ncbi.nlm.nih.gov/books/NBK499909/.

38. Swati Bhardwaj, Santosh Jain Passi, and Anoop Misra, "Overview of Trans Fatty Acids: Biochemistry and Health Effects," *Diabetes & Metabolic Syndrome: Clinical Research & Reviews* 5, no. 3 (July 2011): 161–64, https://doi.org/10.1016/j.dsx.2012.03.002.

39. Anamaria Balić et al., "Omega-3 versus Omega-6 Polyunsaturated Fatty Acids in the Prevention and Treatment of Inflammatory Skin Diseases," *International Journal of Molecular Sciences* 21, no. 3 (January 23, 2020): 741, https://doi.org/10.3390/ijms21030741.

40. Anamaria Balić et al., "Omega-3 versus Omega-6 Polyunsaturated Fatty Acids in the Prevention and Treatment of Inflammatory Skin Diseases," *International Journal of Molecular Sciences* 21, no. 3 (January 23, 2020): 741, https://doi.org/10.3390/ijms21030741.

41. Anamaria Balić et al., "Omega-3 versus Omega-6 Polyunsaturated Fatty Acids in the Prevention and Treatment of Inflammatory Skin Diseases," *International Journal of Molecular Sciences* 21, no. 3 (January 23, 2020): 741, https://doi.org/10.3390/ijms21030741.

42. Priyanka Kajla, Alka Sharma, and Dev Raj Sood, "Flaxseed—a Potential Functional Food Source," *Journal of Food Science and Technology* 52, no. 4 (February 28, 2014): 1857–71, https://doi.org/10.1007/s13197-014-1293-y.

43. Nahid Rahbar, Neda Asgharzadeh, and Raheb Ghorbani, "Effect of Omega-3 Fatty Acids on Intensity of Primary Dysmenorrhea," *International Journal of Gynecology & Obstetrics* 117, no. 1 (January 17, 2012): 45–47, https://doi.org/10.1016/j.ijgo.2011.11.019.

44. V Marchand, "Trans Fats: What Physicians Should Know," *Paediatrics & Child Health* 15, no. 6 (July 1, 2010): 373–75, https://doi.org/10.1093/pch/15.6.373.

45. Chaoyang Li et al., "Global Surveillance of *Trans*-Fatty Acids," *Preventing Chronic Disease* 16 (October 31, 2019), https://doi.org/10.5888/pcd16.190121.

46. Md. Ashraful Islam et al., "Trans Fatty Acids and Lipid Profile: A Serious Risk Factor to Cardiovascular Disease, Cancer and Diabetes," *Diabetes & Metabolic Syndrome: Clinical Research & Reviews* 13, no. 2 (March 21, 2019): 1643–47, https://doi.org/10.1016/j.dsx.2019.03.033.

47. Vandana Dhaka et al., "Trans Fats—Sources, Health Risks and Alternative Approach - A Review," *Journal of Food Science and Technology* 48, no. 5 (January 28, 2011): 534–41, https://doi.org/10.1007/s13197-010-0225-8.

48. J E Chavarro et al., "A Prospective Study of Dietary Carbohydrate Quantity and Quality in Relation to Risk of Ovulatory Infertility," *European Journal of Clinical Nutrition* 63, no. 1 (September 19, 2007): 78–86, https://doi.org/10.1038/sj.ejcn.1602904.

49. Sunni L Mumford et al., "Dietary Fat Intake and Reproductive Hormone Concentrations and Ovulation in Regularly Menstruating Women ," *The American Journal of Clinical Nutrition* 103, no. 3 (March 2016): 868–77, https://doi.org/10.3945/ajcn.115.119321.

50. S. A. Missmer et al., "A Prospective Study of Dietary Fat Consumption and Endometriosis Risk," *Human Reproduction* 25, no. 6 (March 23, 2010): 1528–35, https://doi.org/10.1093/humrep/deq044.

51. S. A. Missmer et al., "A Prospective Study of Dietary Fat Consumption and Endometriosis Risk," *Human Reproduction* 25, no. 6 (March 23, 2010): 1528–35, https://doi.org/10.1093/humrep/deq044.

52. Åsa Nybacka, Per M. Hellström, and Angelica L. Hirschberg, "Increased Fibre and Reduced Trans Fatty Acid Intake Are Primary Predictors of Metabolic Improvement in Overweight Polycystic Ovary Syndrome-Substudy of Randomized Trial between Diet, Exercise and Diet plus Exercise for Weight Control," *Clinical Endocrinology* 87, no. 6 (August 18, 2017): 680–88, https://doi.org/10.1111/cen.13427.

53. Micah Craig, Siva Naga S. Yarrarapu, and Manjari Dimri, "Biochemistry, Cholesterol," essay, in *StatPearls [Internet]* (Treasure Island, FL: StatPearls Publishing, 2023), ncbi.nlm.nih.gov/books/NBK513326/.

54. Victor Cortes et al., "Physiological and Pathological Implications of Cholesterol," *Frontiers in Bioscience* 19, no. 3 (January 1, 2014): 416–28, https://doi.org/10.2741/4216.

55. Uffe Ravnskov et al., "LDL-C Does Not Cause Cardiovascular Disease: A Comprehensive Review of the Current Literature," *Expert Review of Clinical Pharmacology* 11, no. 10 (October 3, 2018): 959–70, https://doi.org/10.1080/17512433.2018.1519391.

56. Winfried März et al., "HDL Cholesterol: Reappraisal of Its Clinical Relevance," *Clinical Research in Cardiology* 106, no. 9 (March 24, 2017): 663–75, https://doi.org/10.1007/s00392-017-1106-1.
Yahya Sohrabi, Dennis Schwarz, and Holger Reinecke, "LDL-C Augments Whereas HDL-C Prevents Inflammatory Innate Immune Memory," *Trends in Molecular Medicine* 28, no. 1 (January 1, 2022): 1–4, https://doi.org/10.1016/j.molmed.2021.11.003.
Philip J. Barter et al., "Antiinflammatory Properties of HDL," *Circulation Research* 95, no. 8 (October 15, 2004): 764–72, https://doi.org/10.1161/01.res.0000146094.59640.13.

57. Winfried März et al., "HDL Cholesterol: Reappraisal of Its Clinical Relevance," *Clinical Research in Cardiology* 106, no. 9 (March 24, 2017): 663–75, https://doi.org/10.1007/s00392-017-1106-1.

58. Seyedeh Negar Assadi, "What Are the Effects of Psychological Stress and Physical Work on Blood Lipid Profiles?," ed. Yung–Hsiang Chen, *Medicine* 96, no. 18 (May 2017): e6816, https://doi.org/10.1097/md.0000000000006816.

59. Ignatius C. Maduka, Emeka E. Neboh, and Silas A. Ufelle, "The Relationship between Serum Cortisol, Adrenaline, Blood Glucose and Lipid Profile of Undergraduate Students under Examination Stress.," *African Health Sciences* 15, no. 1 (March 11, 2015): 131–36, https://doi.org/10.4314/ahs.v15i1.18.

60. Andrew Steptoe and Mika Kivimäki, "Stress and Cardiovascular Disease," *Nature Reviews Cardiology* 9, no. 6 (April 3, 2012): 360–70, https://doi.org/10.1038/nrcardio.2012.45.

61. Winfried März et al., "HDL Cholesterol: Reappraisal of Its Clinical Relevance," *Clinical Research in Cardiology* 106, no. 9 (March 24, 2017): 663–75, https://doi.org/10.1007/s00392-017-1106-1.

62. Zhe Xu, Scott McClure, and Lawrence Appel, "Dietary Cholesterol Intake and Sources among U.S Adults: Results from National Health and Nutrition Examination Surveys (NHANES), 2001–2014," *Nutrients* 10, no. 6 (June 14, 2018): 771, https://doi.org/10.3390/nu10060771.

63. P.M. Clifton and J.B. Keogh, "A Systematic Review of the Effect of Dietary Saturated and Polyunsaturated Fat on Heart Disease," *Nutrition, Metabolism and Cardiovascular Diseases* 27, no. 12 (December 1, 2017): 1060–80, https://doi.org/10.1016/j.numecd.2017.10.010.

64. Kay-Tee Khaw et al., "Randomised Trial of Coconut Oil, Olive Oil or Butter on Blood Lipids and Other Cardiovascular Risk Factors in Healthy Men and Women," *BMJ Open* 8, no. 3 (March 6, 2018): e020167, https://doi.org/10.1136/bmjopen-2017-020167.

65. Merel A. van Rooijen et al., "Dietary Stearic Acid and Palmitic Acid Do Not Differently Affect ABCA1-Mediated Cholesterol Efflux Capacity in Healthy Men and Postmenopausal Women: A Randomized Controlled Trial," *Clinical Nutrition* 40, no. 3 (March 1, 2021): 804–11, https://doi.

org/10.1016/j.clnu.2020.08.016.

M A Denke, "Effects of Cocoa Butter on Serum Lipids in Humans: Historical Highlights," *The American Journal of Clinical Nutrition* 60, no. 6 (December 1, 1994): 1014–16, https://doi.org/10.1093/ajcn/60.6.1014s.

66. Anamaria Balić et al., "Omega-3 versus Omega-6 Polyunsaturated Fatty Acids in the Prevention and Treatment of Inflammatory Skin Diseases," *International Journal of Molecular Sciences* 21, no. 3 (January 23, 2020): 741, https://doi.org/10.3390/ijms21030741.

67. Alyssa L Morris and Shamim S Mohiuddin, "Biochemistry, Nutrients," in *StatPearls [Internet]* (Treasure Island, FL: StatPearls Publishing, 2022), https://www.ncbi.nlm.nih.gov/books/NBK554545/.

68. Victor J. Navarro et al., "Liver Injury from Herbal and Dietary Supplements," *Hepatology* 65, no. 1 (November 17, 2016): 363–73, https://doi.org/10.1002/hep.28813.

69. Pilin Francis and Victor J. Navarro, "Drug Induced Hepatotoxicity," in *StatPearls [Internet],* (Treasure Island, FL: StatPearls Publishing, 2022), https://www.ncbi.nlm.nih.gov/books/NBK557535/.

70. Maura Palmery et al., "Oral Contraceptives and Changes in Nutritional Requirements," *European Review for Medical and Pharmacological Sciences* 17, no. 13 (July 2013): 1804–13, https://pubmed.ncbi.nlm.nih.gov/23852908/.

71. Maura Palmery et al., "Oral Contraceptives and Changes in Nutritional Requirements," *European Review for Medical and Pharmacological Sciences* 17, no. 13 (July 2013): 1804–13, https://pubmed.ncbi.nlm.nih.gov/23852908/.

72. Sareen S. Gropper, Jack L. Smith, and Timothy P. Carr, *Advanced Nutrition and Human Metabolism*, 7th ed. (Boston, MA: Cengage Learning, 2018).

73. Sareen S. Gropper, Jack L. Smith, and Timothy P. Carr, *Advanced Nutrition and Human Metabolism*, 7th ed. (Boston, MA: Cengage Learning, 2018).

74. Sareen S. Gropper, Jack L. Smith, and Timothy P. Carr, *Advanced Nutrition and Human Metabolism*, 7th ed. (Boston, MA: Cengage Learning, 2018).

75. Alyssa L Morris and Shamim S Mohiuddin, "Biochemistry, Nutrients," essay, in *StatPearls [Internet]* (Treasure Island, FL: StatPearls Publishing, 2022), https://www.ncbi.nlm.nih.gov/books/NBK554545/.

76. Elad Tako, "Dietary Trace Minerals," *Nutrients* 11, no. 11 (November 19, 2019): 2823, https://doi.org/10.3390/nu11112823.

77. Kohji Sato, "Why Is Vitamin B6 Effective in Alleviating the Symptoms of Autism?," *Medical Hypotheses* 115 (June 2018): 103–6, https://doi.org/10.1016/j.mehy.2018.04.007.

78. G E Abraham, "Nutritional Factors in the Etiology of the Premenstrual Tension Syndromes," *The Journal of Reproductive Medicine* 28, no. 7 (July 1983): 446–64.

79. Seyedeh Zahra Masoumi, Maryam Ataollahi, and Khodayar Oshvandi, "Effect of Combined Use of Calcium and Vitamin B6 on Premenstrual Syndrome Symptoms: A Randomized Clinical Trial," *Journal of Caring Sciences* 5, no. 1 (March 1, 2016): 67–73, https://doi.org/10.15171/jcs.2016.007.

80. Audrey J. Gaskins et al., "The Impact of Dietary Folate Intake on Reproductive Function in Premenopausal Women: A Prospective Cohort Study," *PLoS ONE* 7, no. 9 (September 26, 2012), https://doi.org/10.1371/journal.pone.0046276.

81. Sarah Long and Jack Goldblatt, "MTHFR Genetic Testing: Controversy and Clinical Implications," *Australian Family Physician* 45, no. 4 (April 2016): 237–40.

82. Maša Vidmar Golja et al., "Folate Insufficiency Due to MTHFR Deficiency Is Bypassed by 5-Methyltetrahydrofolate," *Journal of Clinical Medicine* 9, no. 9 (September 2, 2020): 2836, https://doi.org/10.3390/jcm9092836.

83. Thierry Forges et al., "Impact of Folate and Homocysteine Metabolism on Human Reproductive Health," *Human Reproduction Update* 13, no. 3 (February 16, 2007): 225–38, https://doi.org/10.1093/humupd/dml063.

84. Audrey J. Gaskins et al., "The Impact of Dietary Folate Intake on Reproductive Function in Premenopausal Women: A Prospective Cohort Study," *PLoS ONE* 7, no. 9 (September 26, 2012), https://doi.org/10.1371/journal.pone.0046276.

85. Sareen S. Gropper, Jack L. Smith, and Timothy P. Carr, *Advanced Nutrition and Human Metabolism,* 7th ed. (Boston, MA: Cengage Learning, 2018).

86. Alan R. Gaby, *Nutritional Medicine* (Concord, NH: Fritz Perlberg Publishing, 2017).

87. Sareen S. Gropper, Jack L. Smith, and Timothy P. Carr, *Advanced Nutrition and Human Metabolism,* 7th ed. (Boston, MA: Cengage Learning, 2018).

88. Nur Kesiktas et al., "Is There a Relationship between Vitamin B12 and Stress Urinary Incontinence?," *LUTS: Lower Urinary Tract Symptoms* 4, no. 2 (December 28, 2011): 55–58, https://doi.org/10.1111/j.1757-5672.2011.00116.x.

89. Sareen S. Gropper, Jack L. Smith, and Timothy P. Carr, *Advanced Nutrition and Human Metabolism,* 7th ed. (Boston, MA: Cengage Learning, 2018).

90. Jessica Morales-Gutierrez et al., "Toxicity Induced by Multiple High Doses of Vitamin B12 during Pernicious Anemia Treatment: A Case Report," *Clinical Toxicology* 58, no. 2 (April 24, 2019): 129–31, https://doi.org/10.1080/15563650.2019.1606432.

91. Sareen S. Gropper, Jack L. Smith, and Timothy P. Carr, *Advanced Nutrition and Human Metabolism,* 7th ed. (Boston, MA: Cengage Learning, 2018).

92. Krati Chauhan, Mahsa Shahrokhi, and Martin R. Huecker, "Vitamin D," essay, in *StatPearls [Internet]* (Treasure Island, FL: StatPearls Publishing, 2022), https://www.ncbi.nlm.nih.gov/books/NBK441912/.

93. Mohamad Irani and Zaher Merhi, "Role of Vitamin D in Ovarian Physiology and Its Implication in Reproduction: A Systematic Review," *Fertility and Sterility* 102, no. 2 (August 2014): 460–68, https://doi.org/10.1016/j.fertnstert.2014.04.046.

94. Karolina Łagowska, "The Relationship between Vitamin D Status and the Menstrual Cycle in Young Women: A Preliminary Study," *Nutrients* 10, no. 11 (November 11, 2018): 1729, https://doi.org/10.3390/nu10111729.

95. Roma Pahwa, Amandeep Goyal, and Ishwarlal Jialal, "Chronic Inflammation," essay, in *StatPearls [Internet]* (Treasure Island, FL: StatPearls Publishing, 2022), https://www.ncbi.nlm.nih.gov/books/NBK493173/.

96. Donna Day Baird et al., "Vitamin D and the Risk of Uterine Fibroids," *Epidemiology* 24, no. 3 (May 2013): 447–53, https://doi.org/10.1097/ede.0b013e31828acca0.

97. Kurt A. Kennel, Matthew T. Drake, and Daniel L. Hurley, "Vitamin D Deficiency in Adults: When to Test and How to Treat," *Mayo Clinic Proceedings* 85, no. 8 (August 2010): 752–58, https://doi.org/10.4065/mcp.2010.0138.

98. Jadwiga Malczewska-Lenczowska et al., "The Association between Iron and Vitamin D Status in Female Elite Athletes," *Nutrients* 10, no. 2 (January 31, 2018): 167, https://doi.org/10.3390/nu10020167.

99. Jacquelyn Medina and Vikas Gupta, "Vitamin E," essay, in *StatPearls [Internet]* (Treasure Island, FL: StatPearls Publishing, 2022), https://www.ncbi.nlm.nih.gov/books/NBK557737/.

100. Maret G. Traber and Jeffrey Atkinson, "Vitamin E, Antioxidant and Nothing More," *Free Radical Biology and Medicine* 43, no. 1 (July 1, 2007): 4–15, https://doi.org/10.1016/j.freeradbiomed.2007.03.024. Jacquelyn Medina and Vikas Gupta, "Vitamin E," essay, in *StatPearls [Internet]* (Treasure Island, FL: StatPearls Publishing, 2022), https://www.ncbi.nlm.nih.gov/books/NBK557737/.

101. Siti Mohd Mutalip, Sharaniza Ab-Rahim, and Mohd Rajikin, "Vitamin E as an Antioxidant in Female Reproductive Health," *Antioxidants* 7, no. 2 (January 26, 2018): 22, https://doi.org/10.3390/antiox7020022. Maryam Kashanian et al., "Evaluation of the Effect of Vitamin E on Pelvic Pain Reduction in Women Suffering from Primary Dysmenorrhea," *The Journal of Reproductive Medicine* 58, no. 1–2 (2013): 34–38, https://pubmed.ncbi.nlm.nih.gov/23447916/. Saeideh Ziaei, Anoshirvan Kazemnejad, and Akram Sedighi, "The Effect of Vitamin E on the Treatment of Menstrual Migraine," *Medical Science Monitor : International Medical Journal of Experimental and Clinical Research* 15, no. 1 (January 2009): 16–19, https://pubmed.ncbi.nlm.nih.gov/19114966/.

102. Kristen N. Owen, "Vitamin E Toxicity," essay, in *StatPearls [Internet]*, ed. Olga Dewald (Treasure Island, FL: StatPearls Publishing, 2022), https://www.ncbi.nlm.nih.gov/books/NBK564373/.

103. Maria Laura Colombo, "An Update on Vitamin E, Tocopherol and Tocotrienol—Perspectives," *Molecules* 15, no. 4 (March 24, 2010): 2103–13, https://doi.org/10.3390/molecules15042103.

104. Mary J Allen and Sandeep Sharma, "Magnesium," essay, in *StatPearls [Internet]* (Treasure Island, FL: StatPearls Publishing, 2022), https://www.ncbi.nlm.nih.gov/books/NBK519036/.
    Sareen S. Gropper, Jack L. Smith, and Timothy P. Carr, *Advanced Nutrition and Human Metabolism*, 7th ed. (Boston, MA: Cengage Learning, 2018).

105. Roma Pahwa, Amandeep Goyal, and Ishwarlal Jialal, "Chronic Inflammation," essay, in *StatPearls [Internet]* (Treasure Island, FL: StatPearls Publishing, 2022), https://www.ncbi.nlm.nih.gov/books/NBK493173/.
    B. Seifert et al., "Magnesium--Eine Therapeutische Alternative Bei Der Primären Dysmenorrhoe [Magnesium--a New Therapeutic Alternative in Primary Dysmenorrhea]," *Zentralblatt Fur Gynakologie* 111, no. 11 (January 1, 1989): 755–60, https://pubmed.ncbi.nlm.nih.gov/2675496/.
    Mary J Allen and Sandeep Sharma, "Magnesium," essay, in *StatPearls [Internet]* (Treasure Island, FL: StatPearls Publishing, 2022), https://www.ncbi.nlm.nih.gov/books/NBK519036/.

106. Mohsen Moslehi et al., "The Association between Serum Magnesium and Premenstrual Syndrome: A Systematic Review and Meta-Analysis of Observational Studies," *Biological Trace Element Research* 192, no. 2 (March 18, 2019): 145–52, https://doi.org/10.1007/s12011-019-01672-z.

107. Afsaneh Saeedian Kia, Reza Amani, and Bahman Cheraghian, "The Association between the Risk of Premenstrual Syndrome and Vitamin D, Calcium, and Magnesium Status among University Students: A Case Control Study," *Health Promotion Perspectives* 5, no. 3 (October 25, 2015): 225–30, https://doi.org/10.15171/hpp.2015.027.

108. Jayme Workinger, Robert. Doyle, and Jonathan Bortz, "Challenges in the Diagnosis of Magnesium Status," *Nutrients* 10, no. 9 (September 1, 2018): 1202, https://doi.org/10.3390/nu10091202.

109. Yasmin Ismail, Abbas A. Ismail, and Adel A.A. Ismail, "The Underestimated Problem of Using Serum Magnesium Measurements to Exclude Magnesium Deficiency in Adults; a Health Warning Is Needed for 'Normal' Results," *Clinical Chemistry and Laboratory Medicine* 48, no. 3 (March 1, 2010): 323–27, https://doi.org/10.1515/cclm.2010.077.

110. Mary J Allen and Sandeep Sharma, "Magnesium," essay, in *StatPearls [Internet]* (Treasure Island, FL: StatPearls Publishing, 2022), https://www.ncbi.nlm.nih.gov/books/NBK519036/.

111. Taylor M. Drake and Vikas Gupta, "Calcium," essay, in *StatPearls [Internet]* (Treasure Island, FL: StatPearls Publishing, 2022), https://www.ncbi.nlm.nih.gov/books/NBK557683/.

112. Zinat Ghanbari et al., "Effects of Calcium Supplement Therapy in Women with Premenstrual Syndrome," *Taiwanese Journal of Obstetrics and Gynecology* 48, no. 2 (June 2009): 124–29, https://doi.org/10.1016/s1028-4559(09)60271-0.
Fatemeh Shobeiri et al., "Effect of Calcium on Premenstrual Syndrome: A Double-Blind Randomized Clinical Trial," *Obstetrics & Gynecology Science* 60, no. 1 (January 15, 2017): 100–105, https://doi.org/10.5468/ogs.2017.60.1.100.

113. A. Catharine Ross et al., eds., "Overview of Calcium," essay, in *Dietary Reference Intakes for Calcium and Vitamin D* (Washington, DC: National Academies Press, 2011).

114. Kanjaksha Ghosh, "Non Haematological Effects of Iron Deficiency - A Perspective," *Indian Journal of Medical Sciences* 60, no. 1 (January 2006): 30, https://pubmed.ncbi.nlm.nih.gov/16444088/.
Sergi Puig et al., "The Elemental Role of Iron in DNA Synthesis and Repair," *Metallomics* 9, no. 11 (August 31, 2017): 1483–1500, https://doi.org/10.1039/c7mt00116a.
Nazanin Abbaspour, Richard Hurrell, and Roya Kelishadi, "Review on Iron and Its Importance for Human Health," *Journal of Research in Medical Sciences : The Official Journal of Isfahan University of Medical Sciences* 19, no. 2 (February 2014): 164–74, https://www.ncbi.nlm.nih.gov/pmc/articles/PMC3999603/.

115. Adeline Angeli et al., "Joint Model of Iron and Hepcidin during the Menstrual Cycle in Healthy Women," *The AAPS Journal* 18, no. 2 (February 2, 2016): 490–504, https://doi.org/10.1208/s12248-016-9875-4.

116. Jorge E. Chavarro et al., "Iron Intake and Risk of Ovulatory Infertility," *Obstetrics & Gynecology* 108, no. 5 (November 2006): 1145–52, https://doi.org/10.1097/01.aog.0000238333.37423.ab.

117. Thomas G. DeLoughery, "Iron Deficiency Anemia," *Medical Clinics of North America* 101, no. 2 (March 2017): 319–32, https://doi.org/10.1016/j.mcna.2016.09.004.

118. Alan R. Gaby, *Nutritional Medicine* (Concord, NH: Fritz Perlberg Publishing, 2017).

119. Richard Hurrell and Ines Egli, "Iron Bioavailability and Dietary Reference Values," *The American Journal of Clinical Nutrition* 91, no. 5 (March 3, 2010): 1461–67, https://doi.org/10.3945/ajcn.2010.28674f.

120. Adeline Angeli et al., "Joint Model of Iron and Hepcidin during the Menstrual Cycle in Healthy Women," *The AAPS Journal* 18, no. 2 (February 2, 2016): 490–504, https://doi.org/10.1208/s12248-016-9875-4.

121. Ananda S. Prasad, "Zinc Is an Antioxidant and Anti-Inflammatory Agent: Its Role in Human Health," *Frontiers in Nutrition* 1 (September 1, 2014), https://doi.org/10.3389/fnut.2014.00014.

122. Marzenna Nasiadek et al., "The Role of Zinc in Selected Female Reproductive System Disorders," *Nutrients* 12, no. 8 (August 16, 2020): 2464, https://doi.org/10.3390/nu12082464.

123. Marzenna Nasiadek et al., "The Role of Zinc in Selected Female Reproductive System Disorders," *Nutrients* 12, no. 8 (August 16, 2020): 2464, https://doi.org/10.3390/nu12082464.

124. H A Ronaghy and J A Halsted, "Zinc Deficiency Occurring in Females. Report of Two Cases," *The American Journal of Clinical Nutrition* 28, no. 8 (August 1, 1975): 831–36, https://doi.org/10.1093/ajcn/28.8.831.

125. George A. Eby, "Zinc Treatment Prevents Dysmenorrhea," *Medical Hypotheses* 69, no. 2 (January 2007): 297–301, https://doi.org/10.1016/j.mehy.2006.12.009.

126. G J Fosmire, "Zinc Toxicity," *The American Journal of Clinical Nutrition* 51, no. 2 (February 1, 1990): 225–27, https://doi.org/10.1093/ajcn/51.2.225.

127. Lisa A Houghton et al., "Serum Zinc Is a Major Predictor of Anemia and Mediates the Effect of Selenium on Hemoglobin in School-Aged Children in a Nationally Representative Survey in New Zealand," *The Journal of Nutrition* 146, no. 9 (July 27, 2016): 1670–76, https://doi.org/10.3945/jn.116.235127.

128. Trevor A. Nessel and Vikas Gupta, "Selenium," essay, in *StatPearls [Internet]* (Treasure Island, FL: StatPearls Publishing, 2022), https://www.ncbi.nlm.nih.gov/books/NBK557551/.

129. Izhar Qazi et al., "Selenium, Selenoproteins, and Female Reproduction: A Review," *Molecules* 23, no. 12 (November 22, 2018): 3053, https://doi.org/10.3390/molecules23123053.
     T. Paszkowski et al., "Selenium Dependent Glutathione Peroxidase Activity in Human Follicular Fluid," *Clinica Chimica Acta* 236, no. 2 (May 15, 1995): 173–80, https://doi.org/10.1016/0009-8981(95)98130-9.

130. Alison P. Southern and Sharhabeel Jwayyed, "Iodine Toxicity," essay, in *StatPearls [Internet]* (Treasure Island, FL: StatPearls Publishing, 2022), https://www.ncbi.nlm.nih.gov/books/NBK560770/.

131. Divya M Mathews et al., "Iodine and Fertility: Do We Know Enough?," *Human Reproduction* 36, no. 2 (December 8, 2020): 265–74, https://doi.org/10.1093/humrep/deaa312.
     Jay Rappaport, "Changes in Dietary Iodine Explains Increasing Incidence of Breast Cancer with Distant Involvement in Young Women," *Journal of Cancer* 8, no. 2 (2017): 174–77, https://doi.org/10.7150/jca.17835.

132. Jorge D. Flechas, "Iodine Study #10," Orthoiodosupplementation in a Primary Care Practice, Jorge D. Flechas, M.D., n.d., https://www.optimox.com/iodine-study-10.

133. T. Maruo et al., "A Role for Thyroid Hormone in the Induction of Ovulation and Corpus Luteum Function," *Hormone Research* 37, no. 1 (1992): 12–18, https://doi.org/10.1159/000182338.

134. William L. Stone, Tram Pham, and Shamim S. Mohiuddin, "Biochemistry, Antioxidants," essay, in *StatPearls [Internet]* (Treasure Island, FL: StatPearls Publishing, 2022), https://www.ncbi.nlm.nih.gov/books/NBK541064/.

135. Joseph Pizzorno, "Glutathione!," *Integrative Medicine a Clinician's Journal* 13, no. 1 (February 2014): 8–12, https://www.ncbi.nlm.nih.gov/pmc/articles/PMC4684116/.

136. Joseph Pizzorno, "Glutathione!," *Integrative Medicine a Clinician's Journal* 13, no. 1 (February 2014): 8–12, https://www.ncbi.nlm.nih.gov/pmc/articles/PMC4684116/.
Geoffrey M. Cooper, "Mitochondria," essay, in *The Cell: A Molecular Approach*, 2nd ed. (Sunderland, MA: Sinauer Associates, 2000), https://www.ncbi.nlm.nih.gov/books/NBK9896/.

137. Joseph Pizzorno, "Glutathione!," *Integrative Medicine a Clinician's Journal* 13, no. 1 (February 2014): 8–12, https://www.ncbi.nlm.nih.gov/pmc/articles/PMC4684116/.

138. Oyewopo Adeoye et al., "Review on the Role of Glutathione on Oxidative Stress and Infertility," *JBRA Assisted Reproduction* 22, no. 1 (March 1, 2017): 61–66, https://doi.org/10.5935/1518-0557.20180003.

139. Romilly E. Hodges and Deanna M. Minich, "Modulation of Metabolic Detoxification Pathways Using Foods and Food-Derived Components: A Scientific Review with Clinical Application," *Journal of Nutrition and Metabolism* 2015 (June 15, 2015): 1–23, https://doi.org/10.1155/2015/760689.
Simone Phang-Lyn, "Biochemistry, Biotransformation," essay, in *StatPearls [Internet]*, ed. Valerie A. Llerena (Treasure Island, FL: StatPearls Publishing, 2022), https://www.ncbi.nlm.nih.gov/books/NBK544353/.

140. Cruz E. García-Rodríguez et al., "Does Consumption of Two Portions of Salmon per Week Enhance the Antioxidant Defense System in Pregnant Women?," *Antioxidants & Redox Signaling* 16, no. 12 (June 15, 2012): 1401–6, https://doi.org/10.1089/ars.2012.4508.
Oyewopo Adeoye et al., "Review on the Role of Glutathione on Oxidative Stress and Infertility," *JBRA Assisted Reproduction* 22, no. 1 (March 1, 2017): 61–66, https://doi.org/10.5935/1518-0557.20180003.

141. Joseph Pizzorno, "Glutathione!," *Integrative Medicine a Clinician's Journal* 13, no. 1 (February 2014): 8–12, https://www.ncbi.nlm.nih.gov/pmc/articles/PMC4684116/.
G. Bounous, "Whey Protein Concentrate (WPC) and Glutathione Modulation in Cancer Treatment," *Anticancer Research* 20, no. 6C (2000): 4785–92, https://pubmed.ncbi.nlm.nih.gov/11205219/.

142. Joseph Pizzorno, "The Path Ahead: Persistent Organic Pollutants (POPs)—a Serious Clinical Concern," *Integrative Medicine a Clinician's Journal* 12, no. 2 (April 2013): 8–11.

Himani Sharma et al., "Gene Expression Profiling in Practitioners of Sudarshan Kriya," *Journal of Psychosomatic Research* 64, no. 2 (February 2008): 213–18, https://doi.org/10.1016/j.jpsychores.2007.07.003.

Joseph Pizzorno, "Glutathione!," *Integrative Medicine a Clinician's Journal* 13, no. 1 (February 2014): 8–12, https://www.ncbi.nlm.nih.gov/pmc/articles/PMC4684116/.

Cholsoon Jang et al., "The Small Intestine Converts Dietary Fructose into Glucose and Organic Acids," *Cell Metabolism* 27, no. 2 (February 6, 2018): 351–61, https://doi.org/10.1016/j.cmet.2017.12.016.

143. Mimi L. Tang and Raymond J. Mullins, "Food Allergy: Is Prevalence Increasing?," *Internal Medicine Journal* 47, no. 3 (March 2017): 256–61, https://doi.org/10.1111/imj.13362.

144. Aristo Vojdani, "Detection of IGE, IGG, IGA and IGM Antibodies against Raw and Processed Food Antigens," *Nutrition & Metabolism* 6, no. 1 (May 12, 2009), https://doi.org/10.1186/1743-7075-6-22.

145. Erin Smith et al., "Food Sensitivity Testing and Elimination Diets in the Management of Irritable Bowel Syndrome," *Journal of Osteopathic Medicine* 120, no. 1 (January 1, 2020): 19–23, https://doi.org/10.7556/jaoa.2020.008.

Kirsten Beyer and Suzanne S Teuber, "Food Allergy Diagnostics: Scientific and Unproven Procedures," *Current Opinion in Allergy & Clinical Immunology* 5, no. 3 (June 2005): 261–66, https://doi.org/10.1097/01.all.0000168792.27948.f9.

Aristo Vojdani, "Detection of IGE, IGG, IGA and IGM Antibodies against Raw and Processed Food Antigens," *Nutrition & Metabolism* 6, no. 1 (May 12, 2009), https://doi.org/10.1186/1743-7075-6-22.

146. Aristo Vojdani, "Detection of IGE, IGG, IGA and IGM Antibodies against Raw and Processed Food Antigens," *Nutrition & Metabolism* 6, no. 1 (May 12, 2009), https://doi.org/10.1186/1743-7075-6-22.

147. Zahid Shakoor et al., "Prevalence of IGG-Mediated Food Intolerance among Patients with Allergic Symptoms," *Annals of Saudi Medicine* 36, no. 6 (December 1, 2016): 386–90, https://doi.org/10.5144/0256-4947.2016.386.

148. Kirsten Beyer and Suzanne S Teuber, "Food Allergy Diagnostics: Scientific and Unproven Procedures," *Current Opinion in Allergy & Clinical Immunology* 5, no. 3 (June 2005): 261–66, https://doi.org/10.1097/01.all.0000168792.27948.f9.

Aristo Vojdani, "Detection of IGE, IGG, IGA and IGM Antibodies against Raw and Processed Food Antigens," *Nutrition & Metabolism* 6, no. 1 (May 12, 2009), https://doi.org/10.1186/1743-7075-6-22.

149. Patricia M. Herman and Lisa M. Drost, "Evaluating the Clinical Relevance of Food Sensitivity Tests: A Single Subject Experiment," *Alternative Medicine Review : A Journal of Clinical Therapeutic* 9, no. 2 (June 2004): 198–207, https://pubmed.ncbi.nlm.nih.gov/15253678/.

150. Aristo Vojdani, "Detection of IGE, IGG, IGA and IGM Antibodies against Raw and Processed Food Antigens," *Nutrition & Metabolism* 6, no. 1 (May 12, 2009), https://doi.org/10.1186/1743-7075-6-22.

151. Jaime Uribarri et al., "Advanced Glycation End Products in Foods and a Practical Guide to Their Reduction in the Diet," *Journal of the American Dietetic Association* 110, no. 6 (June 1, 2010): 911–16, https://doi.org/10.1016/j.jada.2010.03.018.
Aristo Vojdani, "Detection of IGE, IGG, IGA and IGM Antibodies against Raw and Processed Food Antigens," *Nutrition & Metabolism* 6, no. 1 (May 12, 2009), https://doi.org/10.1186/1743-7075-6-22.

152. Teresia Goldberg et al., "Advanced Glycoxidation End Products in Commonly Consumed Foods," *Journal of the American Dietetic Association* 104, no. 8 (August 1, 2004): 1287–91, https://doi.org/10.1016/j.jada.2004.05.214.

153. Caroline J Tuck et al., "Food Intolerances," *Nutrients* 11, no. 7 (July 22, 2019): 1684, https://doi.org/10.3390/nu11071684.

154. Caroline J Tuck et al., "Food Intolerances," *Nutrients* 11, no. 7 (July 22, 2019): 1684, https://doi.org/10.3390/nu11071684.

155. Caroline J Tuck et al., "Food Intolerances," *Nutrients* 11, no. 7 (July 22, 2019): 1684, https://doi.org/10.3390/nu11071684.

156. Jacqueline S Barrett, "How to Institute the Low-Fodmap Diet," *Journal of Gastroenterology and Hepatology* 32 (February 28, 2017): 8–10, https://doi.org/10.1111/jgh.13686.
Caroline J Tuck et al., "Food Intolerances," *Nutrients* 11, no. 7 (July 22, 2019): 1684, https://doi.org/10.3390/nu11071684.

157. Alan R. Gaby and David Rakel, "Chapter 31 - Food Allergy and Intolerance," essay, in *Integrative Medicine*, 4th ed. (Elsevier, 2018), 310–18, https://doi.org/10.1016/b978-0-323-35868-2.00031-1.

158. Zahid Shakoor et al., "Prevalence of IGG-Mediated Food Intolerance among Patients with Allergic Symptoms," *Annals of Saudi Medicine* 36, no. 6 (December 1, 2016): 386–90, https://doi.org/10.5144/0256-4947.2016.386.
Sara M. Seifert et al., "Health Effects of Energy Drinks on Children, Adolescents, and Young Adults," *Pediatrics* 127, no. 3 (March 1, 2011): 511–28, https://doi.org/10.1542/peds.2009-3592.
Olukayode Isaac Adeosun et al., "Methanolic Extract of Cola Nitida Elicits Dose-Dependent Diuretic, Natriuretic and Kaliuretic Activities without Causing Electrolyte Impairment, Hepatotoxicity and Nephrotoxicity in Rats," *International Journal of Physiology, Pathophysiology and Pharmacology* 9, no. 6 (December 25, 2017): 231–39, https://www.ncbi.nlm.nih.gov/pmc/articles/PMC5770520/.

159. Ewa B. Posner and Muhammad Haseeb, "Celiac Disease," essay, in *StatPearls [Internet]* (Treasure Island, FL: StatPearls Publishing, 2022), https://www.ncbi.nlm.nih.gov/books/NBK441900/.

160. Rosa Leonôra Salerno Soares, "Irritable Bowel Syndrome, Food Intolerance and Non- Celiac Gluten Sensitivity. A New Clinical Challenge," *Arquivos de Gastroenterologia* 55, no. 4 (December 2018): 417–22, https://doi.org/10.1590/s0004-2803.201800000-88.

161. Anna Roszkowska et al., "Non-Celiac Gluten Sensitivity: A Review," *Medicina* 55, no. 6 (May 28, 2019): 222, https://doi.org/10.3390/medicina55060222.

162. Spencer P Thornton, "Opioids in Milk and Beef," *JOJ Ophthalmology* 4, no. 3 (September 6, 2017), https://doi.org/10.19080/jojo.2017.04.555638.

163. Simon Brooke-Taylor et al., "Systematic Review of the Gastrointestinal Effects of A1 Compared with A2 β-Casein," *Advances in Nutrition: An International Review Journal* 8, no. 5 (September 7, 2017): 739–48, https://doi.org/10.3945/an.116.013953.

164. Massimo Bellini et al., "Low Fodmap Diet: Evidence, Doubts, and Hopes," *Nutrients* 12, no. 1 (January 4, 2020): 148, https://doi.org/10.3390/nu12010148.

165. Wolfgang J. Schnedl and Dietmar Enko, "Histamine Intolerance Originates in the Gut," *Nutrients* 13, no. 4 (April 12, 2021): 1262, https://doi.org/10.3390/nu13041262.

166. Helmut L. Haas, Olga A. Sergeeva, and Oliver Selbach, "Histamine in the Nervous System," *Physiological Reviews* 88, no. 3 (July 1, 2008): 1183–1241, https://doi.org/10.1152/physrev.00043.2007.

167. Oriol Comas-Basté et al., "Histamine Intolerance: The Current State of the Art," *Biomolecules* 10, no. 8 (August 14, 2020): 1181, https://doi.org/10.3390/biom10081181.
    E. Kovacova-Hanuskova et al., "Histamine, Histamine Intoxication and Intolerance," *Allergologia et Immunopathologia* 43, no. 5 (September 2015): 498–506, https://doi.org/10.1016/j.aller.2015.05.001.

168. Oriol Comas-Basté et al., "Histamine Intolerance: The Current State of the Art," *Biomolecules* 10, no. 8 (August 14, 2020): 1181, https://doi.org/10.3390/biom10081181.
    E. Kovacova-Hanuskova et al., "Histamine, Histamine Intoxication and Intolerance," *Allergologia et Immunopathologia* 43, no. 5 (September 2015): 498–506, https://doi.org/10.1016/j.aller.2015.05.001.

169. S Gangi and O Johansson, "A Theoretical Model Based upon Mast Cells and Histamine to Explain the Recently Proclaimed Sensitivity to Electric and/or Magnetic Fields in Humans," *Medical Hypotheses* 54, no. 4 (April 2000): 663–71, https://doi.org/10.1054/mehy.1999.0923.

170. Pio Conti et al., "Mast Cells Activated by SARS-CoV-2 Release Histamine Which Increases IL-1 Levels Causing Cytokine Storm and Inflammatory Reaction in COVID-19," *Journal of Biological Regulators*

and Homeostatic Agents 34, no. 5 (October 20, 2020): 1629–32, https://doi.org/https://doi.org/10.23812/20-2EDIT.

171.   Martin Hrubisko et al., "Histamine Intolerance—the More We Know the Less We Know. A Review," *Nutrients* 13, no. 7 (June 29, 2021): 2228, https://doi.org/10.3390/nu13072228.

172.   Martin Hrubisko et al., "Histamine Intolerance—the More We Know the Less We Know. A Review," *Nutrients* 13, no. 7 (June 29, 2021): 2228, https://doi.org/10.3390/nu13072228.

173.   Sònia Sánchez-Pérez et al., "Biogenic Amines in Plant-Origin Foods: Are They Frequently Underestimated in Low-Histamine Diets?," *Foods* 7, no. 12 (December 14, 2018): 205, https://doi.org/10.3390/foods7120205. Claudia Ruiz-Capillas and Ana Herrero, "Impact of Biogenic Amines on Food Quality and Safety," *Foods* 8, no. 2 (February 8, 2019): 62, https://doi.org/10.3390/foods8020062.

174.   Z. Fan et al., "Estrogen and Estrogen Receptor Signaling Promotes Allergic Immune Responses: Effects on Immune Cells, Cytokines, and Inflammatory Factors Involved in Allergy," *Allergologia et Immunopathologia* 47, no. 5 (September 2019): 506–12, https://doi.org/10.1016/j.aller.2019.03.001.

175.   W. A. Fogel, "Diamine Oxidase (DAO) and Female Sex Hormones," *Agents and Actions* 18, no. 1–2 (April 1986): 44–45, https://doi.org/10.1007/bf01987978.

176.   M. Vasiadi et al., "Progesterone Inhibits Mast Cell Secretion," *International Journal of Immunopathology and Pharmacology* 19, no. 4 (October 1, 2006): 787–94, https://doi.org/10.1177/039463200601900408.

177.   Peter C. Konturek, Thomas Brzozowski, and S. J. Konturek, "Stress and the Gut: Pathophysiology, Clinical Consequences, Diagnostic Approach and Treatment Options," *Journal of Physiology and Pharmacology : An Official Journal of the Polish Physiological Society* 62, no. 6 (December 2011): 591–99, https://pubmed.ncbi.nlm.nih.gov/22314561/.

178.   Peter C. Konturek, Thomas Brzozowski, and S. J. Konturek, "Stress and the Gut: Pathophysiology, Clinical Consequences, Diagnostic Approach and Treatment Options," *Journal of Physiology and Pharmacology : An Official Journal of the Polish Physiological Society* 62, no. 6 (December 2011): 591–99, https://pubmed.ncbi.nlm.nih.gov/22314561/.

179.   Bruno Bordoni and Bruno Morabito, "Symptomatology Correlations between the Diaphragm and Irritable Bowel Syndrome," *Cureus* 10, no. 7 (July 23, 2018), https://doi.org/10.7759/cureus.3036.

MOVEMENT OVERVIEW

1. GranolaJeremy, "USWNT: 12 Stats That Prove Women's Soccer Is the Best in America," UNAFRAID SHOW, July 5, 2019, https://unafraidshow.com/12-uswnt-stats-womens-soccer-america-is-the-best/.

2. Joseph T. Costello, Francois Bieuzen, and Chris M. Bleakley, "Where Are All the Female Participants in Sports and Exercise Medicine Research?," *European Journal of Sport Science* 14, no. 8 (April 25, 2014): 847–51, https://doi.org/10.1080/17461391.2014.911354.

3. Marius Rademaker, "Do Women Have More Adverse Drug Reactions?," *American Journal of Clinical Dermatology* 2, no. 6 (December 2001): 349–51, https://doi.org/10.2165/00128071-200102060-00001.

4. L. J. Tarnopolsky et al., "Gender Differences in Substrate for Endurance Exercise," *Journal of Applied Physiology* 68, no. 1 (January 1, 1990): 302–8, https://doi.org/10.1152/jappl.1990.68.1.302.
    M. A. Tarnopolsky et al., "Carbohydrate Loading and Metabolism during Exercise in Men and Women," *Journal of Applied Physiology* 78, no. 4 (April 1, 1995): 1360–68, https://doi.org/10.1152/jappl.1995.78.4.1360.

5. M. A. Tarnopolsky et al., "Carbohydrate Loading and Metabolism during Exercise in Men and Women," *Journal of Applied Physiology* 78, no. 4 (April 1, 1995): 1360–68, https://doi.org/10.1152/jappl.1995.78.4.1360.

6. J. Lynne Walker et al., "Dietary Carbohydrate, Muscle Glycogen Content, and Endurance Performance in Well-Trained Women," *Journal of Applied Physiology* 88, no. 6 (June 1, 2000): 2151–58, https://doi.org/10.1152/jappl.2000.88.6.2151.

7. Gregory N. Ruegsegger and Frank W. Booth, "Health Benefits of Exercise," *Cold Spring Harbor Perspectives in Medicine* 8, no. 7 (May 15, 2017), https://doi.org/10.1101/cshperspect.a029694.
    Brett A. Dolezal et al., "Interrelationship between Sleep and Exercise: A Systematic Review," *Advances in Preventive Medicine* 2017 (March 26, 2017): 1–14, https://doi.org/10.1155/2017/1364387.

8. Jonathan P. Little et al., "Sprint Exercise Snacks: A Novel Approach to Increase Aerobic Fitness," *European Journal of Applied Physiology* 119, no. 5 (March 7, 2019): 1203–12, https://doi.org/10.1007/s00421-019-04110-z.

9. Thomas R. Baechle and Roger W. Earle, *Essentials of Strength Training and Conditioning*, 3rd ed. (Champaign, IL: Human Kinetics, 2008).

10. Thomas R. Baechle and Roger W. Earle, *Essentials of Strength Training and Conditioning*, 3rd ed. (Champaign, IL: Human Kinetics, 2008).
    P. D. Gollnick and H. Matoba, "Role of Carbohydrate in Exercise," *Clinics in Sports Medicine* 3, no. 3 (July 1984): 583–93, https://pubmed.ncbi.nlm.nih.gov/6571232/.

11. Thomas R. Baechle and Roger W. Earle, *Essentials of Strength Training and Conditioning*, 3rd ed. (Champaign, IL: Human Kinetics, 2008).

12. M. P. Miles and P. M. Clarkson, "Exercise-Induced Muscle Pain, Soreness, and Cramps," *The Journal of Sports Medicine and Physical Fitness* 34, no. 3 (September 1994): 203–16, https://pubmed.ncbi.nlm.nih.gov/7830383/.

13. Paul B. Lewis, Deana Ruby, and Charles A. Bush-Joseph, "Muscle Soreness and Delayed-Onset Muscle Soreness," *Clinics in Sports Medicine* 31, no. 2 (April 1, 2012): 255–62, https://doi.org/10.1016/j.csm.2011.09.009.

14. Kyle L. Flann et al., "Muscle Damage and Muscle Remodeling: No Pain, No Gain?," *Journal of Experimental Biology* 214, no. 4 (February 15, 2011): 674–79, https://doi.org/10.1242/jeb.050112.

15. J E Hilbert, G A Sforzo, and T Swensen, "The Effects of Massage on Delayed Onset Muscle Soreness," *British Journal of Sports Medicine* 37, no. 1 (February 1, 2003): 72–75, https://doi.org/10.1136/bjsm.37.1.72. Gregory E. Pearcey et al., "Foam Rolling for Delayed-Onset Muscle Soreness and Recovery of Dynamic Performance Measures," *Journal of Athletic Training* 50, no. 1 (January 1, 2015): 5–13, https://doi.org/10.4085/1062-6050-50.1.01.

16. Gregory E. Pearcey et al., "Foam Rolling for Delayed-Onset Muscle Soreness and Recovery of Dynamic Performance Measures," *Journal of Athletic Training* 50, no. 1 (January 1, 2015): 5–13, https://doi.org/10.4085/1062-6050-50.1.01.

17. Rudolf E. Noble, "Depression in Women," *Metabolism* 54, no. 5 (May 1, 2005): 49–52, https://doi.org/10.1016/j.metabol.2005.01.014.

18. Peter J. Carek, Sarah E. Laibstain, and Stephen M. Carek, "Exercise for the Treatment of Depression and Anxiety," *The International Journal of Psychiatry in Medicine* 41, no. 1 (January 31, 2011): 15–28, https://doi.org/10.2190/pm.41.1.c.

19. Jan Knapen et al., "Exercise Therapy Improves Both Mental and Physical Health in Patients with Major Depression," *Disability and Rehabilitation* 37, no. 16 (October 24, 2014): 1490–95, https://doi.org/10.3109/09638288.2014.972579.

20. Peter J. Carek, Sarah E. Laibstain, and Stephen M. Carek, "Exercise for the Treatment of Depression and Anxiety," *The International Journal of Psychiatry in Medicine* 41, no. 1 (January 31, 2011): 15–28, https://doi.org/10.2190/pm.41.1.c.

21. Peter J. Carek, Sarah E. Laibstain, and Stephen M. Carek, "Exercise for the Treatment of Depression and Anxiety," *The International Journal of Psychiatry in Medicine* 41, no. 1 (January 31, 2011): 15–28, https://doi.org/10.2190/pm.41.1.c. Brendon Stubbs et al., "Physical Activity and Anxiety: A Perspective from the World Health Survey," *Journal of Affective Disorders* 208 (January 15, 2017): 545–52, https://doi.org/10.1016/j.jad.2016.10.028.

22.   Jan Knapen et al., "Exercise Therapy Improves Both Mental and Physical Health in Patients with Major Depression," *Disability and Rehabilitation* 37, no. 16 (October 24, 2014): 1490–95, https://doi.org/10.3109/09638288.2014.972579.

23.   Manda Null and Manuj Agarwal, "Anatomy, Lymphatic System," essay, in *StatPearls [Internet]* (Treasure Island, FL: StatPearls Publishing, 2022), https://www.statpearls.com/ArticleLibrary/viewarticle/24559.

24.   Manda Null and Manuj Agarwal, "Anatomy, Lymphatic System," essay, in *StatPearls [Internet]* (Treasure Island, FL: StatPearls Publishing, 2022), https://www.statpearls.com/ArticleLibrary/viewarticle/24559.

25.   Lauren Ozdowski, "Physiology, Lymphatic System," essay, in *StatPearls [Internet]*, ed. Vikas Gupta (Treasure Island, FL: StatPearls Publishing, n.d.), https://www.ncbi.nlm.nih.gov/books/NBK557833/.
      Manda Null and Manuj Agarwal, "Anatomy, Lymphatic System," essay, in *StatPearls [Internet]* (Treasure Island, FL: StatPearls Publishing, 2022), https://www.statpearls.com/ArticleLibrary/viewarticle/24559.

26.   Joshua P. Scallan et al., "Lymphatic Pumping: Mechanics, Mechanisms and Malfunction," *The Journal of Physiology* 594, no. 20 (August 2, 2016): 5749–68, https://doi.org/10.1113/jp272088.

27.   Feifei Wang and Szilvia Boros, "The Effect of Physical Activity on Sleep Quality: A Systematic Review," *European Journal of Physiotherapy* 23, no. 1 (June 24, 2019): 11–18, https://doi.org/10.1080/21679169.2019.1623314.

28.   Feifei Wang and Szilvia Boros, "The Effect of Physical Activity on Sleep Quality: A Systematic Review," *European Journal of Physiotherapy* 23, no. 1 (June 24, 2019): 11–18, https://doi.org/10.1080/21679169.2019.1623314.
      Ana Kovacevic et al., "The Effect of Resistance Exercise on Sleep: A Systematic Review of Randomized Controlled Trials," *Sleep Medicine Reviews* 39 (June 2018): 52–68, https://doi.org/10.1016/j.smrv.2017.07.002.

EATING AND MOVING FOR YOUR CYCLE

1.   Gabrielle L. Davidson et al., "The Gut Microbiome as a Driver of Individual Variation in Cognition and Functional Behaviour," *Philosophical Transactions of the Royal Society B: Biological Sciences* 373, no. 1756 (August 13, 2018): p. 20170286, https://doi.org/10.1098/rstb.2017.0286.

2.   Simeng Zhang et al., "Changes in Sleeping Energy Metabolism and Thermoregulation during Menstrual Cycle," *Physiological Reports* 8, no. 2 (January 24, 2020), https://doi.org/10.14814/phy2.14353.

3.   Fiona C. Baker, Felicia Siboza, and Andrea Fuller, "Temperature Regulation in Women: Effects of the Menstrual Cycle," *Temperature* 7, no. 3 (March 22, 2020): pp. 226-262, https://doi.org/10.1080/23328940.2020.1735927.

4. Beverly G Reed and Bruce R Carr, "The Normal Menstrual Cycle and the Control of Ovulation," essay, in *Endotext [Internet]*, ed. Kenneth R Feingold, Bradley Anawalt, and Alison Boyce (South Dartmouth, MA: MDText.com, Inc., 2000), https://www.ncbi.nlm.nih.gov/books/NBK279054/.

5. Beverly G Reed and Bruce R Carr, "The Normal Menstrual Cycle and the Control of Ovulation," essay, in *Endotext [Internet]*, ed. Kenneth R Feingold, Bradley Anawalt, and Alison Boyce (South Dartmouth, MA: MDText.com, Inc., 2000), https://www.ncbi.nlm.nih.gov/books/NBK279054/.

6. Toni Weschler, *Taking Charge of Your Fertility: The Definitive Guide to Natural Birth Control and Pregnancy Achievement* (New York, NY: Quill, 2002).

7. Adeline Angeli et al., "Joint Model of Iron and Hepcidin during the Menstrual Cycle in Healthy Women," *The AAPS Journal* 18, no. 2 (February 2, 2016): pp. 490-504, https://doi.org/10.1208/s12248-016-9875-4.

8. Beverly G Reed and Bruce R Carr, "The Normal Menstrual Cycle and the Control of Ovulation," essay, in *Endotext [Internet]*, ed. Kenneth R Feingold, Bradley Anawalt, and Alison Boyce (South Dartmouth, MA: MDText.com, Inc., 2000), https://www.ncbi.nlm.nih.gov/books/NBK279054/.
   Sandy Jiang and Cassandra L Quave, "A Comparison of Traditional Food and Health Strategies among Taiwanese and Chinese Immigrants in Atlanta, Georgia, USA," *Journal of Ethnobiology and Ethnomedicine* 9, no. 1 (August 27, 2013), https://doi.org/10.1186/1746-4269-9-61.

9. Hadas Rachel Rabinovitz et al., "Big Breakfast Rich in Protein and Fat Improves Glycemic Control in Type 2 Diabetics," *Obesity* 22, no. 5 (December 6, 2013), https://doi.org/10.1002/oby.20654.

10. Juliana Fernandes Matos et al., "Role of Sex Hormones in Gastrointestinal Motility in Pregnant and Non-Pregnant Rats," *World Journal of Gastroenterology* 22, no. 25 (July 7, 2016): pp. 5761-5768, https://doi.org/10.3748/wjg.v22.i25.5761.

11. Nkechinyere Chidi-Ogbolu and Keith Baar, "Effect of Estrogen on Musculoskeletal Performance and Injury Risk," *Frontiers in Physiology* 9 (January 15, 2019), https://doi.org/10.3389/fphys.2018.01834.

12. Beverly G Reed and Bruce R Carr, "The Normal Menstrual Cycle and the Control of Ovulation," essay, in *Endotext [Internet]*, ed. Kenneth R Feingold, Bradley Anawalt, and Alison Boyce (South Dartmouth, MA: MDText.com, Inc., 2000), https://www.ncbi.nlm.nih.gov/books/NBK279054/.

13. Blanca Romero-Moraleda et al., "The Influence of the Menstrual Cycle on Muscle Strength and Power Performance," *Journal of Human Kinetics* 68, no. 1 (August 21, 2019): pp. 123-133, https://doi.org/10.2478/hukin-2019-0061.

14. Toni Weschler, *Taking Charge of Your Fertility: The Definitive Guide to Natural Birth Control and Pregnancy Achievement* (New York, NY: Quill, 2002).

15. Eunsook Sung et al., "Effects of Follicular versus Luteal Phase-Based Strength Training in Young Women," *SpringerPlus* 3, no. 1 (November 11, 2014), https://doi.org/10.1186/2193-1801-3-668.

16. Blanca Romero-Moraleda et al., "The Influence of the Menstrual Cycle on Muscle Strength and Power Performance," *Journal of Human Kinetics* 68, no. 1 (August 21, 2019): 123–33, https://doi.org/10.2478/hukin-2019-0061.

17. JongEun Yim, Jerrold Petrofsky, and Haneul Lee, "Correlation between Mechanical Properties of the Ankle Muscles and Postural Sway during the Menstrual Cycle," *The Tohoku Journal of Experimental Medicine* 244, no. 3 (March 14, 2018): pp. 201-207, https://doi.org/10.1620/tjem.244.201.

18. Beverly G Reed and Bruce R Carr, "The Normal Menstrual Cycle and the Control of Ovulation," essay, in *Endotext [Internet],* ed. Kenneth R Feingold, Bradley Anawalt, and Alison Boyce (South Dartmouth, MA: MDText.com, Inc., 2000), https://www.ncbi.nlm.nih.gov/books/NBK279054/.

19. Toni Weschler, *Taking Charge of Your Fertility: The Definitive Guide to Natural Birth Control and Pregnancy Achievement* (New York, NY: Quill, 2002).

20. Sandy Jiang and Cassandra L Quave, "A Comparison of Traditional Food and Health Strategies among Taiwanese and Chinese Immigrants in Atlanta, Georgia, USA," *Journal of Ethnobiology and Ethnomedicine* 9, no. 1 (August 27, 2013), https://doi.org/10.1186/1746-4269-9-61.

21. Karen J. Auborn et al., "Indole-3-Carbinol Is a Negative Regulator of Estrogen," *The Journal of Nutrition* 133, no. 7 (July 1, 2003): pp. 2470-2475, https://doi.org/10.1093/jn/133.7.2470s.
    J. H. Fowke, C. Longcope, and J. R. Hebert, "Brassica Vegetable Consumption Shifts Estrogen Metabolism in Healthy Postmenopausal Women," *Cancer Epidemiology, Biomarkers & Prevention: a Publication of the American Association for Cancer Research, Cosponsored by the American Society of Preventive Oncology* 9, no. 8 (August 2000): pp. 773-779, https://pubmed.ncbi.nlm.nih.gov/10952093/.

22. JongEun Yim, Jerrold Petrofsky, and Haneul Lee, "Correlation between Mechanical Properties of the Ankle Muscles and Postural Sway during the Menstrual Cycle," *The Tohoku Journal of Experimental Medicine* 244, no. 3 (March 14, 2018): 201–7, https://doi.org/10.1620/tjem.244.201.

23. Blanca Romero-Moraleda et al., "The Influence of the Menstrual Cycle on Muscle Strength and Power Performance," *Journal of Human Kinetics* 68, no. 1 (August 21, 2019): 123–33, https://doi.org/10.2478/hukin-2019-0061.

24. Toni Weschler, *Taking Charge of Your Fertility: The Definitive Guide to*

Natural Birth Control and Pregnancy Achievement (New York, NY: Quill, 2002).

25. Kaitlyn Steward and Avais Raja, "Physiology, Ovulation And Basal Body Temperature," in *StatPearls [Internet]* (Treasure Island, FL: StatPearls Publishing, 2022), https://www.ncbi.nlm.nih.gov/books/NBK546686/. Simeng Zhang et al., "Changes in Sleeping Energy Metabolism and Thermoregulation during Menstrual Cycle," *Physiological Reports* 8, no. 2 (January 24, 2020), https://doi.org/10.14814/phy2.14353.

26. Hadas Rachel Rabinovitz et al., "Big Breakfast Rich in Protein and Fat Improves Glycemic Control in Type 2 Diabetics," *Obesity* 22, no. 5 (December 6, 2013), https://doi.org/10.1002/oby.20654. Allison M. Hodge et al., "Glycemic Index and Dietary Fiber and the Risk of Type 2 Diabetes," *Diabetes Care* 27, no. 11 (November 1, 2004): pp. 2701-2706, https://doi.org/10.2337/diacare.27.11.2701.

27. Dawn M Richard et al., "I-Tryptophan: Basic Metabolic Functions, Behavioral Research and Therapeutic Indications," *International Journal of Tryptophan Research* 2 (March 23, 2009): pp. 45-60, https://doi.org/10.4137/ijtr.s2129.

28. Anne-Laure Tardy et al., "Vitamins and Minerals for Energy, Fatigue and Cognition: A Narrative Review of the Biochemical and Clinical Evidence," *Nutrients* 12, no. 1 (January 16, 2020): p. 228, https://doi.org/10.3390/nu12010228. Kara A. Michels et al., "Folate, Homocysteine and the Ovarian Cycle among Healthy Regularly Menstruating Women," *Human Reproduction* 32, no. 8 (June 23, 2017): pp. 1743-1750, https://doi.org/10.1093/humrep/dex233. Keewan Kim et al., "Dietary Intakes of Vitamin B-2 (Riboflavin), Vitamin B-6, and Vitamin B-12 and Ovarian Cycle Function among Premenopausal Women," *Journal of the Academy of Nutrition and Dietetics* 120, no. 5 (May 1, 2020): pp. 885-892, https://doi.org/10.1016/j.jand.2019.10.013. G E Abraham, "Nutritional Factors in the Etiology of the Premenstrual Tension Syndromes," *The Journal of Reproductive Medicine* 28, no. 7 (July 1983): pp. 446-464.

29. Stephen J. Lewis, Robert E. Oakey, and Kenneth W. Heaton, "Intestinal Absorption of Oestrogen," *European Journal of Gastroenterology &Amp; Hepatology* 10, no. 1 (January 1998): pp. 33-40, https://doi.org/10.1097/00042737-199801000-00007. SJ Lewis et al., "Lower Serum Oestrogen Concentrations Associated with Faster Intestinal Transit," *British Journal of Cancer* 76, no. 3 (August 1, 1997): pp. 395-400, https://doi.org/10.1038/bjc.1997.397.

30. Keewan Kim et al., "Dietary Intakes of Vitamin B-2 (Riboflavin), Vitamin B-6, and Vitamin B-12 and Ovarian Cycle Function among Premenopausal Women," *Journal of the Academy of Nutrition and Dietetics* 120, no. 5 (May 1, 2020): pp. 885-892, https://doi.org/10.1016/j.

jand.2019.10.013.

31. Zahra Mohebbi Dehnavi, Farzaneh Jafarnejad, and Somayeh Sadeghi Goghary, "The Effect of 8 Weeks Aerobic Exercise on Severity of Physical Symptoms of Premenstrual Syndrome: A Clinical Trial Study," *BMC Women's Health* 18, no. 1 (May 31, 2018), https://doi.org/10.1186/s12905-018-0565-5.

32. Ross Julian et al., "The Effects of Menstrual Cycle Phase on Physical Performance in Female Soccer Players," *PLOS ONE* 12, no. 3 (March 13, 2017), https://doi.org/10.1371/journal.pone.0173951.

PROBLEMS WITH YOUR CYCLE

1. Hoyer, J., Burmann, I., Kieseler, M. L., Vollrath, F., Hellrung, L., Arelin, K., Roggenhofer, E., Villringer, A., & Sacher, J. (2013). Menstrual cycle phase modulates emotional conflict processing in women with and without premenstrual syndrome (PMS)--a pilot study. PloS one, 8(4), e59780. https://doi.org/10.1371/journal.pone.0059780

2. "Office on Women's Health," Office on Women's Health, n.d., https://www.womenshealth.gov/.

3. "Premenstrual Syndrome (PMS)," ACOG, May 2021, https://www.acog.org/womens-health/faqs/premenstrual-syndrome?utm_source=redirect&utm_medium=web&utm_campaign=int.

4. "Premenstrual Syndrome (PMS)," ACOG, May 2021, https://www.acog.org/womens-health/faqs/premenstrual-syndrome?utm_source=redirect&utm_medium=web&utm_campaign=int.

5. Lena Seippel and Torbjörn Bäckström, "Luteal-Phase Estradiol Relates to Symptom Severity in Patients with Premenstrual Syndrome1," *The Journal of Clinical Endocrinology & Metabolism* 83, no. 6 (June 1, 1998): pp. 1988-1992, https://doi.org/10.1210/jcem.83.6.4899.

6. Maura Palmery et al., "Oral Contraceptives and Changes in Nutritional Requirements," *European Review for Medical and Pharmacological Sciences* 17, no. 13 (July 2013): 1804–13, https://pubmed.ncbi.nlm.nih.gov/23852908/.

7. Rupa Vani K. et al., "Menstrual Abnormalities in School Going Girls – Are They Related to Dietary and Exercise Pattern?," *JOURNAL OF CLINICAL AND DIAGNOSTIC RESEARCH* 7, no. 11 (November 2013): 2537–40, https://doi.org/10.7860/jcdr/2013/6464.3603.

8. Rupa Vani K. et al., "Menstrual Abnormalities in School Going Girls – Are They Related to Dietary and Exercise Pattern?," *JOURNAL OF CLINICAL AND DIAGNOSTIC RESEARCH* 7, no. 11 (November 2013): 2537–40, https://doi.org/10.7860/jcdr/2013/6464.3603.

9. Judith J. Wurtman et al., "Effect of Nutrient Intake on Premenstrual Depression," *American Journal of Obstetrics and Gynecology* 161, no. 5 (November 1, 1989): 1228–34, https://doi.org/10.1016/0002-

9378(89)90671-6.

10. Daisy Whitbread, "Top 10 Foods Highest in Tryptophan," My Food Data, April 24, 2022, https://www.myfooddata.com/articles/high-tryptophan-foods.php#high-tryptophan-foods.

11. Simon N. Young, "How to Increase Serotonin in the Human Brain without Drugs," *Journal of Psychiatry & Neuroscience : JPN* 32, no. 6 (November 2007): 394–99.

12. Lisa K. Mannix, "Menstrual-Related Pain Conditions: Dysmenorrhea and Migraine," *Journal of Women's Health* 17, no. 5 (June 6, 2008): 879–91, https://doi.org/10.1089/jwh.2007.0440.

13. E. R. Bertone-Johnson et al., "Cigarette Smoking and the Development of Premenstrual Syndrome," *American Journal of Epidemiology* 168, no. 8 (August 12, 2008): 938–45, https://doi.org/10.1093/aje/kwn194.

14. Claude Monneret, "What Is an Endocrine Disruptor?," *Comptes Rendus Biologies* 340, no. 9–10 (2017): 403–5, https://doi.org/10.1016/j.crvi.2017.07.004.

15. David W Singleton and Sohaib A Khan, "Xenoestrogen Exposure and Mechanisms of Endocrine Disruption," *Frontiers in Bioscience* 8, no. 6 (January 3, 2003): 110–18, https://doi.org/10.2741/1010.

16. Victor J. Navarro et al., "Liver Injury from Herbals and Dietary Supplements in the U.S. Drug-Induced Liver Injury Network," *Hepatology* 60, no. 4 (August 25, 2014): 1399–1408, https://doi.org/10.1002/hep.27317.

17. Susan Thys-Jacobs et al., "Calcium Carbonate and the Premenstrual Syndrome: Effects on Premenstrual and Menstrual Symptoms," *American Journal of Obstetrics and Gynecology* 179, no. 2 (August 1, 1998): 444–52, https://doi.org/10.1016/s0002-9378(98)70377-1. Zinat Ghanbari et al., "Effects of Calcium Supplement Therapy in Women with Premenstrual Syndrome," *Taiwanese Journal of Obstetrics and Gynecology* 48, no. 2 (June 2009): 124–29, https://doi.org/10.1016/s1028-4559(09)60271-0. Fatemeh Shobeiri et al., "Effect of Calcium on Premenstrual Syndrome: A Double-Blind Randomized Clinical Trial," *Obstetrics & Gynecology Science* 60, no. 1 (January 15, 2017): 100–105, https://doi.org/10.5468/ogs.2017.60.1.100.

18. Fatemeh Abdi, Gity Ozgoli, and Fatemeh Sadat Rahnemaie, "A Systematic Review of the Role of Vitamin D and Calcium in Premenstrual Syndrome," *Obstetrics & Gynecology Science* 62, no. 2 (March 2019): 73–86, https://doi.org/10.5468/ogs.2019.62.2.73.

19. "A Guide to Calcium-Rich Foods," Bone Health & Osteoporosis Foundation, May 20, 2020, https://www.nof.org/patients/treatment/calciumvitamin-d/a-guide-to-calcium-rich-foods/.

20. Mohamad Irani and Zaher Merhi, "Role of Vitamin D in Ovarian Physiology and Its Implication in Reproduction: A Systematic Review," *Fertility and Sterility* 102, no. 2 (August 2014): 460–68, https://doi.org/10.1016/j.fertnstert.2014.04.046.

21. Arman Arab, Sahar Golpour-Hamedani, and Nahid Rafie, "The Association between Vitamin D and Premenstrual Syndrome: A Systematic Review and Meta-Analysis of Current Literature," *Journal of the American College of Nutrition* 38, no. 7 (May 10, 2019): 648–56, https://doi.org/10.1080/07315724.2019.1566036.

22. Mohsen Moslehi et al., "The Association between Serum Magnesium and Premenstrual Syndrome: A Systematic Review and Meta-Analysis of Observational Studies," *Biological Trace Element Research* 192, no. 2 (March 18, 2019): pp. 145-152, https://doi.org/10.1007/s12011-019-01672-z.

23. Afsaneh Saeedian Kia, Reza Amani, and Bahman Cheraghian, "The Association between the Risk of Premenstrual Syndrome and Vitamin D, Calcium, and Magnesium Status among University Students: A Case Control Study," *Health Promotion Perspectives* 5, no. 3 (October 25, 2015): pp. 225-230, https://doi.org/10.15171/hpp.2015.027.

24. Sara M. Seifert et al., "Health Effects of Energy Drinks on Children, Adolescents, and Young Adults," *Pediatrics* 127, no. 3 (March 1, 2011): pp. 511-528, https://doi.org/10.1542/peds.2009-3592.

25. Antonio Giordano and Giuseppina Tommonaro, "Curcumin and Cancer," *Nutrients* 11, no. 10 (October 5, 2019): p. 2376, https://doi.org/10.3390/nu11102376.

26. Samira Khayat et al., "Curcumin Attenuates Severity of Premenstrual Syndrome Symptoms: A Randomized, Double-Blind, Placebo-Controlled Trial," *Complementary Therapies in Medicine* 23, no. 3 (June 2015): pp. 318-324, https://doi.org/10.1016/j.ctim.2015.04.001.

27. Sahdeo Prasad, Amit K. Tyagi, and Bharat B. Aggarwal, "Recent Developments in Delivery, Bioavailability, Absorption and Metabolism of Curcumin: The Golden Pigment from Golden Spice," *Cancer Research and Treatment* 46, no. 1 (January 15, 2014): pp. 2-18, https://doi.org/10.4143/crt.2014.46.1.2.

28. Mandana Zafari, Fereshteh Behmanesh, and Azar Agha Mohammadi, "Comparison of the Effect of Fish Oil and Ibuprofen on Treatment of Severe Pain in Primary Dysmenorrhea," *Caspian Journal of Internal Medicine* 2, no. 3 (Summer 2011): 279–82, https://www.ncbi.nlm.nih.gov/pmc/articles/PMC3770499/.

29. B. Deutch, "Menstrual Pain in Danish Women Correlated with Low n-3 Polyunsaturated Fatty Acid Intake," *European Journal of Clinical Nutrition* 49, no. 7 (1995): pp. 508-516.

30. Bente Deutch, Eva Bonefeld Jørgensen, and Jens C Hansen, "Menstrual Discomfort in Danish Women Reduced by Dietary Supplements of Omega-3 PUFA and B12 (Fish Oil or Seal Oil Capsules)," *Nutrition*

Research 20, no. 5 (May 2000): pp. 621–631, https://doi.org/10.1016/s0271-5317(00)00152-4.

31.   Maura Palmery et al., "Oral Contraceptives and Changes in Nutritional Requirements," *European Review for Medical and Pharmacological Sciences* 17, no. 13 (July 2013): 1804–13, https://pubmed.ncbi.nlm.nih.gov/23852908/.

32.   K. Wyatt, "Poor-Quality Studies Suggest That Vitamin B6 Use Is Beneficial in Premenstrual Syndrome," *Western Journal of Medicine* 172, no. 4 (April 1, 2000): pp. 245–245, https://doi.org/10.1136/ewjm.172.4.245.

33.   Seyedeh Zahra Masoumi, Maryam Ataollahi, and Khodayar Oshvandi, "Effect of Combined Use of Calcium and Vitamin B6 on Premenstrual Syndrome Symptoms: A Randomized Clinical Trial," J*ournal of Caring Sciences* 5, no. 1 (March 1, 2016): pp. 67–73, https://doi.org/10.15171/jcs.2016.007.

34.   Thomas Guilliams, "Cruciferous Indole Derivatives as Dietary Supplements: Confusion between IC3 and DIM" (Stevens Point, Wisconsin: The Point Institute, April 2006), https://www.pointinstitute.org/wp-content/uploads/2012/10/Cruciferous-Indole-Derivatives-as-Dietary-Supplements.pdf.
J. J. Michnovicz and H. L. Bradlow, "Induction of Estradiol Metabolism by Dietary Indole-3-Carbinol in Humans," *JNCI Journal of the National Cancer Institute* 82, no. 11 (June 6, 1990): pp. 947–949, https://doi.org/10.1093/jnci/82.11.947.

35.   "Calcium-D-Glucarate," *Alternative Medicine Review : a Journal of Clinical Therapeutic* 7, no. 4 (2002): pp. 336–339.

36.   "Calcium-D-Glucarate," *Alternative Medicine Review : a Journal of Clinical Therapeutic* 7, no. 4 (2002): pp. 336–339.

37.   Emma Pearce et al., "Exercise for Premenstrual Syndrome: A Systematic Review and Meta-Analysis of Randomised Controlled Trials," *BJGP Open* 4, no. 3 (June 10, 2020), https://doi.org/10.3399/bjgpopen20x101032.

38.   Zahra Mohebbi Dehnavi, Farzaneh Jafarnejad, and Somayeh Sadeghi Goghary, "The Effect of 8 Weeks Aerobic Exercise on Severity of Physical Symptoms of Premenstrual Syndrome: A Clinical Trial Study," *BMC Women's Health* 18, no. 1 (May 31, 2018), https://doi.org/10.1186/s12905-018-0565-5.

39.   R. Vishnupriya and P. Rajarajeswaram, "Effects of Aerobic Exercise at Different Intensities in Pre Menstrual Syndrome," *The Journal of Obstetrics and Gynecology of India* 61, no. 6 (December 2011): pp. 675–682, https://doi.org/10.1007/s13224-011-0117-5.

40.   Alexandra M. David et al., "Incidência Da Sindrome Pré-Menstrual Na Prática De Esportes," *Revista Brasileira De Medicina Do Esporte* 15, no. 5 (October 2009): pp. 330–333, https://doi.org/10.1590/s1517-86922009000600001.

41.   Amimi S. Osayande and Suarna Mehulic, "Diagnosis and Initial
       Management of Dysmenorrhea," *American Family Physician* 89, no. 5
       (March 1, 2014): pp. 341-346.

42.   Daniel R. Mishell, "Premenstrual Disorders: Epidemiology and Disease
       Burden," *The American Journal of Managed Care* 11, no. 16 (December
       2005): pp. S473-S479.

43.   RL Reid, "Table 1 Diagnostic Criteria for Premenstrual Dysphoric
       Disorder (PMDD)," in *Endotext [Internet],* ed. Kenneth R Feingold et al.
       (South Dartmouth, MA: MDText.com, Inc., 2017), https://www.ncbi.nlm.
       nih.gov/books/NBK279045/table/premenstrual-syndrom.table1diag/.

44.   Corey E. Pilver et al., "Posttraumatic Stress Disorder and Trauma
       Characteristics Are Correlates of Premenstrual Dysphoric Disorder,"
       Archives of Women's Mental Health 14, no. 5 (July 23, 2011): pp. 383-393,
       https://doi.org/10.1007/s00737-011-0232-4.

45.   Susan S. Girdler et al., "Biological Correlates of Abuse in Women
       with Premenstrual Dysphoric Disorder and Healthy Controls,"
       Psychosomatic Medicine 65, no. 5 (September 2003): pp. 849-856,
       https://doi.org/10.1097/01.psy.0000088593.38201.cd.

46.   Sabrina Hofmeister and Seth Bodden, "Premenstrual Syndrome and
       Premenstrual Dysphoric Disorder," *American Family Physician* 94, no. 3
       (August 1, 2016): pp. 236-240.

47.   Farangis Dorani et al., "Prevalence of Hormone-Related Mood Disorder
       Symptoms in Women with ADHD," *Journal of Psychiatric Research* 133
       (January 2021): 10-15, https://doi.org/10.1016/j.jpsychires.2020.12.005.

48.   Miles Berger, John A. Gray, and Bryan L. Roth, "The Expanded Biology
       of Serotonin," *Annual Review of Medicine* 60, no. 1 (February 1, 2009):
       pp. 355-366, https://doi.org/10.1146/annurev.med.60.042307.110802.

49.   Teresa Lanza di Scalea and Teri Pearlstein, "Premenstrual Dysphoric
       Disorder," *Medical Clinics of North America* 103, no. 4 (July 2019):
       613-28, https://doi.org/10.1016/j.mcna.2019.02.007.

50.   Bonnie Spring, "Recent Research on the Behavioral Effects of
       Tryptophan and Carbohydrate," *Nutrition and Health* 3, no. 1-2 (January
       1984): pp. 55-67, https://doi.org/10.1177/026010608400300204.

51.   Glenda Lindseth, Brian Helland, and Julie Caspers, "The Effects of
       Dietary Tryptophan on Affective Disorders," *Archives of Psychiatric
       Nursing* 29, no. 2 (April 2015): pp. 102-107, https://doi.org/10.1016/j.
       apnu.2014.11.008.

52.   David B. Menkes, Diane C. Coates, and J.Paul Fawcett, "Acute
       Tryptophan Depletion Aggravates Premenstrual Syndrome," *Journal of
       Affective Disorders* 32, no. 1 (September 1994): pp. 37-44, https://doi.
       org/10.1016/0165-0327(94)90059-0.

53.   Judith J. Wurtman et al., "Effect of Nutrient Intake on Premenstrual
       Depression," *American Journal of Obstetrics and Gynecology* 161,
       no. 5 (November 1, 1989): 1228-34, https://doi.org/10.1016/0002-
       9378(89)90671-6.

54. Judith J. Wurtman et al., "Effect of Nutrient Intake on Premenstrual Depression," *American Journal of Obstetrics and Gynecology* 161, no. 5 (November 1, 1989): 1228–34, https://doi.org/10.1016/0002-9378(89)90671-6.

55. Daisy Whitbread, "Top 10 Foods Highest in Tryptophan," My Food Data, April 24, 2022, https://www.myfooddata.com/articles/high-tryptophan-foods.php#high-tryptophan-foods.

56. Simon N. Young, "How to Increase Serotonin in the Human Brain without Drugs," *Journal of Psychiatry & Neuroscience : JPN* 32, no. 6 (November 2007): 394–99.

57. Liisa Hantsoo and C. Neill Epperson, "Premenstrual Dysphoric Disorder: Epidemiology and Treatment," *Current Psychiatry Reports* 17, no. 11 (September 16, 2015): 87, https://doi.org/10.1007/s11920-015-0628-3.

58. Lara Tiranini and Rossella E Nappi, "Recent Advances in Understanding/Management of Premenstrual Dysphoric Disorder/Premenstrual Syndrome," *Faculty Reviews* 11 (April 28, 2022): 11, https://doi.org/10.12703/r/11-11.

59. "Period Pains: Can Anti-Inflammatory Drugs Help?," *InformedHealth.org*, November 16, 2007, https://www.ncbi.nlm.nih.gov/books/NBK279323/.

60. R. A. Matyas et al., "Effects of over-the-Counter Analgesic Use on Reproductive Hormones and Ovulation in Healthy, Premenopausal Women," *Human Reproduction* 30, no. 7 (May 6, 2015): pp. 1714-1723, https://doi.org/10.1093/humrep/dev099.

61. Johan Fredrik Skomsvoll et al., "'Reversibel Infertilitet Ved Ikke-Steroide Antiinflammatoriske Midler' [Reversible Infertility from Nonsteroidal Anti-Inflammatory Drugs]," *Tidsskrift for Den Norske Laegeforening : Tidsskrift for Praktisk Medicin, Ny Raekke* 125, no. 11 (June 2, 2006): pp. 1476-1478, https://pubmed.ncbi.nlm.nih.gov/15940311/.

62. Sherif B.Q, Dr.Al-Zohyri A.M, and Dr. Shihab S.S, "Effects of Some Non Steroidal Anti-Inflammatory Drugs on Ovulation in Women with Mild Musculoskeletal Pain (a Clinical Study)," *IOSR Journal of Pharmacy and Biological Sciences* 9, no. 4 (2014): pp. 43-49, https://doi.org/10.9790/3008-09444349.

63. Benjamin J Delgado and Wilfredo Lopez-Ojeda, "Estrogen," in *StatPearls [Internet]* (Treasure Island, FL: StatPearls Publishing, 2022), https://www.ncbi.nlm.nih.gov/books/NBK538260/.
Anita Kumar et al., "Estradiol: A Steroid with Multiple Facets," *Hormone and Metabolic Research* 50, no. 05 (March 22, 2018): pp. 359-374, https://doi.org/10.1055/s-0044-100920.

64. Seema Patel et al., "Estrogen: The Necessary Evil for Human Health, and Ways to Tame It," *Biomedicine & Pharmacotherapy* 102 (June 2018): pp. 403-411, https://doi.org/10.1016/j.biopha.2018.03.078.

65. Maria Emilia Solano and Petra Clara Arck, "Steroids, Pregnancy and Fetal Development," *Frontiers in Immunology* 10 (January 22, 2020),

https://doi.org/10.3389/fimmu.2019.03017.

66. Maria Emilia Solano and Petra Clara Arck, "Steroids, Pregnancy and Fetal Development," *Frontiers in Immunology* 10 (January 22, 2020), https://doi.org/10.3389/fimmu.2019.03017.

67. Claudia S. Plottel and Martin J. Blaser, "Microbiome and Malignancy," *Cell Host & Microbe* 10, no. 4 (October 20, 2011): pp. 324-335, https://doi.org/10.1016/j.chom.2011.10.003.

68. Stephen J. Lewis, Robert E. Oakey, and Kenneth W. Heaton, "Intestinal Absorption of Oestrogen," *European Journal of Gastroenterology &Amp; Hepatology* 10, no. 1 (January 1998): pp. 33-40, https://doi.org/10.1097/00042737-199801000-00007.

69. Arjun Kalra et al., "Physiology, Liver," in *StatPearls [Internet]* (Treasure Island, FL: StatPearls Publishing, 2022), https://www.ncbi.nlm.nih.gov/books/NBK535438/.

70. Yuki Tsuchiya, Miki Nakajima, and Tsuyoshi Yokoi, "Cytochrome p450-Mediated Metabolism of Estrogens and Its Regulation in Human," *Cancer Letters* 227, no. 2 (September 28, 2005): pp. 115-124, https://doi.org/10.1016/j.canlet.2004.10.007.

71. Hamed Samavat and Mindy S. Kurzer, "Estrogen Metabolism and Breast Cancer," *Cancer Letters* 356, no. 2 (January 28, 2015): pp. 231-243, https://doi.org/10.1016/j.canlet.2014.04.018.

72. Richard S. Lord, Bradley Bongiovanni, and J Alexander Bralley, "Estrogen Metabolism and the Diet-Cancer Connection: Rationale for Assessing the Ratio of Urinary Hydroxylated Estrogen Metabolites," *Alternative Medicine Review : a Journal of Clinical Therapeutic* 7, no. 2 (April 2002): pp. 112-129.

73. Shilpi Rajoria et al., "3,3'-Diindolylmethane Modulates Estrogen Metabolism in Patients with Thyroid Proliferative Disease: A Pilot Study," *Thyroid Economy: Regulation, Cell Biology, and Thyroid Hormone Metabolism and Action, Thyroid Economy* 21, no. 3 (March 4, 2011): pp. 299-304, https://doi.org/10.1089/thy.2010.0245.

74. Karen J. Auborn et al., "Indole-3-Carbinol Is a Negative Regulator of Estrogen," *The Journal of Nutrition* 133, no. 7 (July 1, 2003): pp. 2470-2475, https://doi.org/10.1093/jn/133.7.2470s.

75. "How Does the Liver Work?," essay, in *InformedHealth.Org [Internet]* (Cologne, Germany: Institute for Quality and Efficiency in Health Care (IQWiG), 2006), https://www.ncbi.nlm.nih.gov/books/NBK279393/.

76. Raquel Cano et al., "Role of Endocrine-Disrupting Chemicals in the Pathogenesis of Non-Alcoholic Fatty Liver Disease: A Comprehensive Review," *International Journal of Molecular Sciences* 22, no. 9 (May 1, 2021): p. 4807, https://doi.org/10.3390/ijms22094807.
Phillip A Engen et al., "The Gastrointestinal Microbiome: Alcohol Effects on the Composition of Intestinal Microbiota," *Alcohol Research : Current Reviews* 37, no. 2 (2015): pp. 223-236.
Thomas Jensen et al., "Fructose and Sugar: A Major Mediator of Non-

Alcoholic Fatty Liver Disease," *Journal of Hepatology* 68, no. 5 (May 1, 2018): pp. 1063-1075, https://doi.org/10.1016/j.jhep.2018.01.019.
Xiaosen Ouyang et al., "Fructose Consumption as a Risk Factor for Non-Alcoholic Fatty Liver Disease," *Journal of Hepatology* 48, no. 6 (June 2008): pp. 993-999, https://doi.org/10.1016/j.jhep.2008.02.011.
Prasanthi Jegatheesan et al., "Effect of Specific Amino Acids on Hepatic Lipid Metabolism in Fructose-Induced Non-Alcoholic Fatty Liver Disease," *Clinical Nutrition* 35, no. 1 (February 2016): pp. 175-182, https://doi.org/10.1016/j.clnu.2015.01.021.
Moon Do et al., "High-Glucose or -Fructose Diet Cause Changes of the Gut Microbiota and Metabolic Disorders in Mice without Body Weight Change," *Nutrients* 10, no. 6 (June 13, 2018): p. 761, https://doi.org/10.3390/nu10060761.

77. Himani Sharma et al., "Gene Expression Profiling in Practitioners of Sudarshan Kriya," *Journal of Psychosomatic Research* 64, no. 2 (February 2008): pp. 213-218, https://doi.org/10.1016/j.jpsychores.2007.07.003.
Joseph Pizzorno, "Glutathione!," *Integrative Medicine a Clinician's Journal* 13, no. 1 (February 2014): pp. 8-12.

78. Joseph Pizzorno, "Glutathione!," *Integrative Medicine a Clinician's Journal* 13, no. 1 (February 2014): 8–12.

79. G. Bounous, "Whey Protein Concentrate (WPC) and Glutathione Modulation in Cancer Treatment." *Anticancer Research* 20, no. 6C (November 1, 2000): 4785–92.

80. G. Bounous, "Whey Protein Concentrate (WPC) and Glutathione Modulation in Cancer Treatment." *Anticancer Research* 20, no. 6C (November 1, 2000): 4785–92.

81. C. Loguercio et al., "Effect of Alcohol Abuse and Glutathione Administration on the Circulating Levels of Glutathione and on Antipyrine Metabolism in Patients with Alcoholic Liver Cirrhosis," *Scandinavian Journal of Clinical and Laboratory Investigation* 56, no. 5 (February 20, 1996): pp. 441-447, https://doi.org/10.3109/00365519609088799.

82. Lesley A Powell et al., "High Glucose Decreases Intracellular Glutathione Concentrations and Upregulates Inducible Nitric Oxide Synthase Gene Expression in Intestinal Epithelial Cells," *Journal of Molecular Endocrinology* 33, no. 3 (December 2004): pp. 797-803, https://doi.org/10.1677/jme.1.01671.

83. Joseph Pizzorno, "The Path Ahead: Persistent Organic Pollutants (POPs)—a Serious Clinical Concern," *Integrative Medicine a Clinician's Journal* 12, no. 2 (April 2013): pp. 8-11.

84. Claude Monneret, "What Is an Endocrine Disruptor?," *Comptes Rendus Biologies* 340, no. 9–10 (2017): 403–5, https://doi.org/10.1016/j.crvi.2017.07.004.

85. Claude Monneret, "What Is an Endocrine Disruptor?," *Comptes Rendus Biologies* 340, no. 9–10 (2017): 403–5, https://doi.org/10.1016/j.crvi.2017.07.004.

86. Wissem Mnif et al., "Effect of Endocrine Disruptor Pesticides: A Review," *International Journal of Environmental Research and Public Health* 8, no. 6 (June 17, 2011): pp. 2265-2303, https://doi.org/10.3390/ijerph8062265.

87. Syed Wasim Sardar et al., "Occurrence and Concentration of Chemical Additives in Consumer Products in Korea," *International Journal of Environmental Research and Public Health* 16, no. 24 (December 12, 2019): p. 5075, https://doi.org/10.3390/ijerph16245075.
Seema Patel, "Fragrance Compounds: The Wolves in Sheep's Clothings," *Medical Hypotheses* 102 (May 2017): pp. 106-111, https://doi.org/10.1016/j.mehy.2017.03.025.

88. Claude Monneret, "What Is an Endocrine Disruptor?," *Comptes Rendus Biologies* 340, no. 9–10 (2017): 403–5, https://doi.org/10.1016/j.crvi.2017.07.004.

89. David W Singleton and Sohaib A Khan, "Xenoestrogen Exposure and Mechanisms of Endocrine Disruption," *Frontiers in Bioscience* 8, no. 6 (January 3, 2003): pp. 110-118, https://doi.org/10.2741/1010.

90. Cheryl S. Watson, Guangzhen Hu, and Adriana A. Paulucci-Holthauzen, "Rapid Actions of Xenoestrogens Disrupt Normal Estrogenic Signaling," *Steroids* 81 (March 2014): pp. 36-42, https://doi.org/10.1016/j.steroids.2013.11.006.

91. Roger Engeli et al., "Interference of Paraben Compounds with Estrogen Metabolism by Inhibition of 17β-Hydroxysteroid Dehydrogenases," *International Journal of Molecular Sciences* 18, no. 9 (September 19, 2017): p. 2007, https://doi.org/10.3390/ijms18092007.

92. T. Lorand, E. Vigh, and J. Garai, "Hormonal Action of Plant Derived and Anthropogenic Non-Steroidal Estrogenic Compounds: Phytoestrogens and Xenoestrogens," *Current Medicinal Chemistry* 17, no. 30 (October 1, 2010): 3542–74, https://doi.org/10.2174/092986710792927813.

93. "Learn about Dioxin," EPA (Environmental Protection Agency, n.d.), https://www.epa.gov/dioxin/learn-about-dioxin.

94. Kaylon Bruner-Tran, Tianbing Ding, and Kevin Osteen, "Dioxin and Endometrial Progesterone Resistance," *Seminars in Reproductive Medicine* 28, no. 01 (January 2010): pp. 059-068, https://doi.org/10.1055/s-0029-1242995.

95. "Learn about Dioxin," EPA, n.d., https://www.epa.gov/dioxin/learn-about-dioxin.

96. M-J R Howes et al., "Assessment of Estrogenic Activity in Some Common Essential Oil Constituents," *Journal of Pharmacy and Pharmacology* 54, no. 11 (November 2002): pp. 1521-1528, https://doi.org/10.1211/002235702216.

Seema Patel, "Fragrance Compounds: The Wolves in Sheep's Clothings," *Medical Hypotheses* 102 (May 2017): 106–11, https://doi.org/10.1016/j.mehy.2017.03.025.

97. Stephanie L. Brown et al., "Social Closeness Increases Salivary Progesterone in Humans," Hormones and B*ehavior* 56, no. 1 (June 2009): pp. 108-111, https://doi.org/10.1016/j.yhbeh.2009.03.022.

98. Sherwood L. Gorbach and Barry R. Goldin, "Diet and the Excretion and Enterohepatic Cycling of Estrogens," *Preventive Medicine* 16, no. 4 (July 1987): pp. 525-531, https://doi.org/10.1016/0091-7435(87)90067-3.

99. Audrey J. Gaskins et al., "The Impact of Dietary Folate Intake on Reproductive Function in Premenopausal Women: A Prospective Cohort Study," *PLoS ONE* 7, no. 9 (September 26, 2012), https://doi.org/10.1371/journal.pone.0046276.

100. Hirofumi Henmi et al., "Effects of Ascorbic Acid Supplementation on Serum Progesterone Levels in Patients with a Luteal Phase Defect," *Fertility and Sterility* 80, no. 2 (August 2003): pp. 459-461, https://doi.org/10.1016/s0015-0282(03)00657-5.

101. Mostafa I. Waly, Zahir Al-Attabi, and Nejib Guizani, "Low Nourishment of Vitamin C Induces Glutathione Depletion and Oxidative Stress in Healthy Young Adults," *Preventive Nutrition and Food Science* 20, no. 3 (September 30, 2015): pp. 198-203, https://doi.org/10.3746/pnf.2015.20.3.198.

102. Akihisa Takasaki et al., "Luteal Blood Flow and Luteal Function," *Journal of Ovarian Research* 2, no. 1 (January 14, 2009), https://doi.org/10.1186/1757-2215-2-1.

103. Kristen N. Owen, "Vitamin E Toxicity," essay, in *StatPearls [Internet],* ed. Olga Dewald (Treasure Island, FL: StatPearls Publishing, 2022), https://www.ncbi.nlm.nih.gov/books/NBK564373/.

104. Maria Laura Colombo, "An Update on Vitamin E, Tocopherol and Tocotrienol—Perspectives," *Molecules* 15, no. 4 (March 24, 2010): 2103-13, https://doi.org/10.3390/molecules15042103.

105. Benjamin J Delgado and Wilfredo Lopez-Ojeda, "Estrogen," essay, in *StatPearls [Internet]* (Treasure Island, FL: StatPearls Publishing, 2022), https://www.ncbi.nlm.nih.gov/books/NBK538260/.
Anita Kumar et al., "Estradiol: A Steroid with Multiple Facets," *Hormone and Metabolic Research* 50, no. 05 (March 22, 2018): 359–74, https://doi.org/10.1055/s-0044-100920.
Seema Patel et al., "Estrogen: The Necessary Evil for Human Health, and Ways to Tame It," *Biomedicine & Pharmacotherapy* 102 (June 2018): 403-11, https://doi.org/10.1016/j.biopha.2018.03.078.

106. Shital Sawant and Priya Bhide, "Fertility Treatment Options for Women with Polycystic Ovary Syndrome," *Clinical Medicine Insights: Reproductive Health* 13 (December 27, 2019): p. 117955811989086, https://doi.org/10.1177/1179558119890867.

107. Samer El Hayek et al., "Poly Cystic Ovarian Syndrome: An Updated Overview," *Frontiers in Physiology* 7 (April 5, 2016): p. 124, https://doi.org/10.3389/fphys.2016.00124.

108. Samer El Hayek et al., "Poly Cystic Ovarian Syndrome: An Updated Overview," *Frontiers in Physiology* 7 (April 5, 2016): p. 124, https://doi.org/10.3389/fphys.2016.00124.

109. Ricardo Azziz et al., "The Androgen Excess and PCOS Society Criteria for the Polycystic Ovary Syndrome: The Complete Task Force Report," *Fertility and Sterility* 91, no. 2 (February 2009): pp. 456–488, https://doi.org/10.1016/j.fertnstert.2008.06.035.
Bulent O. Yildiz, "Diagnosis of Hyperandrogenism: Clinical Criteria," *Best Practice & Research Clinical Endocrinology & Metabolism* 20, no. 2 (June 2006): pp. 167-176, https://doi.org/10.1016/j.beem.2006.02.004.

110. Daria Lizneva et al., "Androgen Excess: Investigations and Management," *Best Practice & Research Clinical Obstetrics & Gynaecology* 37 (November 2016): pp. 98-118, https://doi.org/10.1016/j.bpobgyn.2016.05.003.

111. Ricardo Azziz et al., "The Androgen Excess and PCOS Society Criteria for the Polycystic Ovary Syndrome: The Complete Task Force Report," *Fertility and Sterility* 91, no. 2 (February 2009): 456–88, https://doi.org/10.1016/j.fertnstert.2008.06.035.
E. Makrantonaki and C. C. Zouboulis, "Hyperandrogenismus, Adrenale Dysfunktion Und Hirsutismus," *Der Hautarzt* 71, no. 10 (August 28, 2020): pp. 752-761, https://doi.org/10.1007/s00105-020-04677-1.

112. Ricardo Azziz et al., "The Androgen Excess and PCOS Society Criteria for the Polycystic Ovary Syndrome: The Complete Task Force Report," *Fertility and Sterility* 91, no. 2 (February 2009): 456–88, https://doi.org/10.1016/j.fertnstert.2008.06.035.

113. Ricardo Azziz et al., "The Androgen Excess and PCOS Society Criteria for the Polycystic Ovary Syndrome: The Complete Task Force Report," *Fertility and Sterility* 91, no. 2 (February 2009): 456–88, https://doi.org/10.1016/j.fertnstert.2008.06.035.

114. Ricardo Azziz et al., "The Androgen Excess and PCOS Society Criteria for the Polycystic Ovary Syndrome: The Complete Task Force Report," *Fertility and Sterility* 91, no. 2 (February 2009): 456–88, https://doi.org/10.1016/j.fertnstert.2008.06.035.

115. Selma Feldman Witchel, Sharon E Oberfield, and Alexia S Peña, "Polycystic Ovary Syndrome: Pathophysiology, Presentation, and Treatment with Emphasis on Adolescent Girls," *Journal of the Endocrine Society* 3, no. 8 (June 14, 2019): 1545–73, https://doi.org/10.1210/js.2019-00078.

116. Lorena I. Rasquin Leon, Catherine Anastasopoulou, and Jane V. Mayrin, "Polycystic Ovarian Disease," in *StatPearls [Internet]* (Treasure Island, FL: StatPearls Publishing, 2022), https://www.ncbi.nlm.nih.gov/books/NBK459251/.

117.	Li Sun et al., "Oxytocin Regulates Body Composition," *Proceedings of the National Academy of Sciences* 116, no. 52 (December 16, 2019): pp. 26808-26815, https://doi.org/10.1073/pnas.1913611116.

118.	Isabel Krug, Sarah Giles, and Chiara Paganini, "Binge Eating in Patients with Polycystic Ovary Syndrome: Prevalence, Causes, and Management Strategies," *Neuropsychiatric Disease and Treatment* 15 (May 16, 2019): 1273–85, https://doi.org/10.2147/ndt.s168944.

119.	Maryam Azizi Kutenaee et al., "The Impact of Depression, Self-Esteem, and Body Image on Sleep Quality in Patients with PCOS: A Cross-Sectional Study," *Sleep and Breathing* 24, no. 3 (October 19, 2019): pp. 1027-1034, https://doi.org/10.1007/s11325-019-01946-9.

120.	Małgorzata Szczuko et al., "Quantitative Assessment of Nutrition in Patients with Polycystic Ovary Syndrome (PCOS)," *Roczniki Panstwowego Zakladu Higieny* 67, no. 4 (2016): pp. 419-426.

121.	Małgorzata Szczuko et al., "Quantitative Assessment of Nutrition in Patients with Polycystic Ovary Syndrome (PCOS)," *Roczniki Panstwowego Zakladu Higieny* 67, no. 4 (2016): 419–26.

122.	Dylan A. Cutler, Sheila M. Pride, and Anthony P. Cheung, "Low Intakes of Dietary Fiber and Magnesium Are Associated with Insulin Resistance and Hyperandrogenism in Polycystic Ovary Syndrome: A Cohort Study," *Food Science & Nutrition* 7, no. 4 (February 27, 2019): pp. 1426-1437, https://doi.org/10.1002/fsn3.977.

123.	Åsa Nybacka, Per M. Hellström, and Angelica L. Hirschberg, "Increased Fibre and Reduced Trans Fatty Acid Intake Are Primary Predictors of Metabolic Improvement in Overweight Polycystic Ovary Syndrome-Substudy of Randomized Trial between Diet, Exercise and Diet plus Exercise for Weight Control," *Clinical Endocrinology* 87, no. 6 (August 18, 2017): pp. 680-688, https://doi.org/10.1111/cen.13427.

124.	"World Famous Fries®: Calories & Nutrition | McDonald's," McDonald's, January 2022, https://www.mcdonalds.com/us/en-us/product/small-french-fries.html.

125.	Małgorzata Szczuko et al., "Quantitative Assessment of Nutrition in Patients with Polycystic Ovary Syndrome (PCOS)," *Roczniki Panstwowego Zakladu Higieny* 67, no. 4 (2016): 419–26.

126.	Marzenna Nasiadek et al., "The Role of Zinc in Selected Female Reproductive System Disorders," *Nutrients* 12, no. 8 (August 16, 2020): p. 2464, https://doi.org/10.3390/nu12082464.

127.	Mehri Jamilian et al., "Effects of Zinc Supplementation on Endocrine Outcomes in Women with Polycystic Ovary Syndrome: A Randomized, Double-Blind, Placebo-Controlled Trial," *Biological Trace Element Research* 170, no. 2 (August 28, 2015): pp. 271-278, https://doi.org/10.1007/s12011-015-0480-7.

128.	Jorge D Flechas, "Iodine Study #10," Orthoiodosupplementation in a Primary Care Practice, Jorge D. Flechas, M.D., n.d., https://www.optimox.com/iodine-study-10.

129. Lubna Pal et al., "Therapeutic Implications of Vitamin D and Calcium in Overweight Women with Polycystic Ovary Syndrome," *Gynecological Endocrinology* 28, no. 12 (July 11, 2012): pp. 965-968, https://doi.org/10.3109/09513590.2012.696753.

130. Maryam Maktabi, Mehri Jamilian, and Zatollah Asemi, "Magnesium-Zinc-Calcium-Vitamin D Co-Supplementation Improves Hormonal Profiles, Biomarkers of Inflammation and Oxidative Stress in Women with Polycystic Ovary Syndrome: A Randomized, Double-Blind, Placebo-Controlled Trial," *Biological Trace Element Research* 182, no. 1 (July 1, 2017): pp. 21-28, https://doi.org/10.1007/s12011-017-1085-0.

131. Bao Shan et al., "Risk Factors of Polycystic Ovarian Syndrome among Li People," *Asian Pacific Journal of Tropical Medicine* 8, no. 7 (July 2015): pp. 590-593, https://doi.org/10.1016/j.apjtm.2015.07.001.

132. M. Eleftheriadou et al., "Exercise and Sedentary Habits among Adolescents with PCOS," *Journal of Pediatric and Adolescent Gynecology* 25, no. 3 (June 2012): pp. 172-174, https://doi.org/10.1016/j.jpag.2011.11.009.

133. Jeffrey D. Covington et al., "Higher Circulating Leukocytes in Women with PCOS Is Reversed by Aerobic Exercise," *Biochimie* 124 (May 2016): pp. 27-33, https://doi.org/10.1016/j.biochi.2014.10.028.
Victoria S. Sprung et al., "Exercise Training in Polycystic Ovarian Syndrome Enhances Flow-Mediated Dilation in the Absence of Changes in Fatness," *Medicine & Science in Sports & Exercise* 45, no. 12 (December 2013): pp. 2234-2242, https://doi.org/10.1249/mss.0b013e31829ba9a1.

134. Jeffrey D. Covington et al., "Higher Circulating Leukocytes in Women with PCOS Is Reversed by Aerobic Exercise," *Biochimie* 124 (May 2016): 27–33, https://doi.org/10.1016/j.biochi.2014.10.028.
Victoria S. Sprung et al., "Exercise Training in Polycystic Ovarian Syndrome Enhances Flow-Mediated Dilation in the Absence of Changes in Fatness," *Medicine & Science in Sports & Exercise* 45, no. 12 (December 2013): 2234–42, https://doi.org/10.1249/mss.0b013e31829ba9a1.
Sujatha Thathapudi et al., "Tumor Necrosis Factor-Alpha and Polycystic Ovarian Syndrome: A Clinical, Biochemical, and Molecular Genetic Study," *Genetic Testing and Molecular Biomarkers* 18, no. 9 (September 3, 2014): pp. 605-609, https://doi.org/10.1089/gtmb.2014.0151.

135. C. L. Harrison et al., "Exercise Therapy in Polycystic Ovary Syndrome: A Systematic Review," *Human Reproduction Update* 17, no. 2 (September 10, 2010): 171–83, https://doi.org/10.1093/humupd/dmq045.

136. B. K. Pedersen and B. Saltin, "Exercise as Medicine - Evidence for Prescribing Exercise as Therapy in 26 Different Chronic Diseases," *Scandinavian Journal of Medicine & Science in Sports* 25, no. S3 (November 25, 2015): pp. 1-72, https://doi.org/10.1111/sms.12581.

137. Risani Mukhopadhyay et al., "Review on Bisphenol A and the Risk of Polycystic Ovarian Syndrome: An Insight from Endocrine and Gene Expression," *Environmental Science and Pollution Research* 29, no. 22 (February 24, 2022): 32631–50, https://doi.org/10.1007/s11356-022-19244-5.

138. Eleni Palioura and Evanthia Diamanti-Kandarakis, "Polycystic Ovary Syndrome (PCOS) and Endocrine Disrupting Chemicals (Edcs)," *Reviews in Endocrine and Metabolic Disorders* 16, no. 4 (December 2015): 365–71, https://doi.org/10.1007/s11154-016-9326-7.
Risani Mukhopadhyay et al., "Review on Bisphenol A and the Risk of Polycystic Ovarian Syndrome: An Insight from Endocrine and Gene Expression," *Environmental Science and Pollution Research* 29, no. 22 (February 24, 2022): 32631–50, https://doi.org/10.1007/s11356-022-19244-5.

139. Evanthia Diamanti-Kandarakis et al., "Increased Levels of Serum Advanced Glycation End-Products in Women with Polycystic Ovary Syndrome," *Clinical Endocrinology* 62, no. 1 (January 2005): pp. 37–43, https://doi.org/10.1111/j.1365-2265.2004.02170.x.
Evanthia Diamanti-Kandarakis et al., "Increased Serum Advanced Glycation End-Products Is a Distinct Finding in Lean Women with Polycystic Ovary Syndrome (PCOS)," *Clinical Endocrinology* 69, no. 4 (October 2008): pp. 634-641, https://doi.org/10.1111/j.1365-2265.2008.03247.x.

140. Jaime Uribarri et al., "Advanced Glycation End Products in Foods and a Practical Guide to Their Reduction in the Diet," *Journal of the American Dietetic Association* 110, no. 6 (June 1, 2010): pp. 911-916, https://doi.org/10.1016/j.jada.2010.03.018.

141. Teresia Goldberg et al., "Advanced Glycoxidation End Products in Commonly Consumed Foods," *Journal of the American Dietetic Association* 104, no. 8 (August 1, 2004): pp. 1287-1291, https://doi.org/10.1016/j.jada.2004.05.214.

142. Elif Inan-Eroglu, Aylin Ayaz, and Zehra Buyuktuncer, "Formation of Advanced Glycation Endproducts in Foods during Cooking Process and Underlying Mechanisms: A Comprehensive Review of Experimental Studies," *Nutrition Research Reviews* 33, no. 1 (November 8, 2019): pp. 77-89, https://doi.org/10.1017/s0954422419000209.
Teresia Goldberg et al., "Advanced Glycoxidation End Products in Commonly Consumed Foods," *Journal of the American Dietetic Association* 104, no. 8 (August 1, 2004): 1287–91, https://doi.org/10.1016/j.jada.2004.05.214.

143. Carla Cerami et al., "Tobacco Smoke Is a Source of Toxic Reactive Glycation Products," *Proceedings of the National Academy of Sciences* 94, no. 25 (December 9, 1997): pp. 13915-13920, https://doi.org/10.1073/pnas.94.25.13915.

144. J Zhang et al., "Environmental Risk Factors for Women with Polycystic Ovary Syndrome in China: a Population-Based Case-Control Study," *Journal of Biological Regulators and Homeostatic Agents* 28, no. 2 (2014): pp. 203-211.

145. Anderson Melo et al., "Hormonal Contraception in Women with Polycystic Ovary Syndrome: Choices, Challenges, and Noncontraceptive Benefits," *Open Access Journal of Contraception* Volume 8 (February 2, 2017): pp. 13-23, https://doi.org/10.2147/oajc.s85543.

146. David A Grimes et al., "Oral Contraceptives for Functional Ovarian Cysts," *Cochrane Database of Systematic Reviews,* April 15, 2009, https://doi.org/10.1002/14651858.cd006134.pub3.

147. Calette Corcoran and Tibb F Jacobs, "Metformin," in *StatPearls [Internet]* (Treasure Island, FL: StatPearls Publishing, 2022), https://www.ncbi.nlm.nih.gov/books/NBK518983/.

148. Parveen Parasar, Pinar Ozcan, and Kathryn L. Terry, "Endometriosis: Epidemiology, Diagnosis and Clinical Management," *Current Obstetrics and Gynecology Reports* 6, no. 1 (January 27, 2017): 34–41, https://doi.org/10.1007/s13669-017-0187-1.
Linda C Giudice and Lee C Kao, "Endometriosis," *The Lancet* 364, no. 9447 (November 13, 2004): 1789–99, https://doi.org/10.1016/s0140-6736(04)17403-5.

149. Yusuf Alimi et al., "The Clinical Anatomy of Endometriosis: A Review," *Cureus* 10, no. 9 (September 25, 2018): e3361, https://doi.org/10.7759/cureus.3361.

150. Yusuf Alimi et al., "The Clinical Anatomy of Endometriosis: A Review," *Cureus* 10, no. 9 (September 25, 2018): e3361, https://doi.org/10.7759/cureus.3361.
Jessica Maddern et al., "Pain in Endometriosis," *Frontiers in Cellular Neuroscience* 14 (October 6, 2020): 590823, https://doi.org/10.3389/fncel.2020.590823.

151. Yusuf Alimi et al., "The Clinical Anatomy of Endometriosis: A Review," *Cureus* 10, no. 9 (September 25, 2018): e3361, https://doi.org/10.7759/cureus.3361.
Jessica Maddern et al., "Pain in Endometriosis," *Frontiers in Cellular Neuroscience* 14 (October 6, 2020): 590823, https://doi.org/10.3389/fncel.2020.590823.

152. Ryan M. Marquardt et al., "Progesterone and Estrogen Signaling in the Endometrium: What Goes Wrong in Endometriosis?," *International Journal of Molecular Sciences* 20, no. 15 (August 5, 2019): 3822, https://doi.org/10.3390/ijms20153822.
Tian-Hong Zhu et al., "Estrogen Is an Important Mediator of Mast Cell Activation in Ovarian Endometriomas," *Reproduction* 155, no. 1 (January 2018): 73–83, https://doi.org/10.1530/rep-17-0457.

153. Practice Committee of the American Society for Reproductive Medicine, "Endometriosis and Infertility: A Committee Opinion," *Fertility and Sterility* 98, no. 3 (September 2012): 591–98, https://doi.org/10.1016/j.fertnstert.2012.05.031.

154. KD Ballard et al., "Can Symptomatology Help in the Diagnosis of Endometriosis? Findings from a National Case-Control Study-Part 1," *BJOG: An International Journal of Obstetrics & Gynaecology* 115, no. 11 (October 2008): 1382–91, https://doi.org/10.1111/j.1471-0528.2008.01878.x.

155. Malin Ek et al., "Gastrointestinal Symptoms among Endometriosis Patients—a Case-Cohort Study," *BMC Women's Health* 15, no. 1 (August 13, 2015), https://doi.org/10.1186/s12905-015-0213-2.

156. Kristin Nicolaus et al., "Cycle-Related Diarrhea and Dysmenorrhea Are Independent Predictors of Peritoneal Endometriosis, Cycle-Related Dyschezia Is an Independent Predictor of Rectal Involvement," *Geburtshilfe Und Frauenheilkunde* 80, no. 03 (March 2020): 307–15, https://doi.org/10.1055/a-1033-9588.

157. Joshua J. Keith et al., "Catamenial Rectal Bleeding Due to Invasive Endometriosis: A Case Report," *Journal of Medical Case Reports* 14, no. 1 (May 26, 2020), https://doi.org/10.1186/s13256-020-02386-w.
C Sciumè et al., "Endometriosi Intestinale: Una Causa Oscura Di Rettorragia Ciclica" [Intestinal Endometriosis: An Obscure Cause of Cyclic Rectal Bleeding]," *Annali Italiani Di Chirurgia* 75, no. 3 (2004): 379–84, https://pubmed.ncbi.nlm.nih.gov/15605531/.
Susanne Shokoohi et al., "Unusual Cause of Rectal Bleeding: Thinking Outside the Colon," *American Journal of Gastroenterology* 111 (October 2016): S642–43, https://doi.org/10.14309/00000434-201610001-01418.
C. Ribeiro et al., "Deep Infiltrating Endometriosis of the Colon Causing Cyclic Bleeding," *Case Reports* 2015, no. bcr2015209464 (April 16, 2015), https://doi.org/10.1136/bcr-2015-209464.

158. Ryan J. Heitmann et al., "Premenstrual Spotting of ≥2 Days Is Strongly Associated with Histologically Confirmed Endometriosis in Women with Infertility," *American Journal of Obstetrics and Gynecology* 211, no. 4 (October 2014): e1–6, https://doi.org/10.1016/j.ajog.2014.04.041.

159. Yuka Ozawa et al., "Management of the Pain Associated with Endometriosis: An Update of the Painful Problems," *The Tohoku Journal of Experimental Medicine* 210, no. 3 (November 2006): 175–88, https://doi.org/10.1620/tjem.210.175.

160. Federica Facchin et al., "The Subjective Experience of Dyspareunia in Women with Endometriosis: A Systematic Review with Narrative Synthesis of Qualitative Research," *International Journal of Environmental Research and Public Health* 18, no. 22 (November 18, 2021): 12112, https://doi.org/10.3390/ijerph182212112.

161. D Ballard et al., "Can Symptomatology Help in the Diagnosis of Endometriosis? Findings from a National Case-Control Study-Part 1," *BJOG: An International Journal of Obstetrics & Gynaecology* 115, no. 11 (October 2008): 1382–91, https://doi.org/10.1111/j.1471-0528.2008.01878.x.

162. Jenny Vennberg Karlsson, Harshida Patel, and Asa Premberg, "Experiences of Health after Dietary Changes in Endometriosis: A Qualitative Interview Study," *BMJ Open* 10, no. 2 (February 25, 2020): e032321, https://doi.org/10.1136/bmjopen-2019-032321.

163. Bedayah Amro et al., "New Understanding of Diagnosis, Treatment and Prevention of Endometriosis," *International Journal of Environmental Research and Public Health* 19, no. 11 (May 31, 2022): 6725, https://doi.org/10.3390/ijerph19116725.

164. İlker Selcuk and Gurkan Bozdag, "Recurrence of Endometriosis; Risk Factors, Mechanisms and Biomarkers; Review of the Literature," *Journal of the Turkish German Gynecological Association* 14, no. 2 (June 10, 2013): 98–103, https://doi.org/10.5152/jtgga.2013.52385.

165. Sukhbir S. Singh et al., "Surgical Outcomes in Patients With Endometriosis: A Systematic Review," *Journal of Obstetrics and Gynaecology Canada* 42, no. 7 (July 2020): 881–88, https://doi.org/10.1016/j.jogc.2019.08.004.

166. Pamela Stratton and Karen J. Berkley, "Chronic Pelvic Pain and Endometriosis: Translational Evidence of the Relationship and Implications," *Human Reproduction Update* 17, no. 3 (November 23, 2010): 327–46, https://doi.org/10.1093/humupd/dmq050.

167. Pamela Stratton and Karen J. Berkley, "Chronic Pelvic Pain and Endometriosis: Translational Evidence of the Relationship and Implications," *Human Reproduction Update* 17, no. 3 (November 23, 2010): 327–46, https://doi.org/10.1093/humupd/dmq050. Tian-Hong Zhu et al., "Estrogen Is an Important Mediator of Mast Cell Activation in Ovarian Endometriomas," *Reproduction* 155, no. 1 (January 2018): 73–83, https://doi.org/10.1530/rep-17-0457.

168. Tian-Hong Zhu et al., "Estrogen Is an Important Mediator of Mast Cell Activation in Ovarian Endometriomas," *Reproduction* 155, no. 1 (January 2018): 73–83, https://doi.org/10.1530/rep-17-0457.

169. Ryan M. Marquardt et al., "Progesterone and Estrogen Signaling in the Endometrium: What Goes Wrong in Endometriosis?," *International Journal of Molecular Sciences* 20, no. 15 (August 5, 2019): 3822, https://doi.org/10.3390/ijms20153822.

170. Nuria Eritja et al., "Long-Term Estradiol Exposure Is a Direct Mitogen for Insulin/EGF-Primed Endometrial Cells and Drives PTEN Loss-Induced Hyperplasic Growth," *The American Journal of Pathology* 183, no. 1 (July 1, 2013): 277–87, https://doi.org/10.1016/j.ajpath.2013.03.008. Serdar Bulun et al., "Role of Estrogen Receptor-β in Endometriosis," *Seminars in Reproductive Medicine* 30, no. 01 (January 2012): 39–45,

https://doi.org/10.1055/s-0031-1299596.

171.   Albert Asante and Robert N. Taylor, "Endometriosis: The Role of Neuroangiogenesis," *Annual Review of Physiology* 73, no. 1 (March 17, 2011): 163–82, https://doi.org/10.1146/annurev-physiol-012110-142158. Serdar Bulun et al., "Role of Estrogen Receptor-β in Endometriosis," *Seminars in Reproductive Medicine* 30, no. 01 (January 2012): 39–45, https://doi.org/10.1055/s-0031-1299596.

172.   Elodie Chantalat et al., "Estrogen Receptors and Endometriosis," *International Journal of Molecular Sciences* 21, no. 8 (April 17, 2020): 2815, https://doi.org/10.3390/ijms21082815.

173.   Richard O. Burney et al., "Gene Expression Analysis of Endometrium Reveals Progesterone Resistance and Candidate Susceptibility Genes in Women with Endometriosis," *Endocrinology* 148, no. 8 (August 1, 2007): 3814–26, https://doi.org/10.1210/en.2006-1692.

174.   Peter Simsa et al., "Increased Exposure to Dioxin-like Compounds Is Associated with Endometriosis in a Case–Control Study in Women," *Reproductive BioMedicine Online* 20, no. 5 (May 1, 2010): 681–88, https://doi.org/10.1016/j.rbmo.2010.01.018.

175.   Kaylon Bruner-Tran, Tianbing Ding, and Kevin Osteen, "Dioxin and Endometrial Progesterone Resistance," *Seminars in Reproductive Medicine* 28, no. 01 (January 2010): 059–068, https://doi.org/10.1055/s-0029-1242995.

176.   "Learn about Dioxin," EPA, n.d., https://www.epa.gov/dioxin/learn-about-dioxin.

177.   Jenny Vennberg Karlsson, Harshida Patel, and Asa Premberg, "Experiences of Health after Dietary Changes in Endometriosis: A Qualitative Interview Study," *BMJ Open* 10, no. 2 (February 25, 2020): e032321, https://doi.org/10.1136/bmjopen-2019-032321.

178.   Mahboubeh Valiani et al., "The Effects of Massage Therapy on Dysmenorrhea Caused by Endometriosis," *Iranian Journal of Nursing and Midwifery Research* 15 (November 10, 2010): 167–71, https://www.ncbi.nlm.nih.gov/pmc/articles/PMC3093183/.
Jessica A. Payne, "Acupuncture for Endometriosis: A Case Study," *Medical Acupuncture* 31, no. 6 (December 1, 2019): 392–94, https://doi.org/10.1089/acu.2019.1379.
Yang Xu et al., "Effects of Acupuncture for the Treatment of Endometriosis-Related Pain: A Systematic Review and Meta-Analysis," *PLOS ONE* 12, no. 10 (October 27, 2017), https://doi.org/10.1371/journal.pone.0186616.

179.   Jenny Vennberg Karlsson, Harshida Patel, and Asa Premberg, "Experiences of Health after Dietary Changes in Endometriosis: A Qualitative Interview Study," *BMJ Open* 10, no. 2 (February 25, 2020): e032321, https://doi.org/10.1136/bmjopen-2019-032321.

180.   Jenny Vennberg Karlsson, Harshida Patel, and Asa Premberg, "Experiences of Health after Dietary Changes in Endometriosis: A Qualitative Interview Study," *BMJ Open* 10, no. 2 (February 25, 2020): e032321, https://doi.org/10.1136/bmjopen-2019-032321.

181.   Joanna Jurkiewicz-Przondziono et al., "Influence of Diet on the Risk of Developing Endometriosis," *Ginekologia Polska* 88, no. 2 (February 28, 2017): 96–102, https://doi.org/10.5603/gp.a2017.0017.
Fabio Parazzini et al., "A Metaanalysis on Alcohol Consumption and Risk of Endometriosis," *American Journal of Obstetrics and Gynecology* 209, no. 2 (August 1, 2013): e1–10, https://doi.org/10.1016/j.ajog.2013.05.039.

182.   Konstantinos S. Kechagias et al., "The Relation between Caffeine Consumption and Endometriosis: An Updated Systematic Review and Meta-Analysis," *Nutrients* 13, no. 10 (September 29, 2021): 3457, https://doi.org/10.3390/nu13103457.

183.   F. Parazzini, "Selected Food Intake and Risk of Endometriosis," *Human Reproduction* 19, no. 8 (June 3, 2004): 1755–59, https://doi.org/10.1093/humrep/deh395.
H R Harris et al., "Fruit and Vegetable Consumption and Risk of Endometriosis," *Human Reproduction* 33, no. 4 (February 1, 2018): 715–27, https://doi.org/10.1093/humrep/dey014.

184.   Britton Trabert et al., "Diet and Risk of Endometriosis in a Population-Based Case–Control Study," *British Journal of Nutrition* 105, no. 3 (September 28, 2010): 459–67, https://doi.org/10.1017/s0007114510003661.

185.   H R Harris et al., "Fruit and Vegetable Consumption and Risk of Endometriosis," *Human Reproduction* 33, no. 4 (February 1, 2018): 715–27, https://doi.org/10.1093/humrep/dey014.

186.   Judith S. Moore et al., "Endometriosis in Patients with Irritable Bowel Syndrome: Specific Symptomatic and Demographic Profile, and Response to the Low Fodmap Diet," *Australian and New Zealand Journal of Obstetrics and Gynaecology* 57, no. 2 (March 17, 2017): 201–5, https://doi.org/10.1111/ajo.12594.

187.   H R Harris et al., "Fruit and Vegetable Consumption and Risk of Endometriosis," *Human Reproduction* 33, no. 4 (February 1, 2018): 715–27, https://doi.org/10.1093/humrep/dey014.

188.   H R Harris et al., "Fruit and Vegetable Consumption and Risk of Endometriosis," *Human Reproduction* 33, no. 4 (February 1, 2018): 715–27, https://doi.org/10.1093/humrep/dey014.

189.   S. A. Missmer et al., "A Prospective Study of Dietary Fat Consumption and Endometriosis Risk," *Human Reproduction* 25, no. 6 (March 23, 2010): 1528–35, https://doi.org/10.1093/humrep/deq044.

190.   F. Parazzini, "Selected Food Intake and Risk of Endometriosis," *Human Reproduction* 19, no. 8 (June 3, 2004): 1755–59, https://doi.org/10.1093/humrep/deh395.

191. Ana Luiza Savaris and Vivian F. do Amaral, "Nutrient Intake, Anthropometric Data and Correlations with the Systemic Antioxidant Capacity of Women with Pelvic Endometriosis," *European Journal of Obstetrics & Gynecology and Reproductive Biology* 158, no. 2 (October 2011): 314–18, https://doi.org/10.1016/j.ejogrb.2011.05.014.

192. Anne Marie Darling et al., "A Prospective Cohort Study of Vitamins B, C, E, and Multivitamin Intake and Endometriosis," *Journal of Endometriosis and Pelvic Pain Disorders* 5, no. 1 (February 5, 2013): 17–26, https://doi.org/10.5301/je.5000151.

193. Anne Marie Darling et al., "A Prospective Cohort Study of Vitamins B, C, E, and Multivitamin Intake and Endometriosis," *Journal of Endometriosis and Pelvic Pain Disorders* 5, no. 1 (February 5, 2013): 17–26, https://doi.org/10.5301/je.5000151.

194. "Thiaman - Fact Sheet for Health Professionals," NIH Office of Dietary Supplements, March 26, 2021, https://ods.od.nih.gov/factsheets/Thiamin-HealthProfessional/#:~:text=Sources%20of%20Thiamin-,Food,cereals%20and%20bread%20%5B8%5D.

195. Anne Marie Darling et al., "A Prospective Cohort Study of Vitamins B, C, E, and Multivitamin Intake and Endometriosis," *Journal of Endometriosis and Pelvic Pain Disorders* 5, no. 1 (February 5, 2013): 17–26, https://doi.org/10.5301/je.5000151.

196. Audrey J. Gaskins et al., "The Impact of Dietary Folate Intake on Reproductive Function in Premenopausal Women: A Prospective Cohort Study," *PLoS ONE* 7, no. 9 (September 26, 2012), https://doi.org/10.1371/journal.pone.0046276.

197. Nalini Santanam et al., "Antioxidant Supplementation Reduces Endometriosis-Related Pelvic Pain in Humans," *Translational Research* 161, no. 3 (March 1, 2013): 189–95, https://doi.org/10.1016/j.trsl.2012.05.001.

198. Tarique Hussain et al., "Oxidative Stress and Inflammation: What Polyphenols Can Do for Us?," *Oxidative Medicine and Cellular Longevity* 2016 (2016): 1–9, https://doi.org/10.1155/2016/7432797.

199. Margreet C.M. Vissers et al., "The Bioavailability of Vitamin C from Kiwifruit," *Nutritional Benefits of Kiwifruit* 68 (2013): 125–47, https://doi.org/10.1016/b978-0-12-394294-4.00007-9.
Nidhi Mishra, Vijay Lakshmi Ta, and Rekha Gupta, "Immunomodulation by Hibiscus Rosa-Sinensis: Effect on the Humoral and Cellular Immune Response of Mus Musculus," *Pakistan Journal of Biological Sciences* 15, no. 6 (March 1, 2012): 277–83, https://doi.org/10.3923/pjbs.2012.277.283.
Shailja Chambial et al., "Vitamin C in Disease Prevention and Cure: An Overview," *Indian Journal of Clinical Biochemistry* 28, no. 4 (September 1, 2013): 314–28, https://doi.org/10.1007/s12291-013-0375-3.

200. Kristen N. Owen, "Vitamin E Toxicity," essay, in *StatPearls [Internet]*, ed. Olga Dewald (Treasure Island, FL: StatPearls Publishing, 2022), https://www.ncbi.nlm.nih.gov/books/NBK564373/.

201. Maria Laura Colombo, "An Update on Vitamin E, Tocopherol and Tocotrienol—Perspectives," *Molecules* 15, no. 4 (March 24, 2010): 2103–13, https://doi.org/10.3390/molecules15042103.

202. Xiao-Xiao Gao et al., "Effects of L-Arginine on Endometrial Estrogen Receptor α/β and Progesterone Receptor Expression in Nutrient-Restricted Sheep," *Theriogenology* 138 (October 15, 2019): 137–44, https://doi.org/10.1016/j.theriogenology.2019.07.018.

203. Anne Marie Darling et al., "A Prospective Cohort Study of Vitamins B, C, E, and Multivitamin Intake and Endometriosis," *Journal of Endometriosis and Pelvic Pain Disorders* 5, no. 1 (February 5, 2013): 17–26, https://doi.org/10.5301/je.5000151.

204. Parvin Mirmiran et al., "The Association of Dietary L-Arginine Intake and Serum Nitric Oxide Metabolites in Adults: A Population-Based Study," *Nutrients* 8, no. 5 (May 20, 2016): 311, https://doi.org/10.3390/nu8050311.

205. Preet K. Dhillon and Victoria L. Holt, "Recreational Physical Activity and Endometrioma Risk," *American Journal of Epidemiology* 158, no. 2 (July 15, 2003): 156–64, https://doi.org/10.1093/aje/kwg122.

206. Eman Awad et al., "Efficacy of Exercise on Pelvic Pain and Posture Associated with Endometriosis: Within Subject Design," *Journal of Physical Therapy Science* 29, no. 12 (December 7, 2017): 2112–15, https://doi.org/10.1589/jpts.29.2112.

207. Mary Lourdes Montenegro et al., "Effect of Physical Exercise on Endometriosis Experimentally Induced in Rats," *Reproductive Sciences* 26, no. 6 (June 2019): 785–93, https://doi.org/10.1177/1933719118799205.

208. Emily Davis, "Abnormal Uterine Bleeding," essay, in *StatPearls [Internet]*, ed. Paul B. Sparzak (Treasure Island, FL: StatPearls Publishing, 2022), https://www.ncbi.nlm.nih.gov/books/NBK532913/.

209. M. K. Oehler and M. C. P. Rees, "Menorrhagia: An Update," *Acta Obstetricia et Gynecologica Scandinavica* 82, no. 5 (May 12, 2003): 405–22, https://doi.org/10.1034/j.1600-0412.2003.00097.x.

210. "Heavy Menstrual Bleeding," Centers for Disease Control and Prevention, August 17, 2022, https://www.cdc.gov/ncbddd/blooddisorders/women/menorrhagia.html.

211. Catharina A.H. Janssen, Piet C. Scholten, and A. Peter M. Heintz, "A Simple Visual Assessment Technique to Discriminate between Menorrhagia and Normal Menstrual Blood Loss," *Obstetrics & Gynecology* 85, no. 6 (June 1995): 977–82, https://doi.org/10.1016/0029-7844(95)00062-v.

212. Andra H. James, "Heavy Menstrual Bleeding: Work-up and Management," *Hematology* 2016, no. 1 (December 2, 2016): 236–42, https://doi.org/10.1182/asheducation-2016.1.236.

213. Kirsten Duckitt and Sally Collins, "Menorrhagia," *BMJ Clinical Evidence* 2008, no. 0805 (September 18, 2008), https://www.ncbi.nlm.nih.gov/pmc/articles/PMC2907973/.

214. Matthew H. Walker, William Coffey, and Judith Borger, "Menorrhagia," essay, in *StatPearls [Internet]* (Treasure Island, FL: StatPearls Publishing, 2022), https://www.ncbi.nlm.nih.gov/books/NBK536910/.

215. M. K. Oehler and M. C. P. Rees, "Menorrhagia: An Update," *Acta Obstetricia et Gynecologica Scandinavica* 82, no. 5 (May 12, 2003): 405–22, https://doi.org/10.1034/j.1600-0412.2003.00097.x.

216. Gunjan Singh and Yana Puckett, "Endometrial Hyperplasia," essay, in *StatPearls [Internet]* (Treasure Island, FL: StatPearls Publishing, 2022), https://www.ncbi.nlm.nih.gov/books/NBK560693/.

217. K. G. Nygren and G. Rybo, "Prostaglandins and Menorrhagia," *Acta Obstetricia et Gynecologica Scandinavica* 62, no. s113 (January 1983): 101–3, https://doi.org/10.3109/00016348309155208.

218. Reinhard Grzanna, Lars Lindmark, and Carmelita G. Frondoza, "Ginger—an Herbal Medicinal Product with Broad Anti-Inflammatory Actions," *Journal of Medicinal Food* 8, no. 2 (July 20, 2005): 125–32, https://doi.org/10.1089/jmf.2005.8.125.
U. Singh, S. Devaraj, and I. Jialal, "Vitamin E, Oxidative Stress, and Inflammation," *Annual Review of Nutrition* 25, no. 1 (August 21, 2005): 151–74, https://doi.org/10.1146/annurev.nutr.24.012003.132446.

219. Anna B. Livdans-Forret, Phyllis J. Harvey, and Susan M. Larkin-Thier, "Menorrhagia: A Synopsis of Management Focusing on Herbal and Nutritional Supplements, and Chiropractic," *The Journal of the Canadian Chiropractic Association* 51, no. 4 (December 2007): 235–46, https://pubmed.ncbi.nlm.nih.gov/18060009/.

220. Reinhard Grzanna, Lars Lindmark, and Carmelita G. Frondoza, "Ginger—an Herbal Medicinal Product with Broad Anti-Inflammatory Actions," *Journal of Medicinal Food* 8, no. 2 (July 20, 2005): 125–32, https://doi.org/10.1089/jmf.2005.8.125.

221. Farzaneh Kashefi et al., "Effect of Ginger (*Zingiber Officinale*) on Heavy Menstrual Bleeding: A Placebo-Controlled, Randomized Clinical Trial," *Phytotherapy Research* 29, no. 1 (October 8, 2014): 114–19, https://doi.org/10.1002/ptr.5235.

222. S. Ziaei, M. Zakeri, and A. Kazemnejad, "A Randomised Controlled Trial of Vitamin E in the Treatment of Primary Dysmenorrhoea," *BJOG: An International Journal of Obstetrics and Gynaecology* 112, no. 4 (April 2005): 466–69, https://doi.org/10.1111/j.1471-0528.2004.00495.x.

223. Kristen N. Owen, "Vitamin E Toxicity," essay, in *StatPearls [Internet]*, ed. Olga Dewald (Treasure Island, FL: StatPearls Publishing, 2022), https://www.ncbi.nlm.nih.gov/books/NBK564373/.

224. Maria Laura Colombo, "An Update on Vitamin E, Tocopherol and Tocotrienol—Perspectives," *Molecules* 15, no. 4 (March 24, 2010): 2103–13, https://doi.org/10.3390/molecules15042103.

225. Emily P. McEldrew, Michael J. Lopez, and Harold Milstein, essay, in *StatPearls [Internet]* (Treasure Island, FL: StatPearls Publishing, 2022), https://www.ncbi.nlm.nih.gov/books/NBK482362/.
Anna B. Livdans-Forret, Phyllis J. Harvey, and Susan M. Larkin-Thier, "Menorrhagia: A Synopsis of Management Focusing on Herbal and Nutritional Supplements, and Chiropractic," *The Journal of the Canadian Chiropractic Association* 51, no. 4 (December 2007): 235–46, https://pubmed.ncbi.nlm.nih.gov/18060009/.

226. "Office of Dietary Supplements - Vitamin A and Carotenoids," NIH Office of Dietary Supplements, June 15, 2022, https://ods.od.nih.gov/factsheets/VitaminA-HealthProfessional/.

227. Anna B. Livdans-Forret, Phyllis J. Harvey, and Susan M. Larkin-Thier, "Menorrhagia: A Synopsis of Management Focusing on Herbal and Nutritional Supplements, and Chiropractic," *The Journal of the Canadian Chiropractic Association* 51, no. 4 (December 2007): 235–46, https://pubmed.ncbi.nlm.nih.gov/18060009/.
Kory Imbrescia and Zbigniew Moszczynski, "Vitamin K," essay, in *StatPearls [Internet]* (Treasure Island, FL: StatPearls Publishing, 2022), https://www.ncbi.nlm.nih.gov/books/NBK551578/.

228. Sarah L. Booth, "Vitamin K: Food Composition and Dietary Intakes," *Food & Nutrition Research* 56, no. 1 (April 2, 2012): 5505, https://doi.org/10.3402/fnr.v56i0.5505.

229. Anna B. Livdans-Forret, Phyllis J. Harvey, and Susan M. Larkin-Thier, "Menorrhagia: A Synopsis of Management Focusing on Herbal and Nutritional Supplements, and Chiropractic," *The Journal of the Canadian Chiropractic Association* 51, no. 4 (December 2007): 235–46, https://pubmed.ncbi.nlm.nih.gov/18060009/.

230. Margreet C.M. Vissers et al., "The Bioavailability of Vitamin C from Kiwifruit," *Nutritional Benefits of Kiwifruit* 68 (2013): 125–47, https://doi.org/10.1016/b978-0-12-394294-4.00007-9.
Nidhi Mishra, Vijay Lakshmi Ta, and Rekha Gupta, "Immunomodulation by Hibiscus Rosa-Sinensis: Effect on the Humoral and Cellular Immune Response of Mus Musculus," *Pakistan Journal of Biological Sciences* 15, no. 6 (March 1, 2012): 277–83, https://doi.org/10.3923/pjbs.2012.277.283.
Shailja Chambial et al., "Vitamin C in Disease Prevention and Cure: An Overview," *Indian Journal of Clinical Biochemistry* 28, no. 4 (September 1, 2013): 314–28, https://doi.org/10.1007/s12291-013-0375-3.

231. Anna B. Livdans-Forret, Phyllis J. Harvey, and Susan M. Larkin-Thier, "Menorrhagia: A Synopsis of Management Focusing on Herbal and Nutritional Supplements, and Chiropractic," *The Journal of the Canadian Chiropractic Association* 51, no. 4 (December 2007): 235–46, https://pubmed.ncbi.nlm.nih.gov/18060009/.

232. Marcel Hrubša et al., "Biological Properties of Vitamins of the B-Complex, Part 1: Vitamins B1, B2, B3, and B5," *Nutrients* 14, no. 3

(January 22, 2022): 484, https://doi.org/10.3390/nu14030484.

Mary J. Brown, Muhammad Atif Ameer, and Kevin Beier, "Vitamin B6 Deficiency," essay, in *StatPearls [Internet]* (Treasure Island, FL: StatPearls Publishing, 2022).

Janos Zempleni, Subhashinee S.K. Wijeratne, and Yousef I. Hassan, "Biotin," *BioFactors* 35, no. 1 (February 8, 2009): 36–46, https://doi.org/10.1002/biof.8.

Brigham J. Merrell and John P. McMurry, "Folic Acid," essay, in *StatPearls [Internet]* (Treasure Island, FL: StatPearls Publishing, 2022), https://www.ncbi.nlm.nih.gov/books/NBK554487/.

Sareen S. Gropper, Jack L. Smith, and Timothy P. Carr, *Advanced Nutrition and Human Metabolism*, 7th ed. (Boston, MA: Cengage Learning, 2018).

233. Anna B. Livdans-Forret, Phyllis J. Harvey, and Susan M. Larkin-Thier, "Menorrhagia: A Synopsis of Management Focusing on Herbal and Nutritional Supplements, and Chiropractic," *The Journal of the Canadian Chiropractic Association* 51, no. 4 (December 2007): 235–46, https://pubmed.ncbi.nlm.nih.gov/18060009/.

234. Tiffany A. Katz et al., "Endocrine-Disrupting Chemicals and Uterine Fibroids," *Fertility and Sterility* 106, no. 4 (September 15, 2016): 967–77, https://doi.org/10.1016/j.fertnstert.2016.08.023.

235. Kyle Barjon and Lyree N. Mikhail, "Uterine Leiomyomata," essay, in *StatPearls [Internet]* (Treasure Island, FL: StatPearls Publishing, 2022), https://www.ncbi.nlm.nih.gov/books/NBK546680/.

T. Maruo et al., "Sex Steroidal Regulation of Uterine Leiomyoma Growth and Apoptosis," *Human Reproduction Update* 10, no. 3 (May 1, 2004): 207–20, https://doi.org/10.1093/humupd/dmh019.

236. Geum Seon Sohn et al., "Current Medical Treatment of Uterine Fibroids," *Obstetrics & Gynecology Science* 61, no. 2 (February 13, 2018): 192–201, https://doi.org/10.5468/ogs.2018.61.2.192.

237. Michelle M. McWilliams and Vargheese M. Chennathukuzhi, "Recent Advances in Uterine Fibroid Etiology," *Seminars in Reproductive Medicine* 35, no. 02 (March 9, 2017): 181–89, https://doi.org/10.1055/s-0037-1599090.

238. Michelle M. McWilliams and Vargheese M. Chennathukuzhi, "Recent Advances in Uterine Fibroid Etiology," *Seminars in Reproductive Medicine* 35, no. 02 (March 9, 2017): 181–89, https://doi.org/10.1055/s-0037-1599090.

239. Jacques Donnez and Marie-Madeleine Dolmans, "Uterine Fibroid Management: From the Present to the Future," *Human Reproduction Update* 22, no. 6 (July 27, 2016): 665–86, https://doi.org/10.1093/humupd/dmw023.

Geum Seon Sohn et al., "Current Medical Treatment of Uterine Fibroids," *Obstetrics & Gynecology Science* 61, no. 2 (February 13, 2018): 192–201, https://doi.org/10.5468/ogs.2018.61.2.192.

240. Lewis Mehl-Madrona, "Complementary Medicine Treatment of Uterine

Fibroids: A Pilot Study," *Alternative Therapies in Health and Medicine* 8, no. 2 (2002): 34–46, https://pubmed.ncbi.nlm.nih.gov/11890384/.

241. Lewis Mehl-Madrona, "Complementary Medicine Treatment of Uterine Fibroids: A Pilot Study," *Alternative Therapies in Health and Medicine* 8, no. 2 (2002): 34–46, https://pubmed.ncbi.nlm.nih.gov/11890384/.

242. Chisato Nagata et al., "Association of Intakes of Fat, Dietary Fibre, Soya Isoflavones and Alcohol with Uterine Fibroids in Japanese Women," *British Journal of Nutrition* 101, no. 10 (October 3, 2008): 1427–31, https://doi.org/10.1017/s0007114508083566.

243. Rose G Radin et al., "Dietary Glycemic Index and Load in Relation to Risk of Uterine Leiomyomata in the Black Women's Health Study," *The American Journal of Clinical Nutrition* 91, no. 5 (March 3, 2010): 1281–88, https://doi.org/10.3945/ajcn.2009.28698.

244. Andrea Tinelli et al., "Uterine Fibroids and Diet," *International Journal of Environmental Research and Public Health* 18, no. 3 (January 25, 2021): 1066, https://doi.org/10.3390/ijerph18031066.

245. O. R. Orta et al., "Dairy and Related Nutrient Intake and Risk of Uterine Leiomyoma: A Prospective Cohort Study," *Human Reproduction* 35, no. 2 (February 22, 2020): 453–63, https://doi.org/10.1093/humrep/dez278.

246. "A Guide to Calcium-Rich Foods," Bone Health & Osteoporosis Foundation, May 20, 2020, https://www.nof.org/patients/treatment/calciumvitamin-d/a-guide-to-calcium-rich-foods/.

247. Donna Day Baird et al., "Vitamin D and the Risk of Uterine Fibroids," *Epidemiology* 24, no. 3 (May 2013): 447–53, https://doi.org/10.1097/ede.0b013e31828acca0.

248. Eman Roshdy et al., "Treatment of Symptomatic Uterine Fibroids with Green Tea Extract: A Pilot Randomized Controlled Clinical Study," *International Journal of Women's Health* 5 (August 7, 2013): 477–86, https://doi.org/10.2147/ijwh.s41021.

249. Hellen A. Oketch-Rabah et al., "United States Pharmacopeia (USP) Comprehensive Review of the Hepatotoxicity of Green Tea Extracts," *Toxicology Reports* 7 (February 15, 2020): 386–402, https://doi.org/10.1016/j.toxrep.2020.02.008.

250. Qun He, Ru-hai Ma, and Yi Tang, "[Determination of Trace Element Cu, Zn, Mg, Cr in Serum of Women with Barrenness and Hysteromyoma Disease]," *Guang Pu Xue Yu Guang Pu Fen Xi* 22, no. 4 (August 2002): 685–86, https://pubmed.ncbi.nlm.nih.gov/12938400/.

251. Donna Day Baird et al., "Vitamin D and the Risk of Uterine Fibroids," *Epidemiology* 24, no. 3 (May 2013): 447–53, https://doi.org/10.1097/ede.0b013e31828acca0.

252. Qun He, Ru-hai Ma, and Yi Tang, "[Determination of Trace Element Cu, Zn, Mg, Cr in Serum of Women with Barrenness and Hysteromyoma Disease]," *Guang Pu Xue Yu Guang Pu Fen Xi* 22, no. 4 (August 2002): 685–86, https://pubmed.ncbi.nlm.nih.gov/12938400/.

253. Tiffany A. Katz et al., "Endocrine-Disrupting Chemicals and Uterine

Fibroids," *Fertility and Sterility* 106, no. 4 (September 15, 2016): 967–77, https://doi.org/10.1016/j.fertnstert.2016.08.023.

254. Kyle Barjon and Lyree N. Mikhail, "Uterine Leiomyomata," essay, in *StatPearls [Internet]* (Treasure Island, FL: StatPearls Publishing, 2022), https://www.ncbi.nlm.nih.gov/books/NBK546680/.
T. Maruo et al., "Sex Steroidal Regulation of Uterine Leiomyoma Growth and Apoptosis," *Human Reproduction Update* 10, no. 3 (May 1, 2004): 207–20, https://doi.org/10.1093/humupd/dmh019.
David W Singleton and Sohaib A Khan, "Xenoestrogen Exposure and Mechanisms of Endocrine Disruption," *Frontiers in Bioscience* 8, no. 6 (January 3, 2003): 110–18, https://doi.org/10.2741/1010

255. Kyle Barjon and Lyree N. Mikhail, "Uterine Leiomyomata," essay, in *StatPearls [Internet]* (Treasure Island, FL: StatPearls Publishing, 2022), https://www.ncbi.nlm.nih.gov/books/NBK546680/.

256. Michelle M. McWilliams and Vargheese M. Chennathukuzhi, "Recent Advances in Uterine Fibroid Etiology," *Seminars in Reproductive Medicine* 35, no. 02 (March 9, 2017): 181–89, https://doi.org/10.1055/s-0037-1599090.

257. Geum Seon Sohn et al., "Current Medical Treatment of Uterine Fibroids," *Obstetrics & Gynecology Science* 61, no. 2 (February 13, 2018): 192–201, https://doi.org/10.5468/ogs.2018.61.2.192.

258. Jacques Donnez and Marie-Madeleine Dolmans, "Uterine Fibroid Management: From the Present to the Future," *Human Reproduction Update* 22, no. 6 (July 27, 2016): 665–86, https://doi.org/10.1093/humupd/dmw023.
Geum Seon Sohn et al., "Current Medical Treatment of Uterine Fibroids," *Obstetrics & Gynecology Science* 61, no. 2 (February 13, 2018): 192–201, https://doi.org/10.5468/ogs.2018.61.2.192.

259. Adeline Angeli et al., "Joint Model of Iron and Hepcidin during the Menstrual Cycle in Healthy Women," *The AAPS Journal* 18, no. 2 (February 2, 2016): 490–504, https://doi.org/10.1208/s12248-016-9875-4.

260. Adeline Angeli et al., "Joint Model of Iron and Hepcidin during the Menstrual Cycle in Healthy Women," *The AAPS Journal* 18, no. 2 (February 2, 2016): 490–504, https://doi.org/10.1208/s12248-016-9875-4.

261. Matthew J. Warner and Muhammad T. Kamran, "Iron Deficiency Anemia," essay, in *StatPearls [Internet]* (Treasure Island, FL: StatPearls Publishing, 2022), https://www.ncbi.nlm.nih.gov/books/NBK448065/.

262. Jake Turner, Meghana Parsi, and Madhu Badireddy, "Anemia," essay, in *StatPearls [Internet]* (Treasure Island, FL: StatPearls Publishing, 2022), https://www.ncbi.nlm.nih.gov/books/NBK499994/.

263. Shersten Killip, John M. Bennett, and Mara D. Chambers, "Iron Deficiency Anemia," *American Family Physician* 75, no. 5 (March 1, 2007): 671–78, https://pubmed.ncbi.nlm.nih.gov/17375513/.

264. Adeline Angeli et al., "Joint Model of Iron and Hepcidin during the Menstrual Cycle in Healthy Women," The *AAPS Journal* 18, no. 2 (February 2, 2016): 490–504, https://doi.org/10.1208/s12248-016-9875-4.

265. Matthew J. Warner and Muhammad T. Kamran, "Iron Deficiency Anemia," essay, in *StatPearls [Internet]* (Treasure Island, FL: StatPearls Publishing, 2022), https://www.ncbi.nlm.nih.gov/books/NBK448065/.

266. Jake Turner, Meghana Parsi, and Madhu Badireddy, "Anemia," essay, in *StatPearls [Internet]* (Treasure Island, FL: StatPearls Publishing, 2022), https://www.ncbi.nlm.nih.gov/books/NBK499994/.

267. Esa T. Soppi, "Iron Deficiency without Anemia - a Clinical Challenge," *Clinical Case Reports* 6, no. 6 (April 17, 2018): 1082–86, https://doi.org/10.1002/ccr3.1529.

268. Esa T. Soppi, "Iron Deficiency without Anemia - a Clinical Challenge," *Clinical Case Reports* 6, no. 6 (April 17, 2018): 1082–86, https://doi.org/10.1002/ccr3.1529.
Sarah H. O'Brien, "Evaluation and Management of Heavy Menstrual Bleeding in Adolescents: The Role of the Hematologist," *Hematology* 2018, no. 1 (November 30, 2018): 390–98, https://doi.org/10.1182/asheducation-2018.1.390.

269. Paul Vaucher et al., "Effect of Iron Supplementation on Fatigue in Nonanemic Menstruating Women with Low Ferritin: A Randomized Controlled Trial," *Canadian Medical Association Journal* 184, no. 11 (July 9, 2012): 1247–54, https://doi.org/10.1503/cmaj.110950.

270. Matthew J. Warner and Muhammad T. Kamran, "Iron Deficiency Anemia," essay, in *StatPearls [Internet]* (Treasure Island, FL: StatPearls Publishing, 2022), https://www.ncbi.nlm.nih.gov/books/NBK448065/.

271. Muhammad Saboor, "Disorders Associated with Malabsorption of Iron; a Critical Review," *Pakistan Journal of Medical Science*s 31, no. 6 (December 31, 1969): 1549–53, https://doi.org/10.12669/pjms.316.8125.

272. Marc Sim et al., "Iron Considerations for the Athlete: A Narrative Review," *European Journal of Applied Physiology* 119, no. 7 (May 4, 2019): 1463–78, https://doi.org/10.1007/s00421-019-04157-y.

273. Stacy T. Sims et al., "High Prevalence of Iron Deficiency Exhibited in Internationally Competitive, Non-Professional Female Endurance Athletes—a Case Study," *International Journal of Environmental Research and Public Health* 19, no. 24 (December 10, 2022): 16606, https://doi.org/10.3390/ijerph192416606.

274. Georgie Bruinvels et al., "The Prevalence and Impact of Heavy Menstrual Bleeding (Menorrhagia) in Elite and Non-Elite Athletes," *PLOS ONE* 11, no. 2 (February 22, 2016): e0149881, https://doi.org/10.1371/journal.pone.0149881.

275. Joann L. Porter and Prashanth Rawla, "Hemochromatosis," essay, in *StatPearls [Internet]* (Treasure Island, FL: StatPearls Publishing, 2022), https://www.ncbi.nlm.nih.gov/books/NBK430862/.

276. Zoe Tolkien et al., "Ferrous Sulfate Supplementation Causes Significant Gastrointestinal Side-Effects in Adults: A Systematic Review and Meta-Analysis," *PLOS ONE* 10, no. 2 (February 20, 2015), https://doi.org/10.1371/journal.pone.0117383.

277. Erik Björn-Rasmussen et al., "Food Iron Absorption in Man Applications of the Two-Pool Extrinsic Tag Method to Measure Heme and Nonheme Iron Absorption from the Whole Diet," *Journal of Clinical Investigation* 53, no. 1 (January 1, 1974): 247–55, https://doi.org/10.1172/jci107545.

278. Fady Moustarah and Sharon F. Daley, "Dietary Iron," essay, in *StatPearls [Internet]* (Treasure Island, FL: StatPearls Publishing, 2022), https://www.ncbi.nlm.nih.gov/books/NBK540969/.

279. Fady Moustarah and Sharon F. Daley, "Dietary Iron," essay, in *StatPearls [Internet]* (Treasure Island, FL: StatPearls Publishing, 2022), https://www.ncbi.nlm.nih.gov/books/NBK540969/.

280. Birgit Teucher, Manuel Olivares, and Héctor Cori, "Enhancers of Iron Absorption: Ascorbic Acid and Other Organic Acids," *International Journal for Vitamin and Nutrition Research* 74, no. 6 (November 1, 2004): 403–19, https://doi.org/10.1024/0300-9831.74.6.403.

281. Leif Hallberg et al., "Inhibition of Haem-Iron Absorption in Man by Calcium," *British Journal of Nutrition* 69, no. 2 (March 9, 1993): 533–40, https://doi.org/10.1079/bjn19930053.

282. Adeline Angeli et al., "Joint Model of Iron and Hepcidin during the Menstrual Cycle in Healthy Women," *The AAPS Journal* 18, no. 2 (February 2, 2016): 490–504, https://doi.org/10.1208/s12248-016-9875-4.

283. Jake Turner, Meghana Parsi, and Madhu Badireddy, "Anemia," essay, in *StatPearls [Internet]* (Treasure Island, FL: StatPearls Publishing, 2022), https://www.ncbi.nlm.nih.gov/books/NBK499994/.
Stacy T. Sims et al., "High Prevalence of Iron Deficiency Exhibited in Internationally Competitive, Non-Professional Female Endurance Athletes—a Case Study," *International Journal of Environmental Research and Public Health* 19, no. 24 (December 10, 2022): 16606, https://doi.org/10.3390/ijerph192416606.

284. Esa T. Soppi, "Iron Deficiency without Anemia - a Clinical Challenge," *Clinical Case Reports* 6, no. 6 (April 17, 2018): 1082–86, https://doi.org/10.1002/ccr3.1529.

285. Fady Moustarah and Sharon F. Daley, "Dietary Iron," essay, in *StatPearls [Internet]* (Treasure Island, FL: StatPearls Publishing, 2022), https://www.ncbi.nlm.nih.gov/books/NBK540969/.

286. Joann L. Porter and Prashanth Rawla, "Hemochromatosis," essay, in *StatPearls [Internet]* (Treasure Island, FL: StatPearls Publishing, 2022), https://www.ncbi.nlm.nih.gov/books/NBK430862/.

287. Walter Milano et al., "Menstrual Disorders Related to Eating Disorders," *Endocrine, Metabolic & Immune Disorders - Drug Targets* 22, no. 5 (January 14, 2022): 471–80, https://doi.org/10.2174/18715303216662106

25145345.

288. Walter Milano et al., "Menstrual Disorders Related to Eating Disorders," *Endocrine, Metabolic & Immune Disorders - Drug Targets* 22, no. 5 (January 14, 2022): 471–80, https://doi.org/10.2174/18715303216662106 25145345.

289. James H. Liu, Bansari Patel, and Gretchen Collins, "Central Causes of Amenorrhea," essay, in *Endotext [Internet]* (South Dartmouth, MA: MDText.com, Inc., 2000), https://www.ncbi.nlm.nih.gov/books/ NBK278939//.
Karina Ryterska, Agnieszka Kordek, and Patrycja Załęska, "Has Menstruation Disappeared? Functional Hypothalamic Amenorrhea— What Is This Story About?," *Nutrients* 13, no. 8 (August 17, 2021): 2827, https://doi.org/10.3390/nu13082827.

290. Chrisandra L. Shufelt, Tina Torbati, and Erika Dutra, "Hypothalamic Amenorrhea and the Long-Term Health Consequences," *Seminars in Reproductive Medicine* 35, no. 03 (2017): 256–62, https://doi. org/10.1055/s-0037-1603581.
Lara Briden, *Period Repair Manual: Every Woman's Guide to Better Periods* (Sydney, N.S.W.: Macmillan, 2018).

291. Aurelia Nattiv et al., "The Female Athlete Triad," *Medicine and Science in Sports and Exercise* 39, no. 10 (November 2007): 1867–82, https://doi. org/10.1249/mss.0b013e318149f111.

292. José L. Areta et al., "Reduced Resting Skeletal Muscle Protein Synthesis Is Rescued by Resistance Exercise and Protein Ingestion Following Short-Term Energy Deficit," *American Journal of Physiology-Endocrinology and Metabolism* 306, no. 8 (April 15, 2014): E989–97, https://doi.org/10.1152/ajpendo.00590.2013.

293. Kathryn E. Ackerman et al., "Low Energy Availability Surrogates Correlate with Health and Performance Consequences of Relative Energy Deficiency in Sport," *British Journal of Sports Medicine* 53, no. 10 (June 2, 2018): 628–33, https://doi.org/10.1136/bjsports-2017-098958.

294. A. Melin et al., "Energy Availability and the Female Athlete Triad in Elite Endurance Athletes," *Scandinavian Journal of Medicine & Science in Sports* 25, no. 5 (May 30, 2014): 610–22, https://doi.org/10.1111/ sms.12261.

295. Margo Mountjoy et al., "The IOC Consensus Statement: Beyond the Female Athlete Triad—Relative Energy Deficiency in Sport (Red-S)," *British Journal of Sports Medicine* 48, no. 7 (March 11, 2014): 491–97, https://doi.org/10.1136/bjsports-2014-093502.

296. Michael Drew et al., "Prevalence of Illness, Poor Mental Health and Sleep Quality and Low Energy Availability Prior to the 2016 Summer Olympic Games," *British Journal of Sports Medicine* 52, no. 1 (October 22, 2017): 47–53, https://doi.org/10.1136/bjsports-2017-098208.

297. Kazuhiro Shimizu et al., "Mucosal Immune Function Comparison between AMENORRHEIC and EUMENORRHEIC Distance Runners,"

Journal of Strength and Conditioning Research 26, no. 5 (May 2012): 1402–6, https://doi.org/10.1519/jsc.0b013e31822e7a6c.

298. Aurelia Nattiv et al., "The Female Athlete Triad," *Medicine and Science in Sports and Exercise* 39, no. 10 (November 2007): 1867–82, https://doi.org/10.1249/mss.0b013e318149f111.

299. Sayaka Nose Ogura et al., "Risk Factors of Stress Fractures Due to the Female Athlete Triad: Differences in Teens and Twenties," *Scandinavian Journal of Medicine & Science in Sports* 29, no. 10 (June 9, 2019): 1501–10, https://doi.org/10.1111/sms.13464.

300. Katie J. Thralls et al., "Body Mass-Related Predictors of the Female Athlete Triad among Adolescent Athletes," *International Journal of Sport Nutrition and Exercise Metabolism* 26, no. 1 (February 2016): 17–25, https://doi.org/10.1123/ijsnem.2015-0072.

301. Jill M. Thein-Nissenbaum et al., "Menstrual Irregularity and Musculoskeletal Injury in Female High School Athletes," *Journal of Athletic Training* 47, no. 1 (January 1, 2012): 74–82, https://doi.org/10.4085/1062-6050-47.1.74.

302. Julie Agel, Elizabeth A. Arendt, and Boris Bershadsky, "Anterior Cruciate Ligament Injury in National Collegiate Athletic Association Basketball and Soccer: A 13-Year Review," *The American Journal of Sports Medicine* 33, no. 4 (April 2005): 524–31, https://doi.org/10.1177/0363546504269937.

303. Julie Agel, Elizabeth A. Arendt, and Boris Bershadsky, "Anterior Cruciate Ligament Injury in National Collegiate Athletic Association Basketball and Soccer: A 13-Year Review," *The American Journal of Sports Medicine* 33, no. 4 (April 2005): 524–31, https://doi.org/10.1177/0363546504269937.

304. Nkechinyere Chidi-Ogbolu and Keith Baar, "Effect of Estrogen on Musculoskeletal Performance and Injury Risk," *Frontiers in Physiology* 9 (January 15, 2019), https://doi.org/10.3389/fphys.2018.01834.

305. JongEun Yim, Jerrold Petrofsky, and Haneul Lee, "Correlation between Mechanical Properties of the Ankle Muscles and Postural Sway during the Menstrual Cycle," *The Tohoku Journal of Experimental Medicine* 244, no. 3 (March 18, 2018): 201–7, https://doi.org/10.1620/tjem.244.201.

306. Todd May, "Stress Fractures," essay, in *StatPearls [Internet]*, ed. Raghavendra Marappa-Ganeshan (Treasure Island, FL: StatPearls Publishing, 2022), https://www.ncbi.nlm.nih.gov/books/NBK554538/.

307. Katherine Herman et al., "The Effectiveness of Neuromuscular Warm-up Strategies, That Require No Additional Equipment, for Preventing Lower Limb Injuries during Sports Participation: A Systematic Review," *BMC Medicine* 10, no. 1 (July 19, 2012), https://doi.org/10.1186/1741-7015-10-75.

308. Daniel Martin et al., "Period Prevalence and Perceived Side Effects of Hormonal Contraceptive Use and the Menstrual Cycle in Elite Athletes," *International Journal of Sports Physiology and Performance* 13, no. 7

(August 1, 2018): 926–32, https://doi.org/10.1123/ijspp.2017-0330.

309. Jaclyn A. Konopka, Lauren J. Hsue, and Jason L. Dragoo, "Effect of Oral Contraceptives on Soft Tissue Injury Risk, Soft Tissue Laxity, and Muscle Strength: A Systematic Review of the Literature," *Orthopaedic Journal of Sports Medicine* 7, no. 3 (March 22, 2019): 232596711983106, https://doi.org/10.1177/2325967119831061.

310. Marci A. Goolsby and Nicole Boniquit, "Bone Health in Athletes," *Sports Health: A Multidisciplinary Approach* 9, no. 2 (November 30, 2016): 108–17, https://doi.org/10.1177/1941738116677732.

311. Kathryn E. Ackerman et al., "Fractures in Relation to Menstrual Status and Bone Parameters in Young Athletes," *Medicine & Science in Sports & Exercise* 47, no. 8 (August 2015): 1577–86, https://doi.org/10.1249/mss.0000000000000574.

312. Cristina Palacios, "The Role of Nutrients in Bone Health, from A to Z," *Critical Reviews in Food Science and Nutrition* 46, no. 8 (December 2006): 621–28, https://doi.org/10.1080/10408390500466174.

313. Katherine L Tucker et al., "Colas, but Not Other Carbonated Beverages, Are Associated with Low Bone Mineral Density in Older Women: The Framingham Osteoporosis Study," *The American Journal of Clinical Nutrition* 84, no. 4 (October 1, 2006): 936–42, https://doi.org/10.1093/ajcn/84.4.936.

314. Lynn Cialdella-Kam et al., "Dietary Intervention Restored Menses in Female Athletes with Exercise-Associated Menstrual Dysfunction with Limited Impact on Bone and Muscle Health," *Nutrients* 6, no. 8 (July 31, 2014): 3018–39, https://doi.org/10.3390/nu6083018.
Mary Jane De Souza et al., "Randomised Controlled Trial of the Effects of Increased Energy Intake on Menstrual Recovery in Exercising Women with Menstrual Disturbances: The 'Refuel' Study," *Human Reproduction* 36, no. 8 (June 24, 2021): 2285–97, https://doi.org/10.1093/humrep/deab149.

315. JongEun Yim, Jerrold Petrofsky, and Haneul Lee, "Correlation between Mechanical Properties of the Ankle Muscles and Postural Sway during the Menstrual Cycle," *The Tohoku Journal of Experimental Medicine* 244, no. 3 (March 18, 2018): 201–7, https://doi.org/10.1620/tjem.244.201.
Simone D. Herzberg et al., "The Effect of Menstrual Cycle and Contraceptives on ACL Injuries and Laxity: A Systematic Review and Meta-Analysis," *Orthopaedic Journal of Sports Medicine* 5, no. 7 (July 1, 2017): 232596711771878, https://doi.org/10.1177/2325967117718781.

FAD DIETS, SUGAR, AND YOUR CYCLE

1. Mandy Spadine and Megan S. Patterson, "Social Influence on FAD Diet Use: A Systematic Literature Review," *Nutrition and Health* 28, no. 3 (January 13, 2022): 369–88, https://doi.

org/10.1177/02601060211072370.

2. Heather Seid and Michael Rosenbaum, "Low Carbohydrate and Low-Fat Diets: What We Don't Know and Why We Should Know It," *Nutrients* 11, no. 11 (November 12, 2019): 2749, https://doi.org/10.3390/nu11112749.

3. Hima J. Challa, Manav Bandlamudi, and Kalyan R. Uppaluri, "Paleolithic Diet," essay, in *StatPearls [Internet]* (Treasure Island, FL: StatPearls Publishing, 2020), ncbi.nlm.nih.gov/books/NBK482457/.

4. Hima J. Challa, Manav Bandlamudi, and Kalyan R. Uppaluri, "Paleolithic Diet," essay, in *StatPearls [Internet]* (Treasure Island, FL: StatPearls Publishing, 2020), ncbi.nlm.nih.gov/books/NBK482457/.

5. Hima J. Challa, Manav Bandlamudi, and Kalyan R. Uppaluri, "Paleolithic Diet," essay, in *StatPearls [Internet]* (Treasure Island, FL: StatPearls Publishing, 2020), ncbi.nlm.nih.gov/books/NBK482457/.

6. Kristine A Whalen et al., "Paleolithic and Mediterranean Diet Pattern Scores Are Inversely Associated with All-Cause and Cause-Specific Mortality in Adults," *The Journal of Nutrition* 147, no. 4 (April 2017): 612–20, https://doi.org/10.3945/jn.116.241919.

7. Angela Genoni et al., "Long-Term Paleolithic Diet Is Associated with Lower Resistant Starch Intake, Different Gut Microbiota Composition and Increased Serum TMAO Concentrations," *European Journal of Nutrition* 59, no. 5 (July 5, 2019): 1845–58, https://doi.org/10.1007/s00394-019-02036-y.
Amy Jamieson-Petonic, "Is the Paleo Diet Good for Athletes?," stack, November 13, 2015, https://www.stack.com/a/is-the-paleo-diet-good-for-athletes.
Angela Genoni et al., "A Paleolithic Diet Lowers Resistant Starch Intake but Does Not Affect Serum Trimethylamine-*n*-Oxide Concentrations in Healthy Women," *British Journal of Nutrition* 121, no. 3 (December 17, 2018): 322–29, https://doi.org/10.1017/s000711451800329x.

8. Amy Jamieson-Petonic, "Is the Paleo Diet Good for Athletes?," stack, November 13, 2015, https://www.stack.com/a/is-the-paleo-diet-good-for-athletes.

9. "Sodium," Centers for Disease Control and Prevention, December 21, 2021, https://www.cdc.gov/heartdisease/sodium.htm.

10. Rhys D Evans et al., "Emerging Evidence of an Effect of Salt on Innate and Adaptive Immunity," *Nephrology Dialysis Transplantation* 34, no. 12 (December 5, 2018): 2007–14, https://doi.org/10.1093/ndt/gfy362.

11. "Sodium," Centers for Disease Control and Prevention, December 21, 2021, https://www.cdc.gov/heartdisease/sodium.htm.

12. Keewan Kim et al., "Dietary Minerals, Reproductive Hormone Levels and Sporadic Anovulation: Associations in Healthy Women with Regular Menstrual Cycles," *British Journal of Nutrition* 120, no. 1 (April 20, 2018): 81–89, https://doi.org/10.1017/s0007114518000818.

13. "Sodium," Centers for Disease Control and Prevention, December 21, 2021, https://www.cdc.gov/heartdisease/sodium.htm.

14.   Wajeed Masood, Pavan Annamaraju, and Kalyan R. Uppaluri, "Ketogenic Diet," essay, in *StatPearls [Internet]* (Treasure Island, FL: StatPearls Publishing, 2022), https://www.ncbi.nlm.nih.gov/books/NBK499830/.
       David S Ludwig, "The Ketogenic Diet: Evidence for Optimism but High-Quality Research Needed," *The Journal of Nutrition* 150, no. 6 (June 1, 2020): 1354–59, https://doi.org/10.1093/jn/nxz308.

15.   Robert Oh, Brian Gilani, and Kalyan R. Uppaluri, "Low Carbohydrate Diet," essay, in *StatPearls [Internet]* (Treasure Island, FL: StatPearls Publishing, 2021), https://www.ncbi.nlm.nih.gov/books/NBK537084/.

16.   Kiranjit K. Dhillon and Sonu Gupta, "Biochemistry, Ketogenesis," essay, in *StatPearls [Internet]* (Treasure Island, FL: StatPearls, 2023), https://ncbi.nlm.nih.gov/books/NBK493179/#:~:text=Ketogenesis%20occurs%20primarily%20in%20the,acetyl%20CoA%20via%20beta-oxidation.
       Wajeed Masood, Pavan Annamaraju, and Kalyan R. Uppaluri, "Ketogenic Diet," essay, in *StatPearls [Internet]* (Treasure Island, FL: StatPearls Publishing, 2022), https://www.ncbi.nlm.nih.gov/books/NBK499830/.
       Lori Laffel, "Ketone Bodies: A Review of Physiology, Pathophysiology and Application of Monitoring to Diabetes," *Diabetes Metabolism Research and Reviews* 15, no. 6 (January 14, 2000): 412–26, https://doi.org/https://doi.org/10.1002/(SICI)1520-7560(199911/12)15:6%3C412::AID-DMRR72%3E3.0.CO;2-8.

17.   Mackenzie A. Mady et al., "The Ketogenic Diet: Adolescents Can Do It, Too," *Epilepsia* 44, no. 6 (June 9, 2003): 847–51, https://doi.org/10.1046/j.1528-1157.2003.57002.x.

18.   Cara B. Ebbeling et al., "Effects of Dietary Composition on Energy Expenditure during Weight-Loss Maintenance," *JAMA* 307, no. 24 (June 27, 2012): 2627–34, https://doi.org/10.1001/jama.2012.6607.

19.   Jonas Burén et al., "A Ketogenic Low-Carbohydrate High-Fat Diet Increases LDL Cholesterol in Healthy, Young, Normal-Weight Women: A Randomized Controlled Feeding Trial," *Nutrients* 13, no. 3 (March 2, 2021): 814, https://doi.org/10.3390/nu13030814.

20.   David S Ludwig, "The Ketogenic Diet: Evidence for Optimism but High-Quality Research Needed," *The Journal of Nutrition* 150, no. 6 (June 1, 2020): 1354–59, https://doi.org/10.1093/jn/nxz308.
       Jian Li et al., "Ketogenic Diet in Women with Polycystic Ovary Syndrome and Liver Dysfunction Who Are Obese: A Randomized, Open label, parallel Group, Controlled Pilot Trial," *Journal of Obstetrics and Gynaecology Research* 47, no. 3 (January 18, 2021): 1145–52, https://doi.org/10.1111/jog.14650.

21.   Françoise Wilhelmi de Toledo et al., "Unravelling the Health Effects of Fasting: A Long Road from Obesity Treatment to Healthy Life Span Increase and Improved Cognition," *Annals of Medicine* 52, no. 5 (June

10, 2020): 147–61, https://doi.org/10.1080/07853890.2020.1770849.

22. Eric Williamson and Daniel R. Moore, "A Muscle-Centric Perspective on Intermittent Fasting: A Suboptimal Dietary Strategy for Supporting Muscle Protein Remodeling and Muscle Mass?," *Frontiers in Nutrition* 8 (June 9, 2021), https://doi.org/10.3389/fnut.2021.640621.

23. "Who Guideline : Sugar Consumption Recommendation," World Health Organization, March 4, 2015, https://www.who.int/news/item/04-03-2015-who-calls-on-countries-to-reduce-sugars-intake-among-adults-and-children.

24. "Atkins Diet: What's behind the Claims?," Mayo Clinic, May 12, 2022, https://www.mayoclinic.org/healthy-lifestyle/weight-loss/in-depth/atkins-diet/art-20048485.

25. Ghanim Salih Mahdi, "The Atkin's Diet Controversy," *Annals of Saudi Medicine* 26, no. 3 (June 1, 2006): 244–45, https://doi.org/10.5144/0256-4947.2006.244.
     Robert Oh, Brian Gilani, and Kalyan R. Uppaluri, "Low Carbohydrate Diet," essay, in *StatPearls [Internet]* (Treasure Island, FL: StatPearls Publishing, 2021), https://www.ncbi.nlm.nih.gov/books/NBK537084/.

26. Robert Oh, Brian Gilani, and Kalyan R. Uppaluri, "Low Carbohydrate Diet," essay, in *StatPearls [Internet]* (Treasure Island, FL: StatPearls Publishing, 2021), https://www.ncbi.nlm.nih.gov/books/NBK537084/.

27. Lisa Hendrickson-Jack and Lara Briden, *The Fifth Vital Sign: Master Your Cycles and Optimize Your Fertility* (Fertility Friday Publishing Inc., 2019).

28. Colton R. Rishor-Olney and Melissa R. Hinson, "Mediterranean Diet," essay, in *StatPearls [Internet]* (Treasure Island, FL: StatPearls Publishing, 2022).

29. Courtney Davis et al., "Definition of the Mediterranean Diet; a Literature Review," *Nutrients* 7, no. 11 (November 5, 2015): 9139–53, https://doi.org/10.3390/nu7115459.

30. Kristine A Whalen et al., "Paleolithic and Mediterranean Diet Pattern Scores Are Inversely Associated with All-Cause and Cause-Specific Mortality in Adults," *The Journal of Nutrition* 147, no. 4 (April 2017): 612–20, https://doi.org/10.3945/jn.116.241919.

31. Silvia Carlos et al., "Mediterranean Diet and Health Outcomes in the Sun Cohort," *Nutrients* 10, no. 4 (March 31, 2018): 439, https://doi.org/10.3390/nu10040439.
     Audrey J. Gaskins et al., "Dietary Patterns and Outcomes of Assisted Reproduction," *American Journal of Obstetrics and Gynecology* 220, no. 6 (June 2019), https://doi.org/10.1016/j.ajog.2019.02.004.

32. Colton R. Rishor-Olney and Melissa R. Hinson, "Mediterranean Diet," essay, in *StatPearls [Internet]* (Treasure Island, FL: StatPearls Publishing, 2022).

33. Surinder Baines, Jennifer Powers, and Wendy J Brown, "How Does the Health and Well-Being of Young Australian Vegetarian and Semi-

Vegetarian Women Compare with Non-Vegetarians?," *Public Health Nutrition* 10, no. 5 (May 2007): 436–42, https://doi.org/10.1017/s1368980007217938.

34. Naomi Fallon and Stephanie A. Dillon, "Low Intakes of Iodine and Selenium amongst Vegan and Vegetarian Women Highlight a Potential Nutritional Vulnerability," *Frontiers in Nutrition* 7 (May 20, 2020), https://doi.org/10.3389/fnut.2020.00072.
Eric Slywitch et al., "Iron Deficiency in Vegetarian and Omnivorous Individuals: Analysis of 1340 Individuals," *Nutrients* 13, no. 9 (August 26, 2021): 2964, https://doi.org/10.3390/nu13092964.
Hercules Sakkas et al., "Nutritional Status and the Influence of the Vegan Diet on the Gut Microbiota and Human Health," *Medicina* 56, no. 2 (February 22, 2020): 88, https://doi.org/10.3390/medicina56020088.

35. Jana Kadrabová et al., "Selenium Status, Plasma Zinc, Copper, and Magnesium in Vegetarians," *Biological Trace Element Research* 50, no. 1 (October 1995): 13–24, https://doi.org/10.1007/bf02789145.

36. Saul R. Powell, "The Antioxidant Properties of Zinc," *The Journal of Nutrition* 130, no. 5 (May 2000): 1447S-1454S, https://doi.org/10.1093/jn/130.5.1447s.
Lisa M. Gaetke and Ching Kaung Chow, "Copper Toxicity, Oxidative Stress, and Antioxidant Nutrients," *Toxicology* 189, no. 1–2 (July 15, 2003): 147–63, https://doi.org/10.1016/s0300-483x(03)00159-8.

37. James F. Collins and Leslie M. Klevay, "Copper," *Advances in Nutrition* 2, no. 6 (November 2011): 520–22, https://doi.org/10.3945/an.111.001222.

38. "Office of Dietary Supplements - Copper," NIH Office of Dietary Supplements, October 18, 2022, https://ods.od.nih.gov/factsheets/Copper-HealthProfessional/#:~:text=Sources%20of%20Copper,-Food&text=The%20richest%20dietary%20copper%20sources,chocolate%20%5B1%2C2%5D.

39. Izhar Qazi et al., "Selenium, Selenoproteins, and Female Reproduction: A Review," *Molecules* 23, no. 12 (November 22, 2018): 3053, https://doi.org/10.3390/molecules23123053.
Mehmet Okan Özkaya et al., "Effects of Multivitamin/Mineral Supplementation on Trace Element Levels in Serum and Follicular Fluid of Women Undergoing in Vitro Fertilization (IVF)," *Biological Trace Element Research* 139, no. 1 (February 24, 2010): 1–9, https://doi.org/10.1007/s12011-010-8637-x.

40. Jana Kadrabová et al., "Selenium Status, Plasma Zinc, Copper, and Magnesium in Vegetarians," *Biological Trace Element Research* 50, no. 1 (October 1995): 13–24, https://doi.org/10.1007/bf02789145.
Naomi Fallon and Stephanie A. Dillon, "Low Intakes of Iodine and Selenium amongst Vegan and Vegetarian Women Highlight a Potential Nutritional Vulnerability," *Frontiers in Nutrition* 7 (May 20, 2020), https://doi.org/10.3389/fnut.2020.00072.

41. Surinder Baines, Jennifer Powers, and Wendy J Brown, "How Does

the Health and Well-Being of Young Australian Vegetarian and Semi-Vegetarian Women Compare with Non-Vegetarians?," *Public Health Nutrition* 10, no. 5 (May 2007): 436–42, https://doi.org/10.1017/s1368980007217938.

42. Hercules Sakkas et al., "Nutritional Status and the Influence of the Vegan Diet on the Gut Microbiota and Human Health," *Medicina* 56, no. 2 (February 22, 2020): 88, https://doi.org/10.3390/medicina56020088.

43. Alan R. Gaby, *Nutritional Medicine* (Concord, NH: Fritz Perlberg Publishing, 2017).

44. Kam Woo, Timothy Kwok, and David Celermajer, "Vegan Diet, Subnormal Vitamin B-12 Status and Cardiovascular Health," *Nutrients* 6, no. 8 (August 19, 2014): 3259–73, https://doi.org/10.3390/nu6083259.

45. Sareen S. Gropper, Jack L. Smith, and Timothy P. Carr, *Advanced Nutrition and Human Metabolism*, 7th ed. (Boston, MA: Cengage Learning, 2018).

46. Hercules Sakkas et al., "Nutritional Status and the Influence of the Vegan Diet on the Gut Microbiota and Human Health," *Medicina* 56, no. 2 (February 22, 2020): 88, https://doi.org/10.3390/medicina56020088.

47. Hana Kahleova et al., "A Plant-Based Diet in Overweight Individuals in a 16-Week Randomized Clinical Trial: Metabolic Benefits of Plant Protein," *Nutrition & Diabetes* 8, no. 1 (November 2, 2018), https://doi.org/10.1038/s41387-018-0067-4.

48. Gavin Yong-Quan Ng et al., "Dietary Restriction and Epigenetics: Part I," *Conditioning Medicine* 2, no. 6 (December 2019): 284–99, https://pubmed.ncbi.nlm.nih.gov/32039345/.
Rafael de Cabo and Mark P. Mattson, "Effects of Intermittent Fasting on Health, Aging, and Disease," *New England Journal of Medicine* 381, no. 26 (December 26, 2019): 2541–51, https://doi.org/10.1056/nejmra1905136.

49. Bo Hye Kim et al., "Effects of Intermittent Fasting on the Circulating Levels and Circadian Rhythms of Hormones," *Endocrinology and Metabolism* 36, no. 4 (August 31, 2021): 745–56, https://doi.org/10.3803/enm.2021.405.

50. "Who Guideline : Sugar Consumption Recommendation," World Health Organization, March 4, 2015, https://www.who.int/news/item/04-03-2015-who-calls-on-countries-to-reduce-sugars-intake-among-adults-and-children.

51. George A Bray, Samara Joy Nielsen, and Barry M Popkin, "Consumption of High-Fructose Corn Syrup in Beverages May Play a Role in the Epidemic of Obesity," *The American Journal of Clinical Nutrition* 79, no. 4 (April 2004): 537–43, https://doi.org/10.1093/ajcn/79.4.537.

52. Michael I. Goran, Stanley J. Ulijaszek, and Emily E. Ventura, "High Fructose Corn Syrup and Diabetes Prevalence: A Global Perspective," *Global Public Health* 8, no. 1 (November 27, 2012): 55–64, https://doi.org/10.1080/17441692.2012.736257.

53. Xiaosen Ouyang et al., "Fructose Consumption as a Risk Factor for Non-Alcoholic Fatty Liver Disease," *Journal of Hepatology* 48, no. 6 (June 2008): pp. 993-999, https://doi.org/10.1016/j.jhep.2008.02.011.

54. "Definition & Facts of NAFLD & Nash in Children," National Institute of Diabetes and Digestive and Kidney Diseases, December 2021, https://www.niddk.nih.gov/health-information/liver-disease/nafld-nash-children/definition-facts.
    Thomas Jensen et al., "Fructose and Sugar: A Major Mediator of Non-Alcoholic Fatty Liver Disease," *Journal of Hepatology* 68, no. 5 (May 2018): 1063–75, https://doi.org/10.1016/j.jhep.2018.01.019.

55. Xiaosen Ouyang et al., "Fructose Consumption as a Risk Factor for Non-Alcoholic Fatty Liver Disease," *Journal of Hepatology* 48, no. 6 (June 2008): pp. 993-999, https://doi.org/10.1016/j.jhep.2008.02.011.

56. Mark A. Febbraio and Michael Karin, "'Sweet Death': Fructose as a Metabolic Toxin That Targets the Gut-Liver Axis," *Cell Metabolism* 33, no. 12 (December 7, 2021): 2316–28, https://doi.org/10.1016/j.cmet.2021.09.004.

57. Cezmi A. Akdis, "Does the Epithelial Barrier Hypothesis Explain the Increase in Allergy, Autoimmunity and Other Chronic Conditions?," *Nature Reviews Immunology* 21, no. 11 (April 12, 2021): 739–51, https://doi.org/10.1038/s41577-021-00538-7.

58. James J. DiNicolantonio, James H. O'Keefe, and Sean C. Lucan, "Added Fructose," *Mayo Clinic Proceedings* 90, no. 3 (March 2015): 372–81, https://doi.org/10.1016/j.mayocp.2014.12.019.

59. Julia Beisner et al., "Fructose-Induced Intestinal Microbiota Shift Following Two Types of Short-Term High-Fructose Dietary Phases," *Nutrients* 12, no. 11 (November 10, 2020): 3444, https://doi.org/10.3390/nu12113444.

60. "Patients & Families: UW Health," Health and Nutrition Facts for You | Patients & Families | UW Health, n.d., https://patient.uwhealth.org/healthfacts.

61. "Patients & Families: UW Health," Health and Nutrition Facts for You | Patients & Families | UW Health, n.d., https://patient.uwhealth.org/healthfacts.

62. Michelle Pearlman, Jon Obert, and Lisa Casey, "The Association between Artificial Sweeteners and Obesity," *Current Gastroenterology Reports* 19, no. 12 (November 21, 2017): 64, https://doi.org/10.1007/s11894-017-0602-9.

63. American Dietetic Association, "Position of the American Dietetic Association: Use of Nutritive and Nonnutritive Sweeteners," *Journal of the American Dietetic Association* 104, no. 2 (February 2004): 255-75, https://doi.org/10.1016/j.jada.2003.12.001.

64. "Sugar Substitutes," familydoctor.org, May 31, 2023, https://familydoctor.org/sugar-substitutes/.

THE BASICS OF HORMONAL BIRTH CONTROL

1. Paul J Yong et al., "CHC for Pelvic Pain in Women with Endometriosis: Ineffectiveness or Discontinuation Due to Side-Effects," *Human Reproduction Open* 2020, no. 2 (February 28, 2020), https://doi.org/10.1093/hropen/hoz040.

2. Michael Edwards and Ahmet S. Can, "Progestin," essay, in *StatPearls [Internet]* (Treasure Island, FL: StatPearls Publishing, 2023), https://www.ncbi.nlm.nih.gov/books/NBK563211/.

3. Morena L. Rocca et al., "Bone Health and Hormonal Contraception," *Minerva Obstetrics and Gynecology* 73, no. 6 (December 2021): 678–96, https://doi.org/10.23736/s2724-606x.20.04688-2.

4. Kimberly Daniels and Joyce C. Abma, "Current Contraceptive Status Among Women Aged 15–49: United States, 2015–2017," Centers for Disease Control and Prevention, February 14, 2019, https://www.cdc.gov/nchs/products/databriefs/db327.htm.

5. Danielle B. Cooper, Preeti Patel, and Heba Mahdy, "Oral Contraceptive Pills," essay, in *StatPearls [Internet]* (Treasure Island, FL: StatPearls Publishing, 2022), https://www.ncbi.nlm.nih.gov/books/NBK430882/.

6. Laura E. Britton et al., "CE: An Evidence-Based Update on Contraception," *AJN, American Journal of Nursing* 120, no. 2 (February 2020): 22–33, https://doi.org/10.1097/01.naj.0000654304.29632.a7.

7. Danielle B. Cooper, Preeti Patel, and Heba Mahdy, "Oral Contraceptive Pills," essay, in *StatPearls [Internet]* (Treasure Island, FL: StatPearls Publishing, 2022), https://www.ncbi.nlm.nih.gov/books/NBK430882/.

8. Danielle B. Cooper, Preeti Patel, and Heba Mahdy, "Oral Contraceptive Pills," essay, in *StatPearls [Internet]* (Treasure Island, FL: StatPearls Publishing, 2022), https://www.ncbi.nlm.nih.gov/books/NBK430882/.

9. Laura E. Britton et al., "CE: An Evidence-Based Update on Contraception," *AJN, American Journal of Nursing* 120, no. 2 (February 2020): 22–33, https://doi.org/10.1097/01.naj.0000654304.29632.a7. Danielle B. Cooper, Preeti Patel, and Heba Mahdy, "Oral Contraceptive Pills," essay, in *StatPearls [Internet]* (Treasure Island, FL: StatPearls Publishing, 2022), https://www.ncbi.nlm.nih.gov/books/NBK430882/.

10. Danielle B. Cooper, Preeti Patel, and Heba Mahdy, "Oral Contraceptive Pills," essay, in *StatPearls [Internet]* (Treasure Island, FL: StatPearls Publishing, 2022), https://www.ncbi.nlm.nih.gov/books/NBK430882/.

11. Carlo Bastianelli et al., "Effects of Progestin-Only Contraceptives on the Endometrium," *Expert Review of Clinical Pharmacology* 13, no. 10 (September 21, 2020): 1103–23, https://doi.org/10.1080/17512433.2020.1821649.

12. Maura Palmery et al., "Oral Contraceptives and Changes in Nutritional Requirements," *European Review for Medical and Pharmacological*

Sciences 17, no. 13 (July 2013): 1804–13, https://pubmed.ncbi.nlm.nih.gov/23852908/.

13. Michael Edwards and Ahmet S. Can, "Progestin," essay, in *StatPearls [Internet]* (Treasure Island, FL: StatPearls Publishing, 2023), https://www.ncbi.nlm.nih.gov/books/NBK563211/.

14. Christina Vrettakos and Tushar Bajaj, "Levonorgestrel," essay, in *StatPearls [Internet]* (Treasure Island, FL: StatPearls Publishing, 2022), https://www.ncbi.nlm.nih.gov/books/NBK539737/.

15. Daniel Martin et al., "Period Prevalence and Perceived Side Effects of Hormonal Contraceptive Use and the Menstrual Cycle in Elite Athletes," *International Journal of Sports Physiology and Performance* 13, no. 7 (August 1, 2018): 926–32, https://doi.org/10.1123/ijspp.2017-0330.

16. Kimberly Daniels and Joyce C. Abma, "Current Contraceptive Status Among Women Aged 15–49: United States, 2015–2017," Centers for Disease Control and Prevention, February 14, 2019, https://www.cdc.gov/nchs/products/databriefs/db327.htm.

17. Emily L. Lanzola and Kari Ketvertis, "Intrauterine Device," essay, in *StatPearls [Internet]* (Treasure Island, FL : StatPearls Publishing, 2022), https://www.ncbi.nlm.nih.gov/books/NBK557403/.

18. Emily L. Lanzola and Kari Ketvertis, "Intrauterine Device," essay, in *StatPearls [Internet]* (Treasure Island, FL : StatPearls Publishing, 2022), https://www.ncbi.nlm.nih.gov/books/NBK557403/.

19. Jim Slattery et al., "Cohort Study of Psychiatric Adverse Events Following Exposure to Levonorgestrel-Containing Intrauterine Devices in UK General Practice," *Drug Safety* 41, no. 10 (May 21, 2018): 951–58, https://doi.org/10.1007/s40264-018-0683-x.

20. Christina Vrettakos and Tushar Bajaj, "Levonorgestrel," essay, in *StatPearls [Internet]* (Treasure Island, FL: StatPearls Publishing, 2022), https://www.ncbi.nlm.nih.gov/books/NBK539737/.

21. Kathleen Ridgeway et al., "Vaginal Ring Acceptability: A Systematic Review and Meta-Analysis of Vaginal Ring Experiences from around the World," *Contraception* 106 (February 2022): 16–33, https://doi.org/10.1016/j.contraception.2021.10.001.

22. Bernadatte G. Gilbert, "Contraceptive Implant Insertion and Removal," *Primary Care: Clinics in Office Practice* 48, no. 4 (December 2021): 545–54, https://doi.org/10.1016/j.pop.2021.07.002.

23. Maurizio Guida et al., "NEXPLANON Subdermal Implant: Assessment of Sexual Profile, Metabolism, and Bleeding in a Cohort of Italian Women," *BioMed Research International* 2019 (January 31, 2019): 1–6, https://doi.org/10.1155/2019/3726957.

24. Rebecca C Ramdhan et al., "Complications of Subcutaneous Contraception: A Review," *Cureus* 10, no. 1 (January 31, 2018), https://doi.org/10.7759/cureus.2132.

25. Mary Stewart and Deborah Bateson, "Choosing Non-Oral, Long-Acting Reversible Contraception," *Australian Prescriber* 39, no. 5 (October 1,

2016): 153–58, https://doi.org/10.18773/austprescr.2016.057.

26. "Depression among Women," Centers for Disease Control and Prevention, May 22, 2023, https://www.cdc.gov/reproductivehealth/depression/index.htm.

27. Christine Anderl, Gu Li, and Frances S. Chen, "Oral Contraceptive Use in Adolescence Predicts Lasting Vulnerability to Depression in Adulthood," *Journal of Child Psychology and Psychiatry* 61, no. 2 (August 28, 2019): 148–56, https://doi.org/10.1111/jcpp.13115.

28. Christine Anderl, Gu Li, and Frances S. Chen, "Oral Contraceptive Use in Adolescence Predicts Lasting Vulnerability to Depression in Adulthood," *Journal of Child Psychology and Psychiatry* 61, no. 2 (August 28, 2019): 148–56, https://doi.org/10.1111/jcpp.13115.

29. Charlotte Wessel Skovlund et al., "Association of Hormonal Contraception with Depression," *JAMA Psychiatry* 73, no. 11 (November 1, 2016): 1154–62, https://doi.org/10.1001/jamapsychiatry.2016.2387.

30. Charlotte Wessel Skovlund et al., "Association of Hormonal Contraception with Depression," *JAMA Psychiatry* 73, no. 11 (November 1, 2016): 1154–62, https://doi.org/10.1001/jamapsychiatry.2016.2387. Lloyd D Hughes and Olwkayode Majekodunmi, "Hormonal Contraception and Suicide: A New Dimension of Risk," *British Journal of General Practice* 68, no. 676 (October 25, 2018): 512–13, https://doi.org/10.3399/bjgp18x699473.

31. Nancy Grossman Barr, "Managing Adverse Effects of Hormonal Contraceptives," *American Family Physician* 82, no. 12 (December 15, 2010): 1499–1506, https://pubmed.ncbi.nlm.nih.gov/21166370/. Barbara L. Parry and A.John Rush, "Oral Contraceptives and Depressive Symptomatology: Biologic Mechanisms," *Comprehensive Psychiatry* 20, no. 4 (July 1979): 347–58, https://doi.org/10.1016/0010-440x(79)90006-3.

32. Barbara L. Parry and A.John Rush, "Oral Contraceptives and Depressive Symptomatology: Biologic Mechanisms," *Comprehensive Psychiatry* 20, no. 4 (July 1979): 347–58, https://doi.org/10.1016/0010-440x(79)90006-3. J. L. Webb, "Nutritional Effects of Oral Contraceptive Use: A Review," *The Journal of Reproductive Medicine* 25, no. 4 (October 1980): 150–56, https://pubmed.ncbi.nlm.nih.gov/7001015/.

33. Barbara L. Parry and A.John Rush, "Oral Contraceptives and Depressive Symptomatology: Biologic Mechanisms," *Comprehensive Psychiatry* 20, no. 4 (July 1979): 347–58, https://doi.org/10.1016/0010-440x(79)90006-3.

34. Elizabeth Hampson, "Oral Contraceptives in the Central Nervous System: Basic Pharmacology, Methodological Considerations, and Current State of the Field," *Frontiers in Neuroendocrinology* 68 (January 2023): 101040, https://doi.org/10.1016/j.yfrne.2022.101040.

35. Anne Almey, Teresa A. Milner, and Wayne G. Brake, "Estrogen

Receptors in the Central Nervous System and Their Implication for Dopamine-Dependent Cognition in Females," *Hormones and Behavior* 74 (August 2015): 125–38, https://doi.org/10.1016/j.yhbeh.2015.06.010.

36. Nicole Petersen et al., "Oral Contraceptive Pill Use Is Associated with Localized Decreases in Cortical Thickness," *Human Brain Mapping* 36, no. 7 (April 2, 2015): 2644–54, https://doi.org/10.1002/hbm.22797. Edmund T. Rolls, "The Cingulate Cortex and Limbic Systems for Emotion, Action, and Memory," *Brain Structure and Function* 224, no. 9 (August 26, 2019): 3001–18, https://doi.org/10.1007/s00429-019-01945-2.

37. Elizabeth Hampson, "Oral Contraceptives in the Central Nervous System: Basic Pharmacology, Methodological Considerations, and Current State of the Field," *Frontiers in Neuroendocrinology* 68 (January 2023): 101040, https://doi.org/10.1016/j.yfrne.2022.101040.

38. Elizabeth Hampson, "Oral Contraceptives in the Central Nervous System: Basic Pharmacology, Methodological Considerations, and Current State of the Field," *Frontiers in Neuroendocrinology* 68 (January 2023): 101040, https://doi.org/10.1016/j.yfrne.2022.101040.

39. Ann E. Caldwell et al., "Impact of Combined Hormonal Contraceptive Use on Weight Loss: A Secondary Analysis of a Behavioral Weight loss Trial," *Obesity* 28, no. 6 (May 22, 2020): 1040–49, https://doi.org/10.1002/oby.22787.

40. Boyoung Park and Jeongseon Kim, "Oral Contraceptive Use, Micronutrient Deficiency, and Obesity among Premenopausal Females in Korea: The Necessity of Dietary Supplements and Food Intake Improvement," *PLOS ONE* 11, no. 6 (June 27, 2016), https://doi.org/10.1371/journal.pone.0158177.

41. Maura Palmery et al., "Oral Contraceptives and Changes in Nutritional Requirements," *European Review for Medical and Pharmacological Sciences* 17, no. 13 (July 2013): 1804–13, https://pubmed.ncbi.nlm.nih.gov/23852908/.

42. Jovana Mihajlovic et al., "Combined Hormonal Contraceptives Are Associated with Minor Changes in Composition and Diversity in Gut Microbiota of Healthy Women," *Environmental Microbiology* 23, no. 6 (May 6, 2021): 3037–47, https://doi.org/10.1111/1462-2920.15517.

43. Xinwei Hua et al., "Longitudinal Analysis of the Impact of Oral Contraceptive Use on the Gut Microbiome," *Journal of Medical Microbiology* 71, no. 4 (April 22, 2022), https://doi.org/10.1099/jmm.0.001512.

44. Maura Palmery et al., "Oral Contraceptives and Changes in Nutritional Requirements," *European Review for Medical and Pharmacological Sciences* 17, no. 13 (July 2013): 1804–13, https://pubmed.ncbi.nlm.nih.gov/23852908/.

45. Fariha Angum et al., "The Prevalence of Autoimmune Disorders in Women: A Narrative Review," *Cureus* 12, no. 5 (May 13, 2020), https://

doi.org/10.7759/cureus.8094.

46.   Fariha Angum et al., "The Prevalence of Autoimmune Disorders in Women: A Narrative Review," *Cureus* 12, no. 5 (May 13, 2020), https://doi.org/10.7759/cureus.8094.

47.   William V. Williams, "Hormonal Contraception and the Development of Autoimmunity: A Review of the Literature," *The Linacre Quarterly* 84, no. 3 (August 2017): 275–95, https://doi.org/10.1080/00243639.2017.1360065.

NON-HORMONAL BIRTH CONTROL

1.   Emily L. Lanzola and Kari Ketvertis, "Intrauterine Device," essay, in *StatPearls [Internet]* (Treasure Island, FL: StatPearls Publishing, 2022), https://www.ncbi.nlm.nih.gov/books/NBK557403/.

2.   Kaitlyn Steward, "Physiology, Ovulation And Basal Body Temperature," essay, in *StatPearls [Internet]*, ed. Avais Raja (Treasure Island, FL: StatPearls Publishing, 2022), https://www.ncbi.nlm.nih.gov/books/NBK546686/.

3.   Toni Weschler, *Taking Charge of Your Fertility: The Definitive Guide to Natural Birth Control and Pregnancy Achievement* (New York, NY: Quill, 2002).

4.   Toni Weschler, *Taking Charge of Your Fertility: The Definitive Guide to Natural Birth Control and Pregnancy Achievement* (New York, NY: Quill, 2002).

5.   Kaitlyn Steward, "Physiology, Ovulation And Basal Body Temperature," essay, in *StatPearls [Internet],* ed. Avais Raja (Treasure Island, FL: StatPearls Publishing, 2022), https://www.ncbi.nlm.nih.gov/books/NBK546686/.

6.   W. Eggert-Kruse et al., "The pH as an Important Determinant of Sperm-Mucus Interaction," *Fertility and Sterility* 59, no. 3 (March 1993): 617–28, https://pubmed.ncbi.nlm.nih.gov/8458467/.
      Jieying Xu et al., "Fertility Factors Affect the Vaginal Microbiome in Women of Reproductive Age," *American Journal of Reproductive Immunology* 83, no. 4 (January 21, 2020), https://doi.org/10.1111/aji.13220.

7.   Emily L. Lanzola and Kari Ketvertis, "Intrauterine Device," essay, in *StatPearls [Internet]* (Treasure Island, FL: StatPearls Publishing, 2022), https://www.ncbi.nlm.nih.gov/books/NBK557403/.

8.   Emily L. Lanzola and Kari Ketvertis, "Intrauterine Device," essay, in *StatPearls [Internet]* (Treasure Island, FL: StatPearls Publishing, 2022), https://www.ncbi.nlm.nih.gov/books/NBK557403/.

9.   Sharon L. Achilles et al., "Impact of Contraceptive Initiation on Vaginal Microbiota," *American Journal of Obstetrics and Gynecology* 218, no. 6 (June 2018), https://doi.org/10.1016/j.ajog.2018.02.017.

10. Daniel Romero Herrero and Antonia Andreu Domingo, "Vaginosis Bacteriana," *Enfermedades Infecciosas y Microbiología Clínica* 34 (July 2016): 14–18, https://doi.org/10.1016/s0213-005x(16)30214-2.

11. Paulette Bagnall and Denise Rizzolo, "Bacterial Vaginosis," *Journal of the American Academy of Physician Assistants* 30, no. 12 (December 2017): 15–21, https://doi.org/10.1097/01.jaa.0000526770.60197.fa.

12. Emily L. Lanzola and Kari Ketvertis, "Intrauterine Device," essay, in *StatPearls [Internet]* (Treasure Island, FL: StatPearls Publishing, 2022), https://www.ncbi.nlm.nih.gov/books/NBK557403/.

13. M. Steiner et al., "The Impact of Lubricants on Latex Condoms during Vaginal Intercourse," *International Journal of STD & AIDS* 5, no. 1 (January 1994): 29–36, https://doi.org/10.1177/095646249400500108.

14. Courtney A. Schreiber et al., "Effects of Long-Term Use of Nonoxynol-9 on Vaginalflora," *Obstetrics & Gynecology* 107, no. 1 (January 2006): 136–43, https://doi.org/10.1097/01.aog.0000189094.21099.4a.

15. Christine K. Mauck et al., "A Phase I Randomized Postcoital Testing and Safety Study of the Caya Diaphragm Used with 3% Nonoxynol-9 Gel, ContraGel or No Gel," *Contraception* 96, no. 2 (August 2017): 124–30, https://doi.org/10.1016/j.contraception.2017.05.016.

16. Nancy King Reame, "Toxic Shock Syndrome and Tampons: The Birth of a Movement and a Research 'Vagenda,'" *The Palgrave Handbook of Critical Menstruation Studies*, 2020, 687–703, https://doi.org/10.1007/978-981-15-0614-7_51.

17. Inês Paciência et al., "A Systematic Review of Evidence and Implications of Spatial and Seasonal Variations of Volatile Organic Compounds (VOC) in Indoor Human Environments," *Journal of Toxicology and Environmental Health, Part B* 19, no. 2 (February 17, 2016): 47–64, https://doi.org/10.1080/10937404.2015.1134371.

18. Nan Lin et al., "Volatile Organic Compounds in Feminine Hygiene Products Sold in the US Market: A Survey of Products and Health Risks," *Environment International* 144 (November 2020): 105740, https://doi.org/10.1016/j.envint.2020.105740.

19. Jessica Singh et al., "Tampon Use, Environmental Chemicals and Oxidative Stress in the Biocycle Study," *Environmental Health* 18, no. 1 (February 11, 2019), https://doi.org/10.1186/s12940-019-0452-z.

20. Jessica Singh et al., "Tampon Use, Environmental Chemicals and Oxidative Stress in the Biocycle Study," *Environmental Health* 18, no. 1 (February 11, 2019), https://doi.org/10.1186/s12940-019-0452-z.

21. Emiliano Panieri et al., "Pfas Molecules: A Major Concern for the Human Health and the Environment," *Toxics* 10, no. 2 (January 18, 2022): 44, https://doi.org/10.3390/toxics10020044.

22. Ketura Persellin, "New Lawsuit Contends Period Products Contain 'Forever Chemicals,'" *EWG News & Insights* 2022, no. 4 (April 26, 2022), https://www.ewg.org/news-insights/news/2022/04/new-lawsuit-contends-period-products-contain-forever-chemicals.

23. Julie Steinberg, "Knix Wear Sued over Pfas Chemicals in Menstrual Underwear," Bloomberg Law, April 5, 2022, https://news.bloomberglaw.com/litigation/knix-wear-sued-over-pfas-chemicals-in-menstrual-underwear.

24. Ketura Persellin, "New Lawsuit Contends Period Products Contain 'Forever Chemicals,'" *EWG News & Insights* 2022, no. 4 (April 26, 2022), https://www.ewg.org/news-insights/news/2022/04/new-lawsuit-contends-period-products-contain-forever-chemicals.

RESTORING YOUR CYCLE

1. J E Chavarro et al., "A Prospective Study of Dietary Carbohydrate Quantity and Quality in Relation to Risk of Ovulatory Infertility," *European Journal of Clinical Nutrition* 63, no. 1 (September 19, 2007): 78–86, https://doi.org/10.1038/sj.ejcn.1602904.

2. Mahsa Shahrokhi and Shivaraj Nagalli, "Probiotics," essay, in *StatPearls [Internet]* (Treasure Island, FL: StatPearls Publishing, 2022), https://www.ncbi.nlm.nih.gov/books/NBK553134/.

3. Dorna Davani-Davari et al., "Prebiotics: Definition, Types, Sources, Mechanisms, and Clinical Applications," *Foods* 8, no. 3 (March 9, 2019): 92, https://doi.org/10.3390/foods8030092.

4. Nathan Donley, "The USA Lags behind Other Agricultural Nations in Banning Harmful Pesticides," *Environmental Health* 18, no. 1 (June 7, 2019), https://doi.org/10.1186/s12940-019-0488-0.

5. Lynn Cialdella-Kam et al., "Dietary Intervention Restored Menses in Female Athletes with Exercise-Associated Menstrual Dysfunction with Limited Impact on Bone and Muscle Health," *Nutrients* 6, no. 8 (July 31, 2014): 3018–39, https://doi.org/10.3390/nu6083018.

6. Yuki Tada et al., "Higher Energy Intake at Dinner Decreases Parasympathetic Activity during Nighttime Sleep in Menstruating Women: A Randomized Controlled Trial," *Physiology & Behavior* 194 (October 2018): 252–59, https://doi.org/10.1016/j.physbeh.2018.06.010. Kimberly A. Bell et al., "Nocturnal Autonomic Nervous System Activity and Morning Proinflammatory Cytokines in Young Adult African Americans," *Journal of Sleep Research* 26, no. 4 (February 17, 2017): 510–15, https://doi.org/10.1111/jsr.12480.

7. Nadia Rachdaoui and Dipak K. Sarkar, "Pathophysiology of the Effects of Alcohol Abuse on the Endocrine System," *Alcohol Research : Current Reviews* 38, no. 2 (2017): 255–76, https://pubmed.ncbi.nlm.nih.gov/28988577/.

8. Szu-Yi Liu, I-Ting Tsai, and Yin-Chou Hsu, "Alcohol-Related Liver Disease: Basic Mechanisms and Clinical Perspectives," *International Journal of Molecular Sciences* 22, no. 10 (May 13, 2021): 5170, https://doi.org/10.3390/ijms22105170.

9. Phillip A. Engen et al., "The Gastrointestinal Microbiome: Alcohol Effects on the Composition of Intestinal Microbiota," *Alcohol Research : Current Reviews* 37, no. 2 (2015): 223–36, https://pubmed.ncbi.nlm.nih.gov/26695747/.

10. Barry M Popkin, Kristen E D'Anci, and Irwin H Rosenberg, "Water, Hydration, and Health," *Nutrition Reviews* 68, no. 8 (July 20, 2010): 439–58, https://doi.org/10.1111/j.1753-4887.2010.00304.x.

11. Barry M Popkin, Kristen E D'Anci, and Irwin H Rosenberg, "Water, Hydration, and Health," *Nutrition Reviews* 68, no. 8 (July 20, 2010): 439–58, https://doi.org/10.1111/j.1753-4887.2010.00304.x.

12. "Phytoestrogens," *Meyler's Side Effects of Drugs,* 2016, 755–57, https://doi.org/10.1016/b978-0-444-53717-1.00151-7.

13. Johanna W. Lampe, "Isoflavonoid and Lignan Phytoestrogens as Dietary Biomarkers," *The Journal of Nutrition* 133, no. 3 (March 2003): 956S-964S, https://doi.org/10.1093/jn/133.3.956s.

14. Johanna W. Lampe, "Isoflavonoid and Lignan Phytoestrogens as Dietary Biomarkers," *The Journal of Nutrition* 133, no. 3 (March 2003): 956S-964S, https://doi.org/10.1093/jn/133.3.956s.

15. William F. Clark et al., "Flaxseed: A Potential Treatment for Lupus Nephritis," *Kidney International* 48, no. 2 (August 1995): 475–80, https://doi.org/10.1038/ki.1995.316.
    Priyanka Kajla, Alka Sharma, and Dev Raj Sood, "Flaxseed—a Potential Functional Food Source," *Journal of Food Science and Technology* 52, no. 4 (February 28, 2014): 1857–71, https://doi.org/10.1007/s13197-014-1293-y.

16. Kailash Prasad, "Hydroxyl Radical-Scavenging Property of Secoisolariciresinol Diglucoside (SDG) Isolated from Flax-Seed," *Molecular and Cellular Biochemistry* 168, no. 1–2 (March 1997): 117–23, https://doi.org/10.1023/a:1006847310741.
    Jasdeep Kaur Saggar et al., "The Effect of Secoisolariciresinol Diglucoside and Flaxseed Oil, Alone and in Combination, on MCF-7 Tumor Growth and Signaling Pathways," *Nutrition and Cancer* 62, no. 4 (2010): 533–42, https://doi.org/10.1080/01635580903532440.
    "Phytoestrogens," *Meyler's Side Effects of Drugs,* 2016, 755–57, https://doi.org/10.1016/b978-0-444-53717-1.00151-7.

17. C. J. Haggans et al., "The Effect of Flaxseed and Wheat Bran Consumption on Urinary Estrogen Metabolites in Premenopausal Women," *Cancer Epidemiology, Biomarkers & Prevention : A Publication of the American Association for Cancer Research, Cosponsored by the American Society of Preventive* 9, no. 7 (July 2000): 719–25, https://pubmed.ncbi.nlm.nih.gov/10919743/.

18. Tina Sicilia et al., "Identification and Stereochemical Characterization of Lignans in Flaxseed and Pumpkin Seeds," *Journal of Agricultural and Food Chemistry* 51, no. 5 (January 28, 2003): 1181–88, https://doi.org/10.1021/jf0207979.

19. Maria Gammone et al., "Omega-3 Polyunsaturated Fatty Acids: Benefits and Endpoints in Sport," *Nutrients* 11, no. 1 (December 27, 2018): 46, https://doi.org/10.3390/nu11010046.

20. R.H. Glew et al., "Amino Acid, Mineral and Fatty Acid Content of Pumpkin Seeds (Cucurbita Spp) and Cyperus Esculentus Nuts in the Republic of Niger," *Plant Foods for Human Nutrition* 61, no. 2 (June 13, 2006): 49–54, https://doi.org/10.1007/s11130-006-0010-z.

21. Silvia Ghisoni et al., "UHPLC-ESI-QTOF-MS Screening of Lignans and Other Phenolics in Dry Seeds for Human Consumption," *Journal of Functional Foods* 34 (July 2017): 229–36, https://doi.org/10.1016/j.jff.2017.04.037.

22. José L. Peñalvo et al., "Dietary Sesamin Is Converted to Enterolactone in Humans," *The Journal of Nutrition* 135, no. 5 (May 2005): 1056–62, https://doi.org/10.1093/jn/135.5.1056.

23. Shuangshuang Guo, Yan Ge, and Kriskamol Na Jom, "A Review of Phytochemistry, Metabolite Changes, and Medicinal Uses of the Common Sunflower Seed and Sprouts (Helianthus Annuus L.)," *Chemistry Central Journal* 11, no. 1 (September 29, 2017), https://doi.org/10.1186/s13065-017-0328-7.

24. Ali Esmail Al-Snafi, "The Pharmacological Effects of Helianthus Annuus-A Review," *INDO AMERICAN JOURNAL OF PHARMACEUTICAL SCIENCES* 5 (March 31, 2018): 1745–56, https://doi.org/https://doi.org/10.5281/zenodo.1210520.

25. Shuangshuang Guo, Yan Ge, and Kriskamol Na Jom, "A Review of Phytochemistry, Metabolite Changes, and Medicinal Uses of the Common Sunflower Seed and Sprouts (Helianthus Annuus L.)," *Chemistry Central Journal* 11, no. 1 (September 29, 2017), https://doi.org/10.1186/s13065-017-0328-7.

26. Maša Knez Hrnčič et al., "Chia Seeds (Salvia Hispanica L.): An Overview—Phytochemical Profile, Isolation Methods, and Application," *Molecules* 25, no. 1 (December 18, 2019): 11, https://doi.org/10.3390/molecules25010011.

27. Priyanka Kajla, Alka Sharma, and Dev Raj Sood, "Flaxseed—a Potential Functional Food Source," *Journal of Food Science and Technology* 52, no. 4 (February 28, 2014): 1857–71, https://doi.org/10.1007/s13197-014-1293-y.

28. "Calcium-D-Glucarate," *Alternative Medicine Review : A Journal of Clinical Therapeutic* 7, no. 4 (August 2002): 336–39, https://pubmed.ncbi.nlm.nih.gov/12197785/.

29. Sahdeo Prasad, Amit K. Tyagi, and Bharat B. Aggarwal, "Recent Developments in Delivery, Bioavailability, Absorption and Metabolism of Curcumin: The Golden Pigment from Golden Spice," *Cancer Research and Treatment* 46, no. 1 (January 15, 2014): 2–18, https://doi.org/10.4143/crt.2014.46.1.2.

30. Kealey J. Wohlgemuth et al., "Sex Differences and Considerations for Female Specific Nutritional Strategies: A Narrative Review," *Journal of the International Society of Sports Nutrition* 18, no. 1 (January 2, 2021), https://doi.org/10.1186/s12970-021-00422-8.

31. F. Parazzini, "Selected Food Intake and Risk of Endometriosis," *Human Reproduction* 19, no. 8 (June 3, 2004): 1755–59, https://doi.org/10.1093/humrep/deh395.
    H R Harris et al., "Fruit and Vegetable Consumption and Risk of Endometriosis," *Human Reproduction* 33, no. 4 (February 1, 2018): 715–27, https://doi.org/10.1093/humrep/dey014.
    Britton Trabert et al., "Diet and Risk of Endometriosis in a Population-Based Case–Control Study," *British Journal of Nutrition* 105, no. 3 (September 28, 2010): 459–67, https://doi.org/10.1017/s0007114510003661.

32. S. A. Missmer et al., "A Prospective Study of Dietary Fat Consumption and Endometriosis Risk," *Human Reproduction* 25, no. 6 (March 23, 2010): 1528–35, https://doi.org/10.1093/humrep/deq044.

33. F. Parazzini, "Selected Food Intake and Risk of Endometriosis," *Human Reproduction* 19, no. 8 (June 3, 2004): 1755–59, https://doi.org/10.1093/humrep/deh395.

34. Ana Luiza Savaris and Vivian F. do Amaral, "Nutrient Intake, Anthropometric Data and Correlations with the Systemic Antioxidant Capacity of Women with Pelvic Endometriosis," *European Journal of Obstetrics & Gynecology and Reproductive Biology* 158, no. 2 (October 2011): 314–18, https://doi.org/10.1016/j.ejogrb.2011.05.014.

35. Joanna Jurkiewicz-Przondziono et al., "Influence of Diet on the Risk of Developing Endometriosis," *Ginekologia Polska* 88, no. 2 (February 28, 2017): 96–102, https://doi.org/10.5603/gp.a2017.0017.
    Fabio Parazzini et al., "A Metaanalysis on Alcohol Consumption and Risk of Endometriosis," *American Journal of Obstetrics and Gynecology* 209, no. 2 (August 1, 2013): e1–10, https://doi.org/10.1016/j.ajog.2013.05.039.

36. "Thiaman - Fact Sheet for Health Professionals," NIH Office of Dietary Supplements, March 26, 2021, https://ods.od.nih.gov/factsheets/Thiamin-HealthProfessional/#:~:text=Sources%20of%20Thiamin-,Food,cereals%20and%20bread%20%5B8%5D.

37. Margreet C.M. Vissers et al., "The Bioavailability of Vitamin C from Kiwifruit," *Nutritional Benefits of Kiwifruit* 68 (2013): 125–47, https://doi.org/10.1016/b978-0-12-394294-4.00007-9.
    Nidhi Mishra, Vijay Lakshmi Ta, and Rekha Gupta, "Immunomodulation by Hibiscus Rosa-Sinensis: Effect on the Humoral and Cellular Immune Response of Mus Musculus," *Pakistan Journal of Biological Sciences* 15, no. 6 (March 1, 2012): 277–83, https://doi.org/10.3923/pjbs.2012.277.283.
    Shailja Chambial et al., "Vitamin C in Disease Prevention and Cure: An Overview," *Indian Journal of Clinical Biochemistry* 28, no. 4 (September

1, 2013): 314–28, https://doi.org/10.1007/s12291-013-0375-3.

38. Maria Laura Colombo, "An Update on Vitamin E, Tocopherol and Tocotrienol—Perspectives," *Molecules* 15, no. 4 (March 24, 2010): 2103–13, https://doi.org/10.3390/molecules15042103.

39. Kristen N. Owen, "Vitamin E Toxicity," essay, in *StatPearls [Internet]*, ed. Olga Dewald (Treasure Island, FL: StatPearls Publishing, 2022), https://www.ncbi.nlm.nih.gov/books/NBK564373/.

40. Parvin Mirmiran et al., "The Association of Dietary L-Arginine Intake and Serum Nitric Oxide Metabolites in Adults: A Population-Based Study," *Nutrients* 8, no. 5 (May 20, 2016): 311, https://doi.org/10.3390/nu8050311.

41. Farzaneh Kashefi et al., "Effect of Ginger *(Zingiber Officinale)* on Heavy Menstrual Bleeding: A Placebo-Controlled, Randomized Clinical Trial," *Phytotherapy Research* 29, no. 1 (October 8, 2014): 114–19, https://doi.org/10.1002/ptr.5235.

42. Maria Laura Colombo, "An Update on Vitamin E, Tocopherol and Tocotrienol—Perspectives," *Molecules* 15, no. 4 (March 24, 2010): 2103–13, https://doi.org/10.3390/molecules15042103.

43. Kristen N. Owen, "Vitamin E Toxicity," essay, in *StatPearls [Internet]*, ed. Olga Dewald (Treasure Island, FL: StatPearls Publishing, 2022), https://www.ncbi.nlm.nih.gov/books/NBK564373/.

44. Lynn Cialdella-Kam et al., "Dietary Intervention Restored Menses in Female Athletes with Exercise-Associated Menstrual Dysfunction with Limited Impact on Bone and Muscle Health," *Nutrients* 6, no. 8 (July 31, 2014): 3018–39, https://doi.org/10.3390/nu6083018.
   Mary Jane De Souza et al., "Randomised Controlled Trial of the Effects of Increased Energy Intake on Menstrual Recovery in Exercising Women with Menstrual Disturbances: The 'Refuel' Study," *Human Reproduction* 36, no. 8 (June 24, 2021): 2285–97, https://doi.org/10.1093/humrep/deab149.

45. Elisabeth Perreau-Linck et al., "In Vivo Measurements of Brain Trapping of C-Labelled Alpha-Methyl-L-Tryptophan during Acute Changes in Mood States," *Journal of Psychiatry & Neuroscience : JPN* 32, no. 6 (November 2007), https://pubmed.ncbi.nlm.nih.gov/18043767/.

46. Marianne O. Klein et al., "Dopamine: Functions, Signaling, and Association with Neurological Diseases," *Cellular and Molecular Neurobiology* 39, no. 1 (November 16, 2018): 31–59, https://doi.org/10.1007/s10571-018-0632-3.

47. Shwetha Nair et al., "Do Slumped and Upright Postures Affect Stress Responses? A Randomized Trial.," *Health Psychology* 34, no. 6 (2015): 632–41, https://doi.org/10.1037/hea0000146.

48. Carissa Wilkes et al., "Upright Posture Improves Affect and Fatigue in People with Depressive Symptoms," *Journal of Behavior Therapy and Experimental Psychiatry* 54 (March 2017): 143–49, https://doi.org/10.1016/j.jbtep.2016.07.015.

49. Miriam Rennung, Johannes Blum, and Anja S. Göritz, "To Strike a Pose: No Stereotype Backlash for Power Posing Women," *Frontiers in Psychology* 7 (September 27, 2016), https://doi.org/10.3389/fpsyg.2016.01463.

50. Joseph P. Simmons and Uri Simonsohn, "Power Posing: *P*-Curving the Evidence," *Psychological Science* 28, no. 5 (May 20, 2017): 687–93, https://doi.org/10.1177/0956797616658563.
Amy J. Cuddy, S. Jack Schultz, and Nathan E. Fosse, "*P*-Curving a More Comprehensive Body of Research on Postural Feedback Reveals Clear Evidential Value for Power-Posing Effects: Reply to Simmons and Simonsohn (2017)," *Psychological Science* 29, no. 4 (March 2, 2018): 656–66, https://doi.org/10.1177/0956797617746749.

51. Hankyu Park and Dongwook Han, "The Effect of the Correlation between the Contraction of the Pelvic Floor Muscles and Diaphragmatic Motion during Breathing," *Journal of Physical Therapy Science* 27, no. 7 (2015): 2113–15, https://doi.org/10.1589/jpts.27.2113.

52. Björn Rasch and Jan Born, "About Sleep's Role in Memory," *Physiological Reviews* 93, no. 2 (April 1, 2013): 681–766, https://doi.org/10.1152/physrev.00032.2012.
Cecilia Castro-Diehl et al., "Sleep Duration and Quality in Relation to Autonomic Nervous System Measures: The Multi-Ethnic Study of Atherosclerosis (MESA)," *Sleep* 39, no. 11 (November 1, 2016): 1927–40, https://doi.org/10.5665/sleep.6218.
Hui-Leng Tan, Leila Kheirandish-Gozal, and David Gozal, "Sleep, Sleep Disorders, and Immune Function," *Allergy and Sleep,* June 2019, 3–15, https://doi.org/10.1007/978-3-030-14738-9_1.
Min Young Chun et al., "Association between Sleep Duration and Musculoskeletal Pain," *Medicine* 97, no. 50 (December 2018), https://doi.org/10.1097/md.0000000000013656.

53. Susan L. Worley, "The Extraordinary Importance of Sleep: The Detrimental Effects of Inadequate Sleep on Health and Public Safety Drive an Explosion of Sleep Research," *P & T : A Peer-Reviewed Journal for Formulary Management* 43, no. 12 (December 2018): 758–63, https://pubmed.ncbi.nlm.nih.gov/30559589/.

54. Ga Eun Nam, Kyungdo Han, and Gyungjoo Lee, "Association between Sleep Duration and Menstrual Cycle Irregularity in Korean Female Adolescents," *Sleep Medicine* 35 (July 2017): 62–66, https://doi.org/10.1016/j.sleep.2017.04.009.

55. Taeryoon Kim et al., "Associations of Mental Health and Sleep Duration with Menstrual Cycle Irregularity: A Population-Based Study," *Archives of Women's Mental Health* 21, no. 6 (June 16, 2018): 619–26, https://doi.org/10.1007/s00737-018-0872-8.

56. Kenneth P. Wright et al., "Influence of Sleep Deprivation and Circadian Misalignment on Cortisol, Inflammatory Markers, and Cytokine Balance," *Brain, Behavior, and Immunity* 47 (July 2015): 24–34, https://

doi.org/10.1016/j.bbi.2015.01.004.

57. Maria Emilia Solano and Petra Clara Arck, "Steroids, Pregnancy and Fetal Development," *Frontiers in Immunology* 10 (2020), https://doi.org/10.3389/fimmu.2019.03017.

58. Wei Yin et al., "Melatonin for Premenstrual Syndrome: A Potential Remedy but Not Ready," *Frontiers in Endocrinology* 13 (January 9, 2023), https://doi.org/10.3389/fendo.2022.1084249.

59. A. Green et al., "Evening Light Exposure to Computer Screens Disrupts Human Sleep, Biological Rhythms, and Attention Abilities," *Chronobiology International* 34, no. 7 (May 26, 2017): 855–65, https://doi.org/10.1080/07420528.2017.1324878.

60. Yvan Touitou, David Touitou, and Alain Reinberg, "Disruption of Adolescents' Circadian Clock: The Vicious Circle of Media Use, Exposure to Light at Night, Sleep Loss and Risk Behaviors," *Journal of Physiology-Paris* 110, no. 4 (November 2016): 467–79, https://doi.org/10.1016/j.jphysparis.2017.05.001.

61. Zizhen Xie et al., "A Review of Sleep Disorders and Melatonin," *Neurological Research* 39, no. 6 (May 1, 2017): 559–65, https://doi.org/10.1080/01616412.2017.1315864.
F. Donath et al., "Critical Evaluation of the Effect of Valerian Extract on Sleep Structure and Sleep Quality," *Pharmacopsychiatry* 33, no. 2 (March 2000): 47–53, https://doi.org/10.1055/s-2000-7972.

62. Yuki Tada et al., "Higher Energy Intake at Dinner Decreases Parasympathetic Activity during Nighttime Sleep in Menstruating Women: A Randomized Controlled Trial," *Physiology & Behavior* 194 (October 2018): 252–59, https://doi.org/10.1016/j.physbeh.2018.06.010.

63. Ana Kovacevic et al., "The Effect of Resistance Exercise on Sleep: A Systematic Review of Randomized Controlled Trials," *Sleep Medicine Reviews* 39 (June 2018): 52–68, https://doi.org/10.1016/j.smrv.2017.07.002.

64. Christopher E. Kline et al., "The Effect of Exercise Training on Obstructive Sleep Apnea and Sleep Quality: A Randomized Controlled Trial," *Sleep* 34, no. 12 (December 2011): 1631–40, https://doi.org/10.5665/sleep.1422.

www.ingramcontent.com/pod-product-compliance
Lightning Source LLC
Chambersburg PA
CBHW070048030426
42335CB00016B/1834